OBSTETRICS AND GYNECOLOGY ADVANCES

CESAREAN SECTION

PROCEDURES, COMPLICATIONS AND RECOVERY

OBSTETRICS AND GYNECOLOGY ADVANCES

Additional books in this series can be found on Nova's website
under the Series tab.

Additional E-books in this series can be found on Nova's website
under the E-book tab.

OBSTETRICS AND GYNECOLOGY ADVANCES

CESAREAN SECTION

PROCEDURES, COMPLICATIONS AND RECOVERY

EYAL SHEINER
EDITOR

Nova Science Publishers, Inc.
New York

For permission to use material from this book please contact us:
Telephone 631-231-7269; Fax 631-231-8175
Web Site: http://www.novapublishers.com

Library of Congress Cataloging-in-Publication Data

Library of Congress Control Number: 2012933169

ISBN: 978-1-62081-214-3

Published by Nova Science Publishers, Inc. † New York

CONTENTS

PREFACE

This book focuses on essential aspects of cesarean delivery: procedures, complications and recovery in a straightforward manner. The book is divided in five parts: the first part is introductory, including basic concepts such as the history and epidemiology of CS. The second part describes specific procedures, tubal ligation (with its benefits and complication) and anesthesia for CS. The third part focuses on maternal as well as neonatal short and long term complications. Recovery is covered in the forth part of the book, including early feeding, wound care, and mobilization to prevent thromboembolism. Controversial issues are covered in the last part of the book including ethics of unindicted cesarean delivery, vaginal births after cesareans delivery and the preferred timing for elective cesarean delivery.

Chapter 1- The cesarean section (CS) rate worldwide has increased substantially in recent years. Actually, the rates reported in the United States increased from 20.7% in 1996 to an all-time high rate of 31.1% in 2006. Nowadays a third of women delivering in the USA do so by CS. Cesarean Section currently is the most common major surgical procedure for women in the United States with more than 1.3 million CS performed annually. During the 1970s until the early 1980s, the CS rate increased dramatically but began to decline in the late 1980s. Between 1989 and 1996, the total cesarean rate decreased as a result of a reduction in the primary CS rate and an increase in the rate of vaginal birth after cesarean (VBAC). Since 1996, these trends have reversed and increased rates were rapid and sustained for primary and repeat CS. Primary CS accounts for sixty percent of the increase in the total CS rate. The epidemiology of CS in the U.S. is thoroughly discussed in chapter 3. The increase in primary cesarean rate reflects increased numbers of multiple gestations secondary to assisted reproductive technology, CS for breech presentation, increased rates of maternal obesity, physician concerns about litigation for adverse obstetric outcome, and a decline in the use of operative vaginal delivery for cephalic presentations. At the same time, the VBAC rate decreased implying a corresponding increase in the repeat cesarean rate, which reached almost 91% in 2004. The decline in VBAC numbers has attracted much recent attention and is the focus of an ongoing process to remedy the situation. Nonetheless, it is likely that, despite these efforts, there will be a further increase in the overall cesarean section rate in the future.

Chapter 2- The procedure of operative opening of the uterus and delivering the fetus known today as cesarean section was probably practiced for ages. Delivery of a living child after the death of its mother (the postmortem procedure) is referred to in the myths and folklore of many ancient societies. Some infants survived, although their mothers did not.

Aside from folklore, the procedure may have had its origins in some society's requirements. It was believed that a dead mother should be buried separately from her dead infant, thus, first cesareans were performed as a part of burial procedure.

The procedure could have come to have medical implications only when those in attendance could notice that the shorter the interval between the maternal death and the removal of the fetus, the better the chance for infant's survival. Once it was clear to ancient birthing attendants that a live infant might be rescued from its dead mother and survive, the neonate's removal became the main medical objective for performing a post mortem cesarean section.

Historically, we do not have a recall on when it had occurred, but it is reasonable to assume that it had happened that way. The optimal time for initiation of a postmortem cesarean, aimed at saving the neonate's life is not well defined. Nonetheless, modern case reports documented fetal survival without demonstrable neurological damage from a fatal maternal injury. On one occasion, a clinically normal child was delivered by a post mortem cesarean 22 minutes after documented maternal cardiopulmonary arrest and 47 minutes from the fatal injury. This case suggests that a postmortem cesarean with saved neonate's child might have occurred in ancient times.

Chapter 3- In 2009, almost 1.4 million American women had a cesarean delivery, and cesarean delivery is currently the most common major surgical procedure for women in the United States. One out of every 3 US births (32.9%) is now delivered by cesarean section, the highest level ever recorded in the United States, and a level that is higher than most other developed countries. The cesarean rate increased dramatically during the 1970's and early 1980's and then plateaued in the late 1980's (based on data from the National Hospital Discharge Survey). Between 1989 and 1996 the total cesarean rate decreased as a result of a decrease in the primary cesarean rate and an increase in the rate of vaginal birth after cesarean (VBAC). However, in 1996, these trends were reversed, and cesarean rates have increased every year from 1996-2009. This chapter uses national vital statistics data to examine recent trends and characteristics of cesarean delivery in the United States from 1996-2009. In addition, the relevant epidemiologic literature is reviewed to examine broader issues surrounding cesarean delivery, such as trends in medical risks and indications, maternal opinions, and birth outcomes.

Chapter 4- Cesarean section (CS) has been practiced for ages, although originally as a universally postmortem procedure. During the last 15 years, the CS rate was increased despite of the recommendations of the World Health Organization (WHO) to keep it below 10-15% (Figure 1). The concept of CS rate limitation has become obsolete. The increase in the CS rate is mainly justified by the decrease in maternal mortality and morbidity following elective CS: surgery-related risks have decreased and the confusion that was made between the risks of vaginal delivery and those of trial of labor (TOL) has to be clarified to show that maternal mortality and morbidity are not increased by elective CS. However, instrumental delivery and CS during labor remain two situations at high-risk both for the mother and her fetus. There is also an association between the increase in the CS rate and the decrease in PNM and morbidity, but this effect would only become clinically significant after a dramatic increase in the CS rate: this is the preventile principle of "marginal death". Numerous articles have been published reporting on the effects of vaginal delivery for the pelvic floor: urinary incontinence, pelvic organ prolapse, and especially fecal incontinence. All these publications concluded that CS has a protective effect. The rising duty to provide information to patients in high-risk obstetrical situations such as a history of CS also contributes to the overall increase in CS rate mainly through the elective CS rate. Indeed, when faced with the alternative choices of potentially severe complications either for themselves or their child, women are likely to choose what appears to be the safest mode of delivery for their child and thus to opt for a CS. Finally, widespread delivery of information to the patients about TOL itself and the risks of vaginal delivery is the first step towards a "principle of preference", which consists in giving an important place to the patient's choice in the decision-making process, and thus to recognize her right to ask for an elective CS.

Chapter 5- Breech presentation, in which the fetus's bottom presents downward toward the cervix, was described as early as about 400 – 600 A.D. in the Moschion manuscript with figures of the fetus, which were adopted by obstetric texts of the 16 to 18th centuries. Leonardo di Vinci described a fetus in complete breech presentation in his notebook. There are three types of breech presentation: frank breech which is the most common in which hips are flexed and knees extended with buttocks presenting and feet near the head, complete breech when hips and knees are flexed with buttocks and feet presenting in a cross-legged position, and footling or incomplete breech, when one or both feet present first.

Chapter 6- Cesarean section (CS) is defined as a surgical birth of a fetus through the abdominal wall (laparotomy) and the uterine wall (hysterotomy).

The percentage of United States CS increased from 20.7% in 1996 to 31.1% in 2006. The rate of CS is steadily rising and in 2008, nearly one-third (32.3%) of US births were by CS. Cesarean section is the most common major surgical procedure for women in the United States, with 1.4 million surgeries annually.

Cesarean section as a surgical procedure confers an increased risk of wound complications, iatrogenic injury to bladder/bowel, anesthetic risk and venous thromboembolism.

Hence, it is mandatory to use the optimal surgical technique to minimize morbidity. Notwithstanding the traditional CS stages (Table 1), several surgical techniques and modifications are being used to perform this common surgical procedure. This chapter reviews the evidence base of some of the procedures used in a CS.

Chapter 7- Most abdominal operations today have an endoscopic alternative, except the Cesarean Section (CS), at a time when its use is increasing. It is therefore important to re-analyze, optimize and simplify this procedure and introduce evidence-based rather than tradition-based steps.

In a process of evaluation and comparison of alternative surgical steps at the Misgav Ladach hospital in Jerusalem, a modified method has been evolved.

In the early 1970s, Joel-Cohen (JC) described a transverse incision alternative to the traditional Pfannenstiel incision based on time and motion studies. The JC incision with some modifications is now used by obstetricians in more than 100 countries. With this method the longitudinal abdominal structures, muscles and blood vessels which have a lateral sway are stretched laterally and will return to their original positions at the end of the operation.

The peritoneum is opened by repeat bi-digital stretching. No abdominal towels are used, and after the delivery the uterus is sutured with one continuous layer. Both peritoneal layers are left un-sutured as a new peritoneum will be formed within short time.

Moreover, the suture of the visceral peritoneum causes a closed pocket between the bladder and the lower uterine segment, leading to bladder flap collection containing blood, edema, exudate, and fibrin, resulting in fibrosis, adhesions and possible urinary symptoms.

The abdomen is closed in 2 layers only, fascia and skin. The worldwide distribution of this method is due to the beneficial outcome, quicker mobility, early hydration, lower febrile morbidity and lower costs, as only 10 instruments and usually only 3 suture materials are needed.

Chapter 8- Tubal ligation during the course of a Caesarean section (CS) is technically simple and safe from the medical point of view, and does not adversely affect breastfeeding. Demand for tubal ligation by the patients is higher when offered in the context of CS instead of, when offered as a single act. However, failure (i.e. pregnancy following the procedure) although extremely rare, is higher in puerperal tubal sterilization than in the interval tubal ligation, especially when using techniques of mechanical tubal occlusion.

Electrocoagulation by laparoscopy is associated with high efficacy, but with a potentially greater risk of complications and difficulties in the reversal of the tubal ligation. Tubal ligation has a number of advantages over other contraceptive methods, which require strict adherence to their use. Candidates for postpartum tubal sterilization should be carefully selected and assessed, since the technique is generally irreversible.

Chapter 9- Cesarean section possesses particular challenges to the anesthesiologist, derived from the unique physiological stare of pregnancy and its associated pathologies, the nature of the procedure, and, ultimately the need to care for two patients simultaneously – the mother and the fetus. Cesarean section may become a source for serious difficulties and complications, leading to increased maternal and fetal morbidity and mortality. Anesthesia, general or regional, induces a physiological imbalance, representing a significant deviation from the normal physiological state, requiring a deep understanding and knowledge of the induced changes, and specific effects of different interventions and treatment. In the present chapter the authors discuss the anesthetic implications of the physiological and pathophysiological changes throughout pregnancy and during delivery, their impact on the outcome, morbidity and mortality, the unique characteristics of the cesarean section candidate, particular anesthetic challenges, associated complications, and practical recommendations for anesthetic management of the cesarean section candidate.

Chapter 10- Cesarean delivery (CD) currently accounts for the most common major surgical procedure for women in the United States. The percentage of deliveries by CD increased substantially in recent years, from 20.7% in 1996 to an all-time high of 31.1% in 2006. The rate of CD increases with maternal age, nearly half of all deliveries in women over 40 years of age are by CD. Whilst in recent years the rate of CD has increased for all gestational ages, the highest rate (46%) is found in premature deliveries prior to 34 weeks while merely one quarter of postdate deliveries (>40 weeks) are cesarean.

Cesarean section has provided a life-saving form of delivery since medieval history. In those times the fetal life saved was at the expense of the mother's life. With development of safe anesthesia and modern surgery, cesarean delivery has become a delivery method of choice. CDs on maternal request are estimated to make up 4% to 18% of all CDs. These are defined as a CD for a singleton pregnancy at term in the absence of medical or obstetric indications, done upon maternal request. In 2006, the National Institute of Child Health and Human Development (NICHD), held a panel in the subject of CD upon maternal request. The panel acknowledged that a large gap exists between current knowledge and clinical practice and expressed concern that this surgery is being chosen without rigorously evaluating the evidence.

Chapter 11- Cesarean delivery increases the risk of abnormal placentation such as placenta previa, placenta accreta and placental abruption in future pregnancy. Furthermore, unexplained stillbirth may occur. Uterine rupture in a subsequent pregnancy is well known, and rupture in term pregnancy with or without trial of labor is well documented as a severe complication with vaginal birth after cesarean section (VBAC). However, it may occur in preterm pregnancy. Today, the authors also know that complications may develop in the scars resulting from hysterotomy or abdominal incision. These complications occur as scar pregnancy, numbness or pain, and incision endometriosis. To date, there is no strong evidence of a causal relationship between cesarean delivery and subfertility. Abdominal surgery including cesarean section (CS) is associated with long-term risk from the development of clinically significant adhesions. Although these adhesions may be completely asymptomatic, they may cause injury during repeat abdominal surgery as well as bowel obstruction and infertility. This paper reviews the long-term complications after CS.

Chapter 12- The comprehensive discussion of cesarean delivery (CD) complications must include fetal- neonatal issues. This unique surgical intervention targets two patients. One is operated upon sometimes for the mere chance of sparing morbidity from the other. Furthermore, maternal and fetal interests may contradict at times. The decision to perform a CD at times of contradiction between fetus and mother may require ethical principals and in extreme occurrences involve legal intervention. The majority of CD indications are fetal indications. Yet the mainstay of informed consent consists of maternal morbidity issues, rarely are fetal complications discussed as main issues to consider. An exception to this practice is the issue of prematurity, especially if iatrogenic (as a result from the elected timing of the cesarean surgery).

In this chapter, a detailed discussion of the fetal aspects of maternal CD will be illuminated.

Chapter 13- Postpartum hemorrhage is a leading cause of maternal mortality in the developed and developing world. Peripartum hysterectomy, although typically performed as a last resort, is often a life saving procedure. When necessary, peripartum hysterectomy is performed emergently, often in the setting of heavy bleeding with poor visualization, and frequently in settings with less than optimal equipment and personal. As such, the procedure is associated with substantial morbidity and not insignificant mortality.

In the United States it is estimated that peripartum hysterectomy occurs in 0.77 per 1000 deliveries. Compared to a primary vaginal delivery without a history of cesarean delivery the odds ratio for peripartum hysterectomy is 2.70 for vaginal birth after cesarean, 6.54 for primary cesarean delivery and 8.90 at the time of a repeat cesarean delivery. In the U.S. the incidence of both postpartum hemorrhage and peripartum hysterectomy are increasing. Population-based studies have demonstrated that postpartum hemorrhage increased 26% from 1994 to 2006 while peripartum hysterectomy increased 15% from 1994 to 2007. Much of the increase in the rates of postpartum hemorrhage and hysterectomy is due to the dramatically rising cesarean delivery rate.

Prior cesarean delivery is the most important risk factor associated with peripartum hysterectomy. The risk for peripartum hysterectomy increases with the number of prior cesarean deliveries.

Chapter 14- Despite many international and institutional efforts to decrease the rise in cesarean sections, the rates continue to escalate, making it an increasingly common form of delivery. The Healthy People 2010 initiative set out to reduce cesarean delivery to 15%

without success. Current estimates reach near 32% of delivereies in the United States. Concerns over this rise are multifactorial. Long-term sequelae of cesarean delivery demonstrate the need to avoid the procedure when possible. In this chapter, the authors examine three primary areas: recovery, early feeding, wound care, and mobilization to prevent thromboembolism. With increasing obesity in the general population, our attention should be drawn to the increased risk for complications including wound infections, and management thereof. Also, chronic pain due to incision wounds presumably increases medical consumption due to ongoing consultations and pain management needs beyond the postpartum hospital stay.

Chapter 15- Timing of elective repeat cesarean section should take into account both fetal and maternal considerations. The percentage of cesarean deliveries has dramatically increased during the last decades. It undoubtedly leads to an increase in the number of women having multiple cesarean sections. While maternal morbidity increases with increased number of cesarean sections, and the risk potential is elevated with gestational age, when compared with their term counterparts late preterm infants face increased morbidity. Establishing the optimal time of delivery for both mother and child is a major challenge faced by clinicians. The aim of this chapter is to better understand neonatal and maternal morbidity and mortality that are associated with elective repeat cesarean section, in order to provide an educated decision regarding the optimal timing for elective repeat cesarean section.

Chapter 16- This century has set record rates of cesarean deliveries. It is the most common surgical procedure for women in the United States (US) with nearly 1.5 million cesarean surgeries performed every year. When the US national rate of cesarean delivery was first measured in 1965, it was 4.5%. Between 1970 and 2007, the cesarean delivery rate in the US increased dramatically to more than 31%. In 2007, 19% of women in Israel, and 32.8% of women in the US were delivered by a cesarean section.

Among 26 industrialized countries that provided data to the Organization for Economic Cooperation and Development, cesarean rates ranged from a low of 14% for the Netherlands to a high of 40% for Italy in 2007. Three countries had rates that were even higher than the US rate (Korea, Turkey and Italy). This worldwide increase in cesarean rates is a result of tremendous changes in the clinical environment, including the introduction of electronic fetal monitoring, and the decrease in vaginal breech deliveries and forceps deliveries.

As the 21st century approached, there emerged a demand for elective primary cesarean delivery on maternal request, without any medical indication. Patient autonomy, safety of the neonate and the perceived safety of the mother, fear of pain, avoidance of pelvic floor damage and esthetics, all may have contributed to this request. Presently, approximately 15% of cesarean deliveries are attributed to elective, non-medical, maternal request.

Chapter 17- Cesarean section (CS) is believed to be the oldest obstetrical surgical operation, though, in the past, excessive maternal mortality rate has limited its application. In 1937, cesarean delivery rate in the United States averaged at 3%. However, this is no longer the case. Cesarean section rate in the United States has risen ten-fold to a formidable 30% in 2005 partly due to evolution in anesthesia and supportive care, which was associated with decrease in maternal and neonatal postoperative complications. This increase in CS rate is a world wide trend shared by both developing and developed countries. Improved surgical techniques and use of antibiotic prophylaxis together with regional anesthesia has caused a dramatic decrease in post operative complications. Notwithstanding this improvement it is imperative to bear in mind that cesarean delivery still carries a significantly higher rate of both short and long term complications in comparison to vaginal delivery. This rise in cesarean section rate is accompanied by a dramatic change in characteristics of pregnant women population. Pregnant women of the 21st century are older and heavier and more likely to experience concurrent medical conditions such as chronic hypertension and diabetes.

Chapter 18- There are currently 33.3 million people worldwide with HIV or AIDS, of which 15.8 million are women and 2.5 million are children.

Maternal to child transmission (MTCT) is the most common source for pediatric infection with more than 2000 children infected through this method on a daily basis, totaling nearly 750,000 a year. Thus, preventing it is of vital importance to curb the spread of HIV.

Without medical intervention, the MTCT rate is between 15-25 percent; including breastfeeding this rate is as high as 40 percent.

Chapter 19- Peritoneal adhesions are a predictable side-effect of cesarean section (CS) and other abdominal and pelvic surgery. Though most are asymptomatic, adhesions are implicated in a spectrum of disease including chronic pelvic pain, infertility, bowel obstruction and a higher risk of organ injury at repeat cesarean or other abdomino-pelvic operation.

This chapter focuses on the pathogenesis of adhesions; the size of the problem and on strategies that might be employed to reduce the burden of morbidity caused by adhesions due to one of the most commonly performed surgical procedures in the world – cesarean section.

Chapter 20- Maternal-choice cesarean delivery has become controversial throughout the world. In the United States, for example, the American College of Obstetrics and Gynecologists (ACOG) stated in a committee opinion in 2003 that while, the right of patients to refuse unwanted surgery is well known, less clear is the right of patients to have a surgical procedure when scientific evidence supporting it is incomplete, of poor quality, or totally lacking.The committee concluded that the evidence to support the benefit of elective cesarean is still incomplete and that there is not yet extensive morbidity and mortality data to compare elective cesarean delivery with planned vaginal delivery. In addition, the United States National Institutes of Health (NIH) convened a 2006 conference regarding this issue that concluded that there is insufficient evidence to evaluate fully the benefits and risks of primary elective cesarean delivery as compared to vaginal delivery, and that more research is needed. The NIH conference concluded: “The magnitude of cesarean delivery on maternal request is difficult to quantify. There is insufficient evidence to evaluate fully the benefits and risks of cesarean delivery on maternal request compared with planned vaginal delivery. Any decision to perform a cesarean delivery on maternal request should be carefully individualized and consistent with ethical principles.”

In: Cesarean Section: Procedures, Complications and Recovery ISBN: 978-1-62081-214-3
Editor: Eyal Sheiner

Chapter I

Introduction: Caesarean Section: Procedures Complications and Recovery

Eyal Sheiner*

Department of Obstetrics and Gynecology, Soroka University Medical Center, Faculty of Health Sciences, Ben-Gurion University of the Negev, Beer-Sheva, Israel

Cesarean Section: Procedures, Complications and Recovery

The cesarean section (CS) rate worldwide has increased substantially in recent years [1-5]. Actually, the rates reported in the United States increased from 20.7% in 1996 to an all-time high rate of 31.1% in 2006 [6-7]. Nowadays a third of women delivering in the USA do so by CS [8]. Cesarean Section currently is the most common major surgical procedure for women in the United States [9] with more than 1.3 million CS performed annually [10]. During the 1970s until the early 1980s, the CS rate increased dramatically but began to decline in the late 1980s. Between 1989 and 1996, the total cesarean rate decreased as a result of a reduction in the primary CS rate and an increase in the rate of vaginal birth after cesarean (VBAC). Since 1996, these trends have reversed and increased rates were rapid and sustained for primary and repeat CS [7, 10]. Primary CS accounts for sixty percent of the increase in the total CS rate. The epidemiology of CS in the U.S. is thoroughly discussed in chapter 3. The increase in primary cesarean rate reflects increased numbers of multiple gestations secondary to assisted reproductive technology, CS for breech presentation, increased rates of maternal obesity, physician concerns about litigation for adverse obstetric outcome [8], and a decline in the use of operative vaginal delivery for cephalic presentations [11]. At the same time, the VBAC rate decreased implying a corresponding increase in the repeat cesarean rate, which

* Corresponding author: Eyal Sheiner MD, PhD. Department of Obstetrics and Gynecology, Soroka University Medical Center, Faculty of Health Sciences, Ben-Gurion University of the Negev, Beer-Sheva, Israel. E-mail: sheiner@bgu.ac.il.

reached almost 91% in 2004 [10]. The decline in VBAC numbers has attracted much recent attention and is the focus of an ongoing process to remedy the situation [12, 13]. Nonetheless, it is likely that, despite these efforts, there will be a further increase in the overall cesarean section rate in the future.

The increase in cesarean rate may also be explained by improved techniques to control hemorrhage, infection, and thromboembolism which enhanced the safety of the procedure, although studies examining changes in the medical risk profile of mothers over time have found little evidence to suggest that the rising CS rates are due to such changes [14-16].

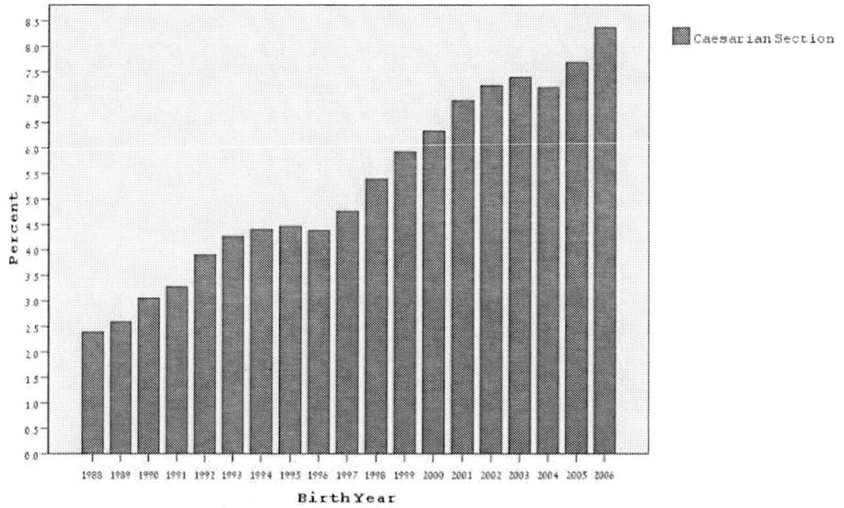

Figure 1. Distribution of all cesarean section cases over the years (% of total cesarean deliveries); data from Soroka University Medical Center.

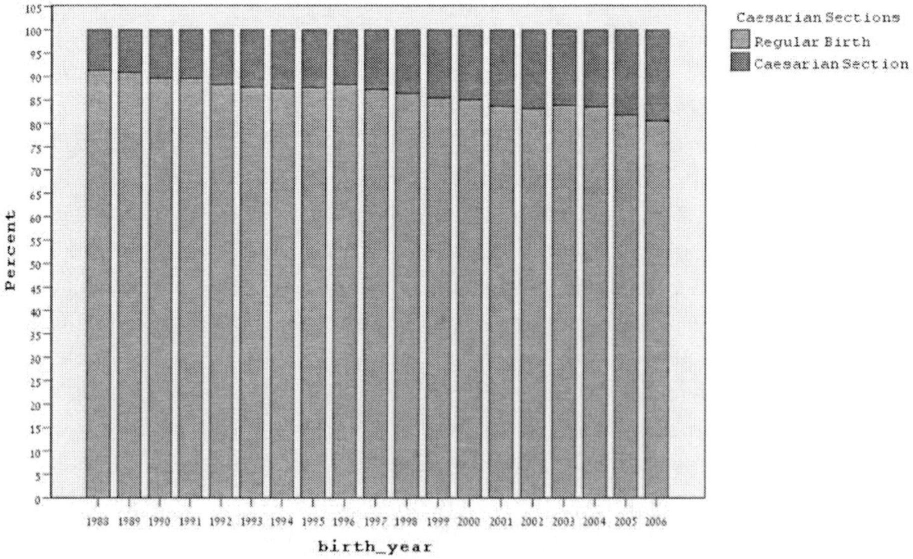

Figure 2. Cesarean section rates over the years (% for each year); data from Soroka University Medical Center.

Needless to say, although the cesarean mode of delivery may at first glance appear to provide a relatively safe and certain outcome, it should not be regarded as a risk free procedure. The involvement of anesthesia and laparotomy increase the risk for maternal morbidity and mortality.

Table 1. Demographic and Obstetrical characteristics of women with Classical CS, Low transverse segment CS and partus spontaneous

	No CS (%)	Low transverse segment C/S (%)	Classical CS (%)	P
Nulliparous women	23.1	26.6	3.5	<0.001
Gestational age ≤36 weeks	6.8	21.2	41.6	<0.001
37-41weeks	88.7	75.0	57.7	<0.001
42+weeks	4.5	3.8	0.8	<0.001
Previous CS	7.2	40.3	83.6	<0.001
Severe PET	0.6	4.5	4.5	<0.001
Chronic hypertension	1.2	3.9	5.3	<0.001
Diabetes mellitus	4.8	11.8	14.5	<0.001
Obesity	0.8	2.4	2.9	<0.001
Multiple gestational	1	6.7	2.5	<0.001
NRFHR patterns	2.6	18.8	5.5	<0.001
Dysticia, 1st stage	0.1	12.8	1.8	<0.001
Dysticia, 2nd stage	1.2	3.8	1.6	<0.001
Placental abruption	0.3	3.7	3.1	<0.001
Placenta previa	0	2.6	9.1	<0.001
Cord prolapse	0.1	2.2	1.7	<0.001
Malpresentations	1.8	30.1	26.0	<0.001
Uterine rupture	0.01	0.3	1.2	<0.001

PET- Preeclampsia toxemia, NRFHR- non-reassuring fetal heart rate.

Table 2. Perinatal outcomes of women with Classical CS, Low transverse segment CS and partus spontaneous

	No CS (%)	Low transverse segment C/S (%)	Classical CS (%)	P
Perinatal mortality	1.3	1.9	4.9	<0.001
Low Apgar 1 min	4.7	18.6	30.9	<0.001
Low Apgar 5 min	3.1	3.1	5.5	0.082
Birth weight < 2500 grams	7.1	20.3	29.1	<0.001
2500-3999 grams	88.6	72.1	67.2	<0.001
≥ 4000 grams	4.3	7.5	3.8	<0.001

According to all these data, the number of women having multiple CS will increase, and hence the importance of understanding its implications. This trend, however, is not inherent only to the United States; a detail which is illustrated by the fact that the worldwide CS birth rate has quadrupled in less than two decades [2, 17, 18]. The same trend is noted at the Soroka University Medical Center where the rates were as low as 8% in 1988, but increased tremendously during the last decade (figures 1 and 2).

CLASSICAL VS. LOW TRANSVERSE CESAREAN SECTION

The so called "classical" (i.e. corporeal incision) cesarean section is rarely used. A recent study compared the frequency, obstetrical characteristics and perinatal outcome of corporeal vs. low transverse segment (LTS) CS. This retrospective study included deliveries occurring at the Soroka University Medical Center between the years 1988 and 2010 [19].

Out of 246,525 deliveries that occurred during the study period, 0.4% (n=895) had a corporeal CS and 13.6% (n=33,457) had LTS CS. Corporeal incision was more common in patients with complications such as previous CS (83.6% vs. 40.3%; P<0.001), chronic hypertension (5.3% vs. 3.9%; P<0.001), diabetes mellitus (either gestation and pregestational, 14.5% vs. 11.8%; P<0.001), placenta previa (9.1% vs. 2.6%; P<0.001) and preterm deliveries (<37 weeks gestation, 41.6% vs. 21.2%; P<0.001; Table 1). These women had higher rates of severe complications such as uterine rupture (1.2% vs. 0.3%; P<0.001) and the need for blood transfusions (10.9%, vs. 4.2%; P<0.001). Patients with corporeal CS had higher rates of adverse perinatal outcomes including low birth-weight (<2500 grams, 29.1% vs. 20.3%; P<0.001) and perinatal mortality (4.9% vs. 1.9%; P<0.001; Table 2).

After reviewing the data it is concluded that corporeal CS is hardly ever used and is reserved for complicated pregnancies. Accordingly, it is associated with adverse maternal and perinatal outcomes.

IN THIS BOOK

This book is aimed to give a wide perspective of the growing epidemic of cesarean deliveries. It includes five sections:

1) *Introduction:* The procedure of operative opening of the uterus and delivering the fetus was probably practiced for ages. [20-24] The first part includes basic concepts such as the history of CS. The chapter describes in a meticulous manner, the history of cesarean delivery from ancient times and until today. The updated epidemiology of CS and breech delivery as well as indications for CS are all presented in the following chapters of the introduction section.
2) *Procedures:* This section gives insights of specific procedures, with a focus on the Misgav Ladach or Stark procedure. Tubal ligation with its benefits and complication as well as CS anesthesia issues are covered.
3) *Complications:* Despite advances in technology, the cesarean mode of delivery should not be regarded as a risk free procedure. It carries risks for both mother and child. The need for anesthesia and laparotomy increases the risk of maternal morbidity and mortality. In this section short and long term maternal consequences

are thoroughly discussed as well as possible perinatal complications. A separate chapter is devoted to cesarean hysterectomy.

4) *Recovery:* This section examines three primary aspects of recovery: early feeding, wound care, and mobilization to prevent thromboembolism. With increasing obesity in the general population, attention should be drawn to the increased risk of complications including wound infections, and management thereof. Also, chronic pain due to incision wounds presumably increases medical consumption due to ongoing consultations and pain management needs beyond the postpartum hospital stay.
5) *Controversy issues*: The last part of the book sheds light on specific updated issues such as ethics of unindicted cesarean delivery. Maternal-choice cesarean delivery has become controversial throughout the world. The degree to which cesarean deliveries and vaginal births after cesareans are affecting public health remains a subject of continued controversy and uncertainty. A specific chapter discusses different aspects relating to trial of labor after a cesarean section. The chapter includes benefits, risks and success rates of vaginal birth after a cesarean section, patient eligibility issues, appropriate counseling, and factors affecting maternal decision-making. Other chapters in this section discuss the preferred timing for elective cesarean delivery, the possibility to decrease adhesions, the association between diabetes mellitus and CS, and whether cesarean is the preferred mode in order to reduce HIV transmission.

REFERENCES

[1] Miller ES, Grobman WA. Interbirth interval with frequency of cesarean delivery. *Obstet. Gynecol.* 2011;118(1):39-42.

[2] Sheiner E, Shoham-Vardi I, Hershkovitz R, Katz M, Mazor M. Infertility treatment is an independent risk factor for cesarean section among nulliparous women aged 40 and above. *Am. J. Obstet. Gynecol.* 2001 Oct;185(4):888-92.

[3] Barber EL, Lundsberg LS, Belanger K, Pettker CM, Funai EF, Illuzzi JL. Indications contributing to the increasing cesarean delivery rate. *Obstet. Gynecol.* 2011 Jul;118(1):29-38.

[4] Zhang J, Troendle J, Reddy UM, Laughon SK, Branch DW, Burkman R, Landy HJ, Hibbard JU, Haberman S, Ramirez MM, Bailit JL, Hoffman MK, Gregory KD, Gonzalez-Quintero VH, Kominiarek M, Learman LA, Hatjis CG, van Veldhuisen P; Consortium on Safe Labor. Contemporary cesarean delivery practice in the United States. *Am. J. Obstet. Gynecol.* 2010 Oct;203(4):326.e1-326.e10.

[5] Blanchette H. The rising cesarean delivery rate in America: what are the consequences? *Obstet. Gynecol.* 2011 Sep;118(3):687-90.

[6] Hamilton BE, Martin JA, Ventura SJ. Births: preliminary data for 2005. *Natl. Vital. Stat. Rep.* 2006;55:1-18.

[7] Hamilton BE, Martin JA, Ventura SJ, Sutton PD, Menacker F. Births: preliminary data for 2004. *Natl. Vital. Stat. Rep.* 2005;54:1-17.

[8] Zhang J, Troendle J, Reddy UM. Contemporary cesarean delivery practice in the United States. *Am. J. Obstet. Gynecol.* 2010;203(4):326.

[9] DeFrances CJ, Hall MJ. 2005 National Hospital Discharge Survey. *Advance data from vital and health statistics*; 2007 Jul 12;(385):1-19.

[10] MacDorman MF, Menacker F, Declercq E. Cesarean Birth in the United States: Epidemiology, Trends, and Outcomes. *Clin. Perinatol.* 2008;35:293-307.

[11] Goetzinger KR, Macones GA. Operative vaginal delivery: current trends in obstetrics. *Women's Health* (Lond Engl) 2008;4(3):281–90.

[12] ACOG Practice bulletin no. 115: vaginal birth after previous cesarean delivery. *Obstet. Gynecol.* 2010;116(2 Pt 1):450–63.

[13] National Institutes of Health Consensus Development conference statement: vaginal birth after cesarean: new insights March 8–10, 2010. *Obstet. Gynecol.* 2010;115(6):1279–95.

[14] Menacker F, Declercq E, Macdorman MF. Cesarean delivery: background, trends, and epidemiology. *Semin. Perina*tol. 2006;30: 235-41.

[15] Reddy UM, Spong DY. Introduction. *Semin. Perinatol.* 2006;30:233–4.

[16] Declercq E, Menacker F. MacDorman MF. Maternal risk profiles and the primary cesarean rate in the United States 1991–2002. *Am. J. Public Health* 2006;96:867–72.

[17] Bulger T, Howden-Chapman P, Stone P. A cut above: the rising cesarean section rate in New Zealand. *N. Z. Med. J.* 1998;11:30-3.

[18] Murray SF, Serani-Pradenas F. *Cesarean birth trends in Chile,* 1986 to 1994. Birth 1997; 24:258-63.

[19] Steiner N, Weintraub AY, Wiznitzer A, Sheiner E. Corporeal versus low transverse cesarean delivery: *Frequency, characteristics and outcome.* Presented at the COGI Conference, November 2011, Bangkok, Thailand.

[20] Lurie S. The changing motives of cesarean section from ancient times to 21st century. *Arch. Gynecol. Obstet.* 2005;271:281-5.

[21] Lurie et Y. " Yotzeh dofen": cesarean section in the days of the Mishna and the Talmud. *Isr. J. Obstet. Gynecol.* 2001;12:111-3.

[22] Blumenfeld-Kosinski R. *Not of woman born.* Cornell University Press, Ithaca and London. 1990; pp.1-47.

[23] Greenhill JP. Obstetrics 11th ed. Philadelphia, WB Saunders Co., 1955; pp.986-1033.

[24] Boley JP. The history of caesarean section. *Can. Med. Assoc. J.* 1991;145: 319-22.

In: Cesarean Section: Procedures, Complications and Recovery ISBN: 978-1-62081-214-3
Editor: Eyal Sheiner

Chapter II

The History of Cesarean Section

Samuel Lurie
Department of Obstetrics and Gynecology, Edith Wolfson Medical Center, Holon, and the Sackler School of Medicine, Tel Aviv University, Israel

Introduction

The procedure of operative opening of the uterus and delivering the fetus known today as cesarean section was probably practiced for ages. [1] Delivery of a living child after the death of its mother (the postmortem procedure) is referred to in the myths and folklore of many ancient societies, [2, 3, 4, 5]. Some infants survived, although their mothers did not. Aside from folklore, the procedure may have had its origins in some society's requirements. [1] It was believed that a dead mother should be buried separately from her dead infant, thus, first cesareans were performed as a part of burial procedure. [1]

The procedure could have come to have medical implications only when those in attendance could notice that the shorter the interval between the maternal death and the removal of the fetus, the better the chance for infant's survival. Once it was clear to ancient birthing attendants that a live infant might be rescued from its dead mother and survive, the neonate's removal became the main medical objective for performing a post mortem cesarean section.

Historically, we do not have a recall on when it had occurred, but it is reasonable to assume that it had happened that way. The optimal time for initiation of a postmortem cesarean, aimed at saving the neonate's life is not well defined. Nonetheless, modern case reports documented fetal survival without demonstrable neurological damage from a fatal maternal injury. [6, 7] On one occasion, [6] a clinically normal child was delivered by a post mortem cesarean 22 minutes after documented maternal cardiopulmonary arrest and 47 minutes from the fatal injury. This case suggests that a postmortem cesarean with saved neonate's child might have occurred in ancient times.

Myths

The myths of cesarean delivery may be an accurate reflection of normal medical practice in the culture that tells them, or it may be an expression of glorification of a certain hero. [1] Since, the outcome of cesarean section was poor, so that if a newborn sustained the operation, than, "unquestionably", the Gods must have intended for this person a special destiny. Virgil (Publius Vergilius Maro) (70BC-19BC), a classical Roman poet, describes the epic of a legendary Trojan hero Aeneas in Aeneid. Aeneas kills Lichas, "'*who had been cut of his dead mother's womb and then made scared*". [3] Virgil dramatizes the contemporary Roman cultural belief and mystery surrounding cesarean birth by signifying the fortune of a person born in such a way. Buddha, too, is believed to be delivered from the right flank of his mother Maya (i.e, cesarean delivery). [8]

The best example of myth designated those born by a cesarean is Asclepius, the Greek God of medicine, who, according to Greek Mythology, was born by a cesarean section, after the death of Coronis, his mother. [9] The "surgeon" was Apollo, Asclepius's father and it happened after Apollo had slain Coronis once he learned that she was unfaithful, and the "operation" occurred on the funeral pyre, when Asclepius removed his unborn son Asclepius from Coronis's body. In Roman writings, there are number of heroes who are ascribed to be born by a cesarean delivery. Scipio Africanus, the Roman general who defeated Hannibal, was conceivably born by a postmortem cesarean section in 237 BC. [5] Gaius Plinius Secundus, known as Pliny the Elder, in addition to Scipio Africanus, notes that first of the Caesars and Manilius who entered Carthage were also born by a postmortem cesarean (*Auspicatius enecta (v.l. e necata) parente gignuntur, sicut Scipio Africanus prioir natus primusque Caesarum a caeseo matris dictus, qua de causa et Caesones appellati, simili modo natus et Maniliu, qui Carthaginem cum exercitu intravit.)*. [10] The phrase "the first of the Caesars" was misunderstood by latter readers as referring to Julius Caesar. This connection was once thought to be the origin of the name "cesarean operation". It is incorrect, mainly because Aurelia, Julius's mother was still alive when he invaded Britain, [11] and because cesarean delivery was universally performed postmortem in Roman Empire. Also, Pliny the Elder probably refers to some earlier Julius Caesar, such as Sextus Julius Caesar who was praetor in 208 BC. [12]

Another example of glorification of a certain hero appears in Persian mythology. Rustam, the most famous hero of the great Persian epic of the kings was conceivably born by a cesarean section. [13] Although not really dateable as a historic person, he lived somewhere in the 6th century, and he had served a succession of Persian monarchs: Kay Kobad, Kay Kaus and Kay Khosrau. [14] He also fought many mythical monsters such as the dragon and the White Demon.

Ancient World

Although cesarean delivery was probably practiced for ages, [1] no ancient medical documents mentioning the techniques or exact indication for cesarean section are extant. The evidence that cesarean section was performed arises from legal texts: a cuneiform tablet dealing with the adoption of a small boy during the 23rd year of the renowned king

Hammurabi of Babylon (1795-1750 BC), [15] "Lex Regia" (the Law of the Kings) proclaimed by Numa Pompilius, an ancient Roman king (716-673 BC), [12] and Mishna, the collection of ancient Jewish laws (2nd century BC – 6th century AD). [2, 16]

"Ibiq-Iltum, the son of Sin-Magir, adopted the male child, born through cesarean section [lit. pulled out of the womb], the son of the deceased woman Atkasim, from his [the child's] older brother Samas-Nasir and his wife [text: sister] Taris-Matum. Ibiq-Iltum handed over one shekel of silver and the nursing expenses for two years [consisting of] barley, oil and wool, to Samas-Nasir and Taris-Matum.". [15] This legal text, dating to the 23rd year of Hammurabi of Babylon (1795-1750 BC), is probably the very first documented evidence of cesarean section. The Akkadian expression silip remim (pulled out of the womb) could mean either cesarean section or forceps delivery. The use of obstetrical forceps is not attested until at least the medieval period. [17] Therefore it is generally presumed that this expression refers to a cesarean section done on a dead or dying mother. Interestingly, the expression silip remim (pulled out of the womb) is only known from Old Babylonian city of Sippar, and then only during a limited time span. [18] Thus, it could be speculated that the knowledge of performing postmortem cesarean was known in the city of Sippar during the reign of Hammurabi (who laid the city wall foundations in his 23rd year) and vanished thereafter.

Cesarean section on dead women was probably done by ancient Egyptians. [5] Sage Susruta, who practiced around 600 BC and is one of the founders of ancient Hindu medicine, refers to a postmortem cesarean delivery in his medical treatise, "Susruta Samhita". [19] He states that after the mother has died, the operation should be done quickly since a delay may cause the death of the child, too.

"Neget lex regia mulierem, quae praegnans mortua sit, humari, antequam partus ei excidatur; qui contra fecerit, spem animantis cum gravida videtur" ("A royal law forbids the burial of a pregnant woman before the child is extracted from the womb <antequam partus ei excidatur>; whoever violates this law is deemed to have destroyed the child's expectancy of life along with the mother.") It was *Numa Pompilius, an ancient Roman king (716-673* BC*), who* issued this ruling in his "*Lex Regia,*" the Law of the Kings. [20] This law of *Numa Pompilius is, in fact, the very first legal reference that established a postmortem delivery of a child* through an incision in the abdomen. Once ancient Rome became the Roman Empire, the "*Lex Regia*" turned into the "*Lex Cesarea.*" From this latter designation, the operation of laparotomy and hysterotomy to deliver a fetus may have taken its name, the cesarean section. A passage in Justinian's "*Corpus Iuris Civilis*" refers to Numa *Pompilius's* "Lex Regia" (527-565 AD). [21] This passage enables legal postmortem cesarean after the fall of the Western Roman Empire.

Interestingly, although legally enabled in the Roman World, cesarean section does not exist as an option for terminating protracted labor in the most important gynecological treatise of Roman World, the Soranus of Ephesos's *Gynecology* (1st -2nd centuries AD). [3, 22] Likewise, in Greek and Byzantine medical writings cesarean section is not mentioned. [3] One possible explanation could be that as in early medieval period, postmortem cesarean were presumptively performed by the clergy, the priests and not by medical professionals, and therefore does not appear in the Soranus's *Gynecology*. [1]

The *first reliable evidence that* a cesarean section *was performed* on living women who survived the operation comes from ancient Jewish writings of the Mishna and the Talmud, i.e. 2nd century BC – 6th century AD. [2, 16] Mishna *is the arranged and edited tractate of Oral Laws in contrast to Mikra, the Written Law.* Initially, cesarean delivery was performed on animals [23] and afterwards on living women with a fair degree of success. A postmortem cesarean delivery was also allowed: *"If a woman was in labor and died on the Sabbath, a knife is brought, her abdomen is opened, and the child extracted "*. [24] In the Talmudic writings, there is a description of a woman whose first child was born by cesarean section and who subsequently delivered again, probably via the vaginal route: "*Neither Yotze dofen, nor the after coming one can receive the rights of primogeniture either concerning property or the payment of redemption fee to the priest; Rabbi Shimon says: ... the first as to inheritance and the second as to five slai'm".*[25] "*Yotze dofen" is the only term which is used for caesarean section in the Mishna and the Talmud.* [2] "Slai'm" *is a form of currency.* If the parturient necessarily dies during cesarean section than there is no need for announcing legal regulation regarding two important aspects of the institution of primogeniture: the redemption of the firstborn and the inheritance of property. We have additional evidence that caesarean delivery on living women was practiced at the time of the Talmud: "*In the case of Yotzeh dofen, we do not observe either the days of ritual uncleanness or the days of purification [Niddah]* ". [26] Niddah are laws that forbid sexual relations of a woman with her husband during and for some time after her menses. These days are considered as days of ritual uncleanness or the days of purification. The blood discharge after childbirth is considered to be in the same category as the blood of menstruation (Leviticus XII, 1-8). If the parturient always dies during caesarean section, there is no need for a regulation stipulating what should be done during the period of purification (the Niddah). It is concerned, that these passages are of theoretical nature, due to known tendency of the Jewish writings to provide commentaries for even the most unlikely cases and since there is no medical writings to support maternal survival in the ancient Jewish world. It appears, however, that there is different terminology used for theoretical and concrete passages in the Mishna and the Talmud. Thus, it is apparent, that the relevant passages use the concrete terminology.

Medieval Period

A 10th century (AD) abbot of Saint Gallen was born by a postmortem cesarean: "*[The mother's] time drew near; she fell into a sore sickness before her time, and died a fortnight before the expected birth. The child was cut from her corpse and wrapped in the fat of a new-born pig, until his skin should grow...The brethren called him "The Unborn"...*". [27] This text indicates that a postmortem cesarean procedure was practiced in the early medieval period at least in Benedictine abbeys of Germany or Switzerland. The story furthers the ancient notion that those born by a cesarean are destined for special future. Also, since no physician is mentioned to be involved in the procedure, it might be assumed that the procedure was done by clergy, may be, though, specifically trained for that. In 1215, at the Fourth Lateran Council, the members of secular clergy were forbidden to practice surgery involving cutting and burning, and thus, perhaps, the postmortem "cutting" (as in cesarean) might have been left to midwives. [3]

By the middle ages, the Catholic Church required execution of obligatory postmortem cesarean section in order to save the soul of the child through baptism. [3, 28] As late as 1749, a Sicilian physician was condemned to death because of his failure to follow this law. [28] It seems that the Parisian archbishop Odon de Sully (1196-1208) was the first church official to recommend a cesarean if the fetus was alive after the death of the mother. [29] Albeit this recommendation, it is apparent that cesarean section as a medical procedure was not performed in medieval Europe before the early 14th century. [3] As a medical procedure, it was Bernard of Gordon, a Montpellier physician who mentions a postmortem cesarean in 1305. [30] Bernard states that even though the mother dies, the fetus may survive and thus an incision should be made in her abdomen (he does not indicate were), and the fetus should be extracted. He also advises that the cervix should be held open to assure the influx of air during the operation. [3]

Another important issue was raised: if baptism was of such paramount importance, whether the imminent death of the mother might be hastened and the mother sacrificed to save her otherwise doomed child? Saint Thomas Aquinas (1225-1274) clearly stated that one should not kill the mother in order to baptize the child. [3]

Islamic religious authorities also favored postmortem cesarean section, as evident from juridical doctrines written by the Imam Abu Hanifah (699-767 AD). [31] In fact, the first known drawing of a cesarean section is in a 14th century (1307-1308) Arabic manuscript al-Athar al Bagiya, [1, 8] which is a late transcription of a medical manuscript by Al-Biruni (973-1048 AD). Still, there is no evidence of cesarean section in writings of Albucasis (Abul Qasim Al-Zahrawi, 936-1013), who is mainly famous for his treatises on surgery, "Kitab Al-tasrif li man aiaz an-il-talif" (*English:* "The Book of enabling him to manage who cannot cope with the complications"), [32] which was the leading textbook on surgery in Europe for about 500 years.

It could be therefore affirmed that cesarean section in the medieval period was performed only for postmortem indication. In contrary to ancient times, there is no evidence for performing a cesarean section on living women. Thus cesarean birth in medieval period was a cultural rather than medical event.

Renaissance and Modern Ages

Probably, the first documented authentic successful cesarean section on a living woman who survived the operation was done upon his wife by Jacob Nufer, a Swiss sow-gelder in 1500. [23] However, the case is not entirely accepted by some historians because it was not reported until the year 1581. Perhaps, a more straightforward report is by a Saxonian surgeon Jeremias Trautmann on April 21, 1610. [8] The mother survived 25 days reflecting the poor maternal outcome in those days and also in the next following centuries. For example, in Paris, out of 24 cesareans performed between 1750-1800 no mother survived. [8] This caused enormous opposition against performing a cesarean on a living woman. Francois Mauriceau, the most famous obstetrician of the 17th century, stated: "*I do not know that there was ever any law, Christian or civil in which both ordain the martyring and killing the mother to save the child*". [33]

In 1581, Francois Rousset, publishes a revolutionary work with self-speaking subtitle: "*The extraction of the child through a lateral incision of the abdomen and the uterus of a pregnant woman who cannot otherwise give birth. And that without endangering the life of the one or the other and without preventing subsequent fertility*". [34] In this book, perhaps, for the first time, the concept of cesarean birth shifted from cultural to medical event. The indications for Cesarean according to Rousset: were large fetus, malformed fetus, dead fetus, twins, malpresentation, extremely young or old mother, too narrow mother, or not elastic enough. In contrary to medieval objective of religious context or of saving the child after his mother's death, these indications reflect emerging of awareness of maternal and fetal safety. So, it was during the Renaissance times, that cesarean section emerged as a medical procedure.

The cesarean section attributed mortality rate in USA during the 19th century, as calculated by Robert Harris, was around 75%. [35] The main reasons for maternal death were "exhaustion", peritonitis, septicemia, hemorrhage and eclampsia. The main indication for cesarean delivery was obstructed labor, typically for days with an intrauterine fetal death. [36, 37, 38] It appears, therefore, that most cesareans in the 19th centuries were performed in a possible milieu of severe infection, sepsis, and even disseminated intravascular coagulation as it is apparent from the case performed in June 1828 in Virginia, USA and reported later by Dr Weems. [38] The operation was performed after weeks of uterine contractions, with offensive discharge from the vagina, and the uterus contained remains of a fetus in half dissolved state. [38]

Anecdotally, one of the first cesareans in USA was performed in 1822 by the patient herself, a 14-yeares-old servant, who made an "L" shaped incision through the abdominal wall and the uterus while lying in a snow bank and recovered the operation. [39] As odd as it might be, a similar case was described in 1996 in Turkey, when a 32-years old woman cut her own abdomen and the uterus and removed the baby and the placenta. [40] The woman was then found by her 11-years old son who called an ambulance and that is how she was saved. It was postulated that in such circumstances, reduced serotonin activity may enable a self-operation. [40]

With introduction of improved surgical techniques, asepsis, modern transfusion techniques and Harris's principle of early operation prior to possible infection, the mortality rates improved to 0.1% between the years 1943-1952. [4] These factors also permitted the shift towards the modern objective of cesarean, which is directed to safety and health of both the mother and the child. A turning point in providing maternal safety was the introduction of the concept of uterine closure towards the end 19th century. [41] Prior to the understanding that suturing of the uterus is essential, the only reasonable solution to obviate the risk of death from hemorrhage and infection was offered by Eduardo Porro in 1876, who suggested performing a subtotal hysterectomy after delivery of the fetus. [42] According to Porro, the mother's life was saved at the expense of her future fertility.

20TH CENTURY

During the 20th century we observed a tremendous rise in the rate of cesarean sections, for example, in the USA, it rose from <1% in 1910 to about 30% in 2006. [43] The main indications for cesarean section during the 20th century can be broadly grouped in protracted labor, non-reassuring fetal heart rate pattern (i.e fetal distress), malpresentation of the fetus, previously scarred uterus, placental abnormalities with heavy bleeding, and maternal reasons. [44] During the 20th century, the definitions of each sub-group as well as absolute and relative indications for cesarean have changed dramatically with the introduction of electronic fetal monitoring, scalp pH monitoring, tremendous improvement of neonatal care, and evidence based medicine concept. Edwin Craigin, in 1916, stated the most quoted dictum in obstetrics: "*Once a cesarean, always a cesarean*". [45] The dictum was valid as long as the typical cesarean section included a classical (upper-segment) incision in the uterus. With the introduction of the transverse lower uterine segment incision by John Munro Kerr, [46] and recognition that this type of incision is not associated with an excessively high rate of uterine rupture during labor, a trial of vaginal birth after one previous cesarean section became the most accepted policy. In 2000, cesarean section became the favorite method of delivery in term breech presentation following publication of a randomized multicentre trial that indicated strongly that planned caesarean section is to be preferred than planned vaginal birth for the term fetus in the breech presentation with similar serious maternal complications rate. [47] Postmortem cesarean is still performed today and perimortem cesarean has emerged as a variation of this ancient indication. [48]

Finally, towards the end of the 20th century, two important issues regarding the objective of cesarean section have emerged, namely cesarean section on patients request [49] and forced cesarean. [50] Nevertheless, there are ethical questions that are still disputed regarding cesarean section on patients' request. Is a vaginal delivery a medical treatment? If so, than by virtue of the concept of informed consent a woman has a legitimate right to choose between the two treatments, the vaginal and the cesarean delivery. If a woman is refused for cesarean section because there are no medical indications, does that imply that she will have a "forced" vaginal birth? Has a physician the right to refuse to perform a cesarean that is requested by a woman without medical indication? In any case, it appears that in the beginning of the 21st century, the focus among practitioners is moving towards supporting maternal choice for delivery. [51, 52]

The History of Cesarean Tecnique

In the context of vanished ancient cesarean section techniques, it is of interest to mention a cesarean section witnessed by a missionary British doctor, R.W. Felkin, in Kahura, Uganda in 1879. [41] The surgical technique could have been used by the Banyoro tribe surgeons for centuries: [8] "*The woman [a 20-year-old primigravida] lay upon an inclined bed.... She was liberally supplied with banana wine, and was in a state of semi-intoxication. She was perfectly naked. A band of mbugu or bark cloth fastened her thorax to the bed, another band of cloth fastened down her thighs, and a man held her ankles. Another man, standing on her right steadied her abdomen...The operator stood....on her left side...holding his knife aloft...and muttering an incantation.... He washed his hands and the patient's abdomen, first with banana wine and then water. Then, having uttered a shrill cry, ... he proceeded to make a rapid cut in the middle line .... The whole abdominal wall and part of the uterine wall were severed by this incision, and the liquor amnii escaped; a few bleeding-points in the abdominal wall were touched with red-hot iron by an assistant...The child was next rapidly removed...after the cord had been cut ... the operator...seized the contracting uterus with both hands and gave it a squeeze or two. He next put his right hand into the uterine cavity... dilated the cervix within outwards. He then cleaned uterus from clots... No sutures were put into the uterine wall ....A porous grass mat was placed over the wound and secured there...the edges of the wound... were brought into close apposition, seven thin iron spikes... being used for the purpose, and fastened by string made from bark cloth. A paste prepared by chewing two different roots and spitting the pulp into a bowel was then quickly plastered over the wound, a banana life warned over the fire being placed on the top of that, and finally a firm bandage of mbugu cloth ... Eleven days after the operation the wound was entirely heaked."* The salient points of the cesarean technique of the Banyoro tribe surgeons are anesthesia (banana wine), antisepsis (banana wine), low midline abdominal incision, good hemostasis (red hot iron), blunt incision of the uterus (minimizing hemorrhage), non-suturing of the uterus with its manual massage and cautery of uterine incision bleeding points (minimizing hemorrhage), suture of abdominal wall, and wound care (root paste). [41] At present, uterine suture is thought to reduce the amount of blood loss and to enhance uterine healing. [53] Non-suture of the uterus is apparently associated with greater hemorrhage that may lead even to exsanguination. Conversely, recent experimental data in dogs reveal that non-closure of a low transverse uterine incision after safe hemostasis and administration of uterotropins is associated with good outcome and might even be preferable in appropriate cases. [54]

One of the first explicit instructions on how to perform a cesarean section dates from about 1480 AD, from southern Germany: [3, 55] " *...the skillful midwife has to open up one side, but not the right one; for in men the heart is located on the left side, but in women the right side. She shall start cutting in the lower part of the belly around the pubic bone, about the width of one hand. With her oiled hand she must carefully move aside all the entrails. The sick women should lie on her back with her head tilted back so that she can reach the uterus. After the opening of the uterus, the women should be tilted to one side .... The child should be freed from the membranes. But the woman, if she still seems to be alive, should be turned again on her back. The wound should be closed with three or four ligatures by means of a needle and a silk or other thread. On top of this should be placed a plaster made from three eggs and some fabric of strong hemp to which one may add .... some Armenian clay. .... The woman receives a sip of the best wine. Should she survive and regain consciousness, give her a drink made of the roots of salsify and of mountain albanum sautéed in wine*." Note that the instructions are addressed to a midwife (perhaps in accordance with Fourth Lateran Council of 1215), the ignorance regarding anatomy (location of heart in men versus women), the special care of intestine (oiled hand), the use of Trendelenburg's position (to improve exposition of the uterus), the use of analgesia (best wine), non-suturing of the uterus, and emphasis on postoperative wound care.

Abdominal Incision

Almost any abdominal area was suggested for abdominal incision for cesarean section. [56] At first, the incision was made on the right or on the left side along the linea alba. [3] An oblique incision was also reported. [38] The next improvement was a midline incision through the linea alba, which was originated by Levret, [57] Solayres, Platner, or Guenin. [56] The apparent advantages of midline incision were reduced bleeding and good healing, while the disadvantage was the risk of injury to the bladder. James Blundell (1790-1878) suggested a high longitudinal incision to minimize the risk of bladder injury and adhesion formation, once the uterus contracted away from abdominal wall. [56, 58]

Blundell's suggestion was not accepted, perhaps because of heavier bleeding and poorer healing. Pfannenstiel introduced the next improvement in 1900. [59] At the turn of the 19th century gynecologists began to incise the skin transversely but still cut the fascia longitudinally. [60] Pfannenstiel's crucial contribution was to incise the fascia transversely. The transverse abdominal incision was modified by Alfred Maylard [61] in 1907 and by Joel-Cohen [62] in 1972. The advantages of the Pfannenstiel incision are potentially more secure closure, less postoperative pain and better cosmetic appearance. Today, apparently, the Pfannenstiel incision is the most commonly used. Still, for most of us, the choice of abdominal incision for cesarean section is determined by surgeon's comfort and habit. [53]

Uterine Incision

Most of the early surgeons used a longitudinal (vertical) incision for opening the uterine cavity. [56] The vertical uterine incision avoids dangerous lateral dissection and allows a sufficiently enlarged aperture for safe delivery. [53, 56] The disadvantages include more severe bleeding, the possibility of downward extension of the incision into the bladder and the vagina and a substantial risk of uterine rupture during subsequent pregnancies. [53, 56] Kehrer in 1882 suggested the low transverse incision at the level of internal cervical os. [63] He believed that placing the incision at the level of the internal os would improve the morbidity because of the natural tendency of uterus to anteflexy. Kehrer's incision did not become popular as well as Fritsch's suggestion for transverse fundal incision. [56] The next development was one of the most dramatic advances in cesarean technique. In 1926, Monro Kerr made popular the transverse lower uterine segment incision as opposed to the upper classical variety. [64] In fact several surgeons had suggested this approach in the 18th and early 19th century, [56] but, it did not become popular until its introduction by Kerr. The apparent advantages are less bleeding and reduced risk of uterine rupture during subsequent trials of vaginal delivery. When a larger uterine incision is needed for the delivery of the fetus, the transverse lower uterine segment incision may be extended upward in the bilateral "J" shape or inverted "T" incision. [41]

Uterine Closure

In the 15th-19th centuries, and even later, the prevailing notion was that the uterine wound at cesarean section required no treatment except for cleansing. There was a perception that contraction and relaxation of the uterus would make the placement of uterine sutures ineffective, if not impossible. [5] In those days sutures had to be removed and it was considered impossible to remove the sutures after the abdomen was closed. For example, Andre Levret (1703-1780) had taught that uterine sutures in cesarean section: "were not only prejudicial but were absolutely useless because of the prodigious contractions which the uterine muscle undergoes following delivery". [39, 57] Lebas, in 1769, suggested using sutures to close the uterine incision. [5, 53, 65] The non-absorbable sutures of silk or linen were left protruding from the wound for later removing. In view of the ignorance of asepsis in the 18th century, this, of course, increased maternal mortality from infection.

A turning point in the evolution of cesarean technique came with the appearance of Max Sanger's monograph in 1882. Max Sanger insisted that suturing of the uterus was essential, and introduced a truly efficient silver suture that produced minimal tissue reaction. [66] Now, in contrary to Porro suggestion, [42] the mother's life could be saved without prejudice to her future fertility. Actually, Robert Harris may have precedence over Max Sanger. Robert Harris was an American surgeon who suggested the use of uterine sutures four years prior to Max Sanger in 1878. [67] However, Harris did not advocate application of uterine sutures in every cesarean section, but only in certain selected cases. Furthermore, Max Sanger certainly deserves the credit for awakening the obstetric community to the importance of uterine sutures. [68] There were two other improvements aimed at obviating infection, which however did not become popular. In 1906, Frank introduced an extra-peritoneal cesarean technique. The principle of this operation was to unite the cut edges of parietal and visceral peritoneum before uterine incision. [69] In 1923, Portes performed a two-step operation. [70] During the first step, the fetus was delivered, the abdominal incision was closed around the exteriorized uterus at the cervical level, and the uterus was closed, and left outside the abdomen. If infection was noted, a hysterectomy was performed. If no infection was noted, a second operation was performed, returning the involuted uterus into the pelvic cavity. Eventually, the incidence of infection attributed to cesarean delivery was reduced by using aseptic technique and prophylactic antibiotics. [71]

Recent Developments

There is a current notion towards simplifying cesarean techniques in order to reduce intraoperative blood loss and operating time. Blunt expansion of the uterine incision in low isthmic transverse cesarean was shown to be associated with better protection of the uterine vessels and decreased blood loss. [72] Not closing the visceral peritoneum was shown to be associated with fewer postoperative complications and to be more cost effective and less painful. [73, 74] Non-closure of subcutaneous tissue was not associated with increased risk of wound infection. [75] A modified Joel-Cohen technique was shown to be associated with reduced intraoperative blood loss and operating time. [76] A single-layer uterine closure was shown to be of similar safety and efficacy as two-layer closure. [77]

The salient points of the "Misgav Ladach" method include Joel-Cohen incision, single-layer repair of the low uterine segment transverse incision, and non-suturing of the visceral and parietal peritoneum and subcutaneous tissue. [75, 78] The result is a more speedy recovery with early ambulation and resumption of drinking and eating. [75, 78] The salient points of the "Laniado" method are Pfannenstiel incision, blunt expansion of subcutaneous tissue and the fascia, blunt opening of parietal peritoneum, blunt expansion of the uterus in the lower uterine segment, and non-suturing of visceral and parietal peritoneum and subcutaneous tissue. [79] In countries with a high prevalence of HIV virus, this technique might decrease the potential exposure of the surgeons because of minimized contact with sharp objects during surgery.

REFERENCES

[1] Lurie S. The changing motives of cesarean section from ancient times to 21st century. *Arch. Gynecol. Obstet.* 2005;271:281-5.

[2] Lurie S, Mamet Y. " Yotzeh dofen": cesarean section in the days of the Mishna and the Talmud. *Isr. J. Obstet. Gynecol.* 2001;12:111-3.

[3] Blumenfeld-Kosinski R. *Not of woman born.* Cornell University Press, Ithaca and London. 1990; pp.1-47.

[4] Greenhill JP. *Obstetrics* 11th ed. Philadelphia, WB Saunders Co., 1955; pp.986-1033.

[5] Boley JP. The history of caesarean section. *Can. Med. Assoc. J.* 1991;145: 319-22 (1935;32:557-9).

[6] Lopez-Zeno JA, Carlo WA, O'Grady JP, Fanaroff AA. Infant survival following delayed postmortem cesarean delivery. *Obstet. Gynecol.* 1990;76:91-2.

[7] Awwad JT, Azar GB, Aouad AT, Raad J, Karam KS. Postmortem cesarean section following maternal blast injury: case report. *J. Trauma* 1994;36:260-1.

[8] Speert H. Obstetrics and Gynecology. *A history and Iconography.* 3rg ed. Parthenon Publishing Group, New York. 2004; pp. 297-309.

[9] Pinsent J. *Greek Mythology*. Hamlyn Publishing, London. 1969; p.82.

[10] Gaius Plinius Secundus. *Natural History*. 77 CE (VII, ix,47).

[11] Galbert HA, Bey M. History and development of cesarean operation. *Obstet. Gynecol. Clin. North Am.* 1988;15:591-605.

[12] Trolle D. *The history of cesarean section.* Reitzel CA, Copenhagen, 1982; p.15,25.

[13] Sahname-i Firdevsi. 1549. Reproduced in Nil Sari. *Turkish medical history through miniature pictures exhibition.* Istanbul, Turkey. 2002; pp. 104-111.

[14] Ehrhard FK, Friedrichs K,. Diener MS, Fischer-Schreiber I, Schuhmacher S. *Encyclopedia of Eastern Philosophy and Religion.* Boston, Shambhala Publications, Inc. 1994.

[15] Oppenheim AL. A cesarean section in the second millennium B.C. J. *Hist. Med.* 1960;15:292-294.

[16] Lurie S. Vaginal delivery after cesarean delivery in the days of the Talmud (2nd century b.c.e.- 6th century c.e.) *Vesalius* 2006;12:23-4.

[17] Luire S. The forceps of Albucasis. *Bull. Isr. Soc. Obstet. Gynecol.* 2004;2:41-2.

[18] Stol M. *Birth in Babylonia and the bible.* SIYX publications, Groningen. 2000; p.128.

[19] Pundel J. L' *Histoire de l'operation cesarienne.* Presses Academiques Europeennes, Brussels. 1969; p.57.

[20] *The laws of the kings.* Rome, 8th/7th cent. B.C. (FIRA 2, vol. 1, p. 3. Tr. ARS, rev. L).

[21] Justinian. *Corpus Iuris Civilis.* Digest. 11,8,2. 533 CE.

[22] Soranus of Ephesos. *Soranus' Gyneclogy.* Trans. Owsei Temkin. Johns Hopkins University Press, Baltimore. 1956.

[23] Schaffer J. "Born from the flank"- discussion concerning "cesarean section" in animals in the Talmud. *Sud. Arch. Z. Wissen.* 1996;80:198-204.

[24] Gmarah, Erchin, chapter 1, page 7,folio 1.

[25] Mishnah, Bechoroth, chapter 2, page 47.

[26] Gmara, Niddah. Chapters 5, page 40, folio 1.

[27] Coulton G. *Life in the middle ages*. Cambridge University Press, Cambridge. 1930; v4, pp.80-1.
[28] Speert H. Historical highlights. In: *Obstetrics and Gynecology*.5th ed. Danforth DN, Scott JR ed. Lippincott Co, Philadelphia. 1986; pp. 2-22.
[29] Patrologiae cursus completes. *Series latina*. ed Migne JP. Paris, 1844-1864. 212, col 63, no 6.
[30] Bernard of Gordon. *Practica sive lilium medicinae*. Lyons, 1498.
[31] Radd-Ul-Muchtar. Cairo, Egypt. 1844.
[32] Albucasis, On Surgery and Instruments. *A definitive edition of the Arabic text with English translation and commentary by Spink MS and Lewis GL*. London, The Welcome Institute of the History of Medicine,1973.
[33] Mauriceau F. *The diseases of women with child, and in child-bed* (English translation. 2nd edition. Hugh Chamberlain). London, John Darby. 1683.
[34] Rousset F. Traitte nouveau de l'hysterotomotokie, ou enfantment Caesarien. *Denys du Val*, Paris, 1581.
[35] Harris RP. Special statistics of the cesarean operation in the United States, showing the success and failures in each state. *Am. J. Obstet.* 1881:144:341-61.
[36] Miller JL. Cesarean section in Virginia in the pre-aseptic era. 1794-1879. *Ann. Med. Hist.* 1938;20:23-35.
[37] Lungren SS. A case of cesarean section twice successfully performed on the same patient, with remarks on the time, indications, and details of the operation. *Am. J. Obstet.* 1881;14:78-94.
[38] Weems ML. *Am. J. Med. Scien.* 1836;8:257.
[39] Eastman NJ. The role of frontier America in the development of cesarean section. *Am. J. Obstet. Gynecol.* 1932;24:919-29.
[40] Yoldas Z, Iscan A, Yoldas T, Ermete L, Akyurek C. A woman who did her own caesarean section. *Lancet* 1996;348:135.
[41] Lurie S, Glezerman M. History of cesarean technique. *Am. J. Obstet. Gynecol.* 2003;189:1803-6.
[42] Porro E. Della amputazione utero-ovarica come complemento di taglio cesareo. *Ann. Univ. Med. Chir.* (Milan) 1876:237:289-350.
[43] Wolf J. Deliver me from pain. *Anesthesia and Birth in America*.The John Hopkins University Press, Baltimore. 2009;p.179.
[44] Cunnigham FG, MacDonald PC, Gant NF, Levono KJ, Gilstrap III LC, Hankins GDV and Clark SL. Williams Obstetrics. 20th ed., Stamford, Connecticut: *Appleton and Lange*, 1997 pp. 509-32.
[45] Craigin EB. Conservatism in obstetrics. *N Y Med. J.* 1916;104:1-3.
[46] Kerr JMM. The technique of cesarean section, with special reference to the lower uterine segment incision. *Am. J. Obstet. Gynecol.* 1926;12:729-34.
[47] Hannah ME, Hannah WJ, Hewson SA, Hodnett ED, Saigal S, Willan AR. Planned caesarean section versus planned vaginal birth for breech presentation at term: a randomized multicentre trial. Term Breech Trial Collaborative Group. *Lancet* 2000;356:375-83.
[48] Lurie S, Mamet Y. Cesarean delivery during maternal cardiopulmonary resuscitation for status asthmaticus. *Emerg. Med. J.* 2003;20:296-7.
[49] Wagner M. Choosing cesarean section. *Lancet* 2000;356:677-80.

[50] Ikemoto LC. Forced cesareans. *Curr. Opin. Obstet. Gynecol.* 1998;10:465-8.

[51] Paterson-Brown S, Fisk N. Cesarean section: every woman's right to choose? *Curr. Opin. Obstet. Gynecol.* 1997;9:351-8.

[52] Husslein P. Elective caesarean section versus vaginal delivery. Whither the end of traditional obstetrics? *Arch. Gynecol. Obstet.* 2001;265:169-74.

[53] Field CS. Surgical techniques for cesarean section. *Obstet. Gynecol. Clin. North Am.* 1988;15:657-72.

[54] Gul A, Kotan C, Ugras S, Alan M, Gul T. Transverse uterine incision: non-closure versus closure: an experimental study in dogs. *Eur. J. Obstet. Gynecol.* 2000;88:95-9.

[55] Ketsch P. *Frauen im Mittelalter*. Schwann-Bagel, Duseldorf. 1983. I:286.

[56] Galbert HA, Bey M. History and development of cesarean operation. *Obstet. Gynecol. Clin. North Am.* 1988;15:591-605 .

[57] Levret A. *L'Art des Accouchements*. Paris, Le Prieur. 1753.

[58] Blundell J. *Principles and practice of Obstetricy*. E Cox, London. 1834.

[59] Pfannenstiel HJ. Uber die Vortheile des Suprasymphysaren Fascienquerschnitts fur die Gynakolodischen Koliotomien zugleich ein Beitrag zu der Iindikationsstellung der Operationswege. *Samml. Klin. Vortr. Lepzig.* 1900;268:1735-56.

[60] Baskett TE. On the shoulders of giants. *Eponyms and names in Obstetrics and Gynecology*. RCOG Press, London. 1996.

[61] Maylard AE. Direction of abdominal incisions. *Br. Med. J.* 1907;2:895-901.

[62] Joel-Cohen S. Abdominal and vaginal hysterectomy. *New techniques based on time and motion studies.* William Heinemann Medical Books, 1972, p170.

[63] Kehrer FA. Uber ein modifiziertes Verfahren beim Kaiserschnitt. *Arch. Gynekol. Bd.* 1882;19:117.

[64] Kerr JMM. The technique of cesarean section, with special reference to the lower uterine segment incision. *Am. J. Obstet. Gynecol.* 1926;12:729-34.

[65] Garrigues HJ. The improved cesarean section. *Am. J. Obstet.* 1883;16:33 .

[66] Sanger M. Der Kaiserschnitt. *Arch. Gynak.* 1882;19:370.

[67] Harris RP. The operation of gastro-hysterotomy (true cesarean section), viewed in the light of American experience and success; with the history and results of sewing up the uterine wound; and a full tabular record of the cesarean operation performed in the United States, many of them not hitherto reported. *Am. J. Med. Scien.* 1878;75:313-42.

[68] Sanger M. My work in reference to the cesarean operation. A word in protest in reply to Doctor Henry J Garrigues. *Am. J. Obstet.* 1887;20:593.

[69] DeLee JB. An illustrated history of the low or cervical cesarean section. *Am. J. Obstet. Gynecol.* 1925;10:503.

[70] Young JH. *The History of Cesarean Sections*. London, HK Lewis. 1944.

[71] Wilson JR. The conquest of cesarean section-related infections: a progress report. *Obstet. Gynecol.* 1988;72:519-32.

[72] Rodrigez AI, Porter KB, O'Brien WF. Blunt versus sharp expansion of the uterine incision in low-segment transverse cesarean section. *Am. J. Obstet. Gynecol.* 1994;171:1022-5.

[73] Orion O, Luzuy F, Beguin F. Nonclosure of the visceral and parietal peritoneum at cesarean section: a randomised controlled trial. *Br. J. Obstet. Gynaecol.* 1996;106:103:690-4.

[74] Hackmon-Ram R, Piura B. To close or not to close the peritoneum in abdominal gynecologic and obstetric operations. *Harefuah* 1999;137:474-7.

[75] Stark M, Finkel AR. Comparison between the Joel-Cohen and Pfannenstiel incisions in cesarean section. *Eur. J. Obstet. Gynecol.* 1994;53:121-2.

[76] Wallin G, Fall O. Modified Joel-Cohen technique for cesarean delivery. *Br. J. Obstet. Gynaecol.* 1999;106:221-6.

[77] Enkin MW, Wilkinson C. Single versus two layer suturing for closure the uterine incision at cesarean section. *Cochrane Database Syst. Rev.* 2000;2:CD0192.

[78] Federici D, Lacelli B, Muggiasca L, Agarosi A, Cipolla, Conti M. Cesarean section using the Misgav Ladach method. *Int. J. Gynecol. Obstet.* 1997;57:273-9.

[79] Lurie S, Feinstein M, Mamet Y. Assessment of a newer technique for cesarean section. *Arch. Gynecol. Obstet.* 2002; 266:195-7.

In: Cesarean Section: Procedures, Complications and Recovery ISBN: 978-1-62081-214-3
Editor: Eyal Sheiner

Chapter III

THE EPIDEMIOLOGY OF CESAREAN DELIVERY IN THE UNITED STATES: TRENDS, CHARACTERISTICS, AND OUTCOMES

Marian F. MacDorman[1,*], Michelle J. K. Osterman[1] and Eugene Declercq[2]

[1]Reproductive Statistics Branch, Division of Vital Statistics, National Center for Health Statistics, Centers for Disease Control and Prevention, Hyattsville, Maryland, US
[2]Department of Community Health Sciences, Boston University School of Public Health, Boston, Massachusetts, US

ABSTRACT

In 2009, almost 1.4 million American women had a cesarean delivery, [1] and cesarean delivery is currently the most common major surgical procedure for women in the United States. [2] One out of every 3 US births (32.9%) is now delivered by cesarean section, the highest level ever recorded in the United States, and a level that is higher than most other developed countries. [1, 3-4] The cesarean rate increased dramatically during the 1970's and early 1980's and then plateaued in the late 1980's (based on data from the National Hospital Discharge Survey). [5] Between 1989 and 1996 the total cesarean rate decreased as a result of a decrease in the primary cesarean rate and an increase in the rate of vaginal birth after cesarean (VBAC). [6, 8] However, in 1996, these trends were reversed, and cesarean rates have increased every year from 1996-2009. [1, 7] This chapter uses national vital statistics data to examine recent trends and characteristics of cesarean delivery in the United States from 1996-2009. In addition, the relevant epidemiologic literature is reviewed to examine broader issues surrounding cesarean delivery, such as trends in medical risks and indications, maternal opinions, and birth outcomes.

* Corresponding author: Marian F. MacDorman, Ph.D. Division of Vital Statistics, National Center for Health Statistics, 3311 Toledo Rd. Room 7318, Hyattsville, Maryland 20782. Phone: (301)458-4356. Email: mfm1@cdc.gov.

Keywords: Cesarean delivery; vaginal delivery, birth certificate, United States, international comparisons

METHODS

Data on cesarean delivery used in this paper are based on the method of delivery as reported on the more than 4 million birth certificates filed each year in the United States and compiled by the National Center for Health Statistics. Cesarean data became available from birth certificates in 1989 and was reported by all US states except Louisiana, Maryland, Nebraska, Nevada, and Oklahoma. In 1990 all states except Oklahoma reported this information, and by 1991 all states reported this information. Prior to 1989, data from the National Hospital Discharge Survey were used to track trends in cesarean delivery. [2, 5]

Several measures of cesarean delivery are used, and are computed as follows. The *total cesarean* rate (also known simply as the cesarean rate) is the percent of cesarean births out *of all births* in a given year. The *primary cesarean rate* is the percent of cesarean births to women in a given year who *have not* had a previous cesarean delivery. The rate of *repeat cesarean delivery* is the percent of births by cesarean to women who *have had* a previous cesarean. A related measure, the rate of *vaginal birth after previous cesarean (VBAC)* is defined as the percent of vaginal births to women who *have had* a previous cesarean. National data on total cesarean rates are available for the entire period from 1990-2009 (except that Oklahoma did not provide data in 1990). However, national primary, repeat, and VBAC rates are only available from 1990-2003 due to a change in the question about prior cesareans on the 2003 revision of the US Standard Certificate of birth and the fact that different states have adopted this revision at different times. [8, 9] For example, in 2008, revised primary cesarean and VBAC data were available for 27 states representing 65% of US births. [9] Until all states adopt the revised birth certificate national levels cannot be produced for primary and repeat cesareans and VBACs. Consequently, Figure 1 presents total cesarean rates for 1990-2009 and primary cesarean and VBAC rates only for 1990-2003.

Data Analysis

National trends in total cesarean rates are examined from 1990-2009 (1990 data excludes Oklahoma). Changes in cesarean rates from 1996-2009 are examined by maternal age, race/ethnicity, live birth order, gestational age, plurality, state, and for selected medical risk factors and complications. 1996 was chosen as the base year for the more detailed analysis since 1996 was the year when the previous downwards trend in cesarean section reversed itself. Trends in national primary and repeat cesarean rates are examined from 1990-2003 and compared with 2008 data from 27 revised states. Trends in cesarean delivery are also discussed in light of recent research on changes in the medical risk profile of births, maternal opinions regarding cesarean delivery, and maternal and neonatal outcomes.

Results

Trends

The percentage of United States' births delivered by cesarean has increased by 59% over a 13-year period, from 20.7% of all US births in 1996 to 32.9% in 2009 (Table 1 and Figure 1). The increase in the cesarean rate since 1996 reflects two concurrent trends: an increase in the primary cesarean rate and a decline in the VBAC rate. The primary cesarean rate increased from 14.6% in 1996 to 19.1% in 2003. About 58% of the increase in the total cesarean rate from 1996-2003 was due to increases in primary cesareans. At the same time, the VBAC rate decreased from 28.3% to 10.6%. A decrease in the VBAC rate implies a corresponding increase in the repeat cesarean rate, which reached almost 90% in 2003. [8] Thus, the adage, "once a cesarean, always a cesarean" appears to now apply to 90% of US women.

National estimates of primary cesarean and VBAC rates cannot be computed after 2003 as the number of states with revised and unrevised birth certificates changed from year to year; accordingly trend analysis of these data are compromised by the changing composition of the revised and unrevised reporting areas. However, vital statistics data suggest a continued increase in the primary cesarean rate and a continued decline in the VBAC rate after 2003. [9-11] In 2009, the primary cesarean rate was 24.0 for the 27 revised states, and 22.3 for the 23 unrevised states; in 2003 the primary cesarean rate was 19.3 for the same 23 states. [10] The VBAC rate was 8.3 for the 27 revised states and 6.8 for the 23 unrevised states; in 2003 the VBAC rate was 11.1 for the same 23 states. [10] The US cesarean rate is high compared to that in most industrialized countries (Figure 2); however most developed countries have also experienced increases in cesarean delivery over the past decade. [3, 12]

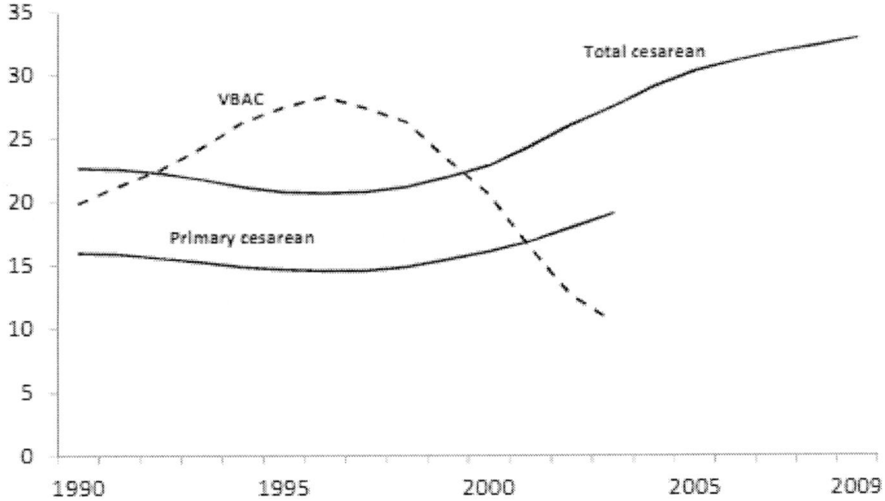

Source: Birth data from the National Vital Statistics System, CDC/NCHS; see references 1 and 8.
Note: 1990 data excludes Oklahoma.

Figure 1. US total cesarean rate 1990-2009, and primary cesarean and VBAC rates 1990-2003.

Table 1. Cesarean rates by selected characteristics, United States, 1996 and 2009, and percent change in cesarean rates, 1996-2009

	1996	2009	Percent change 1996-2009
Total	20.7	32.9	59
Maternal age			
<20	14.5	23.1	59
20-24	17.4	28.5	64
25-29	20.6	31.7	54
30-34	23.8	36.3	53
35-39	27.4	42.8	56
40+	31.6	49.5	57
Maternal race/ethnicity			
Non-Hispanic white	20.8	32.8	58
Non-Hispanic black	21.7	35.4	63
American Indian	18.1	28.5	57
Asian or Pacific Islander	18.6	33.1	78
Hispanic:*	20.0	31.6	58
Mexican	19.4	30.3	56
Puerto Rican	20.8	34.3	65
Cuban	30.3	48.8	61
Central or South American	21.3	32.6	53
Live birth order			
1	22.0	32.4	47
2-3	20.2	34.2	69
4+	17.6	28.9	64
Gestational age (weeks)			
<32	39.7	55.0	39
32-33	35.3	52.2	48
34-36	26.8	42.3	58
37-41	19.5	31.2	60
37-38	21.8	35.1	61
39	20.1	32.7	63
40-41	17.6	25.9	47
42+	20.1	29.3	46
Plurality			
Single birth	19.7	31.3	59
Multiple birth	55.4	76.3	38
Selected medical risk factors			
Diabetes	35.2	47.6	35
Chronic hypertension	38.6	53.5	39
Pregnancy-associated hypertension	36.1	48.9	35

* Includes additional Hispanic ethnicities not shown separately.

Source: Birth data from the National Vital Statistics System, CDC, NCHS.

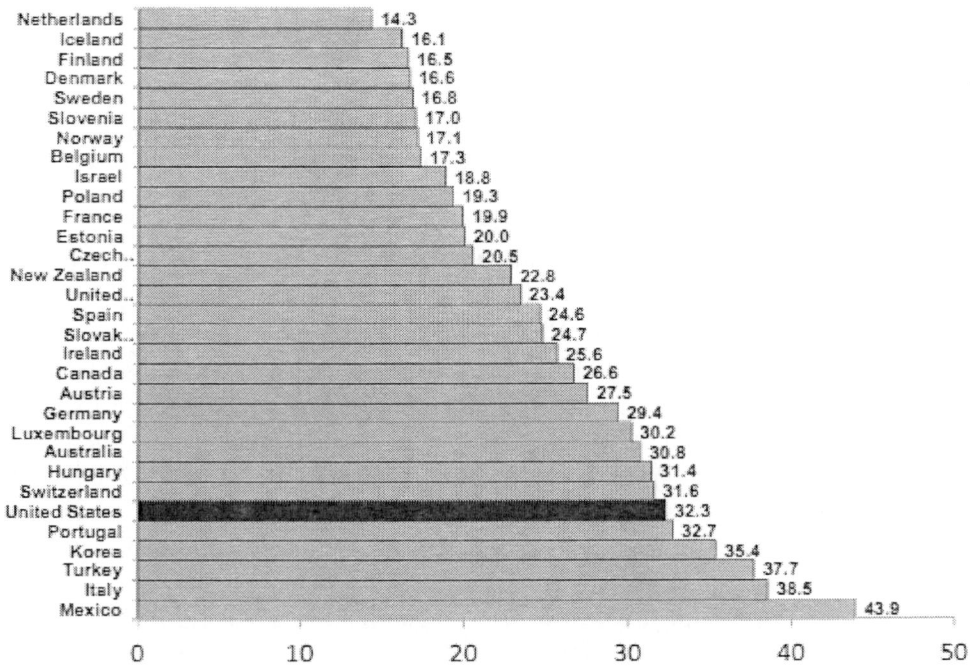

Source: Organization for Economic Cooperation and Development data base, 2011.
Note: Data for Belgium are for 2007.

Figure 2. Percentage of cesarean births, OECD countries, 2008.

Variations by Selected Characteristics

Age-- Cesarean rates increase with increasing maternal age. In 2009, half (49.5%) of births to women aged 40 and over were delivered by cesarean, compared to 23.1% of teen births (Table 1). [1] Prior research had found that higher cesarean rates for older mothers were related to higher rates of cesarean without a trial of labor, induction of labor, and failure to progress and fetal distress during labor. [13] From 1996-2009, cesarean rates increased by 53-64% for women in all age groups, but most rapidly (by 59-64%) for women under age 25 (Table 1).

Race/Ethnicity-- In 2009, nearly one-half (48.8%) of Cuban mothers had a cesarean delivery, the highest cesarean rate among the race/ethnic groups. [1] Non-Hispanic black mothers had the next-highest cesarean rates (35.4%) followed by Puerto Rican (34.3), Asian or Pacific Islander (33.1) and non-Hispanic white women (32.8). Cesarean rates were lowest for Mexican women (30.3). From 1996-2009, cesarean rates increased most rapidly for Asian or Pacific Islander women (78%), followed by Puerto Rican (65%), non-Hispanic black (63%) and Cuban (61%) women. The smallest increases (although still over 50%) were for Central and South American (53%) and Mexican (56%) women.

Live Birth Order--From 1996-2009, cesarean rates increased by 47% for women having a first live birth, by 69% for women having a second or third live birth, and by 64% for women having a 4th or greater live birth. Cesarean rates were highest for women having a second or third live birth, and lowest for women with a live birth order of 4 or more.

Gestational Age--Cesarean rates increased for births at all gestational ages between 1996 and 2009. From 1996-2009, cesarean rates rose by 39-63% for each gestational age category. The largest increases (58-63%) were for gestational ages between 34 and 39 weeks of gestation. However, the highest cesarean rates in 2009 were for the earliest gestational ages. More than half of very preterm (<32 weeks of gestation) and moderately preterm (32-33 weeks of gestation) births were delivered by cesarean, compared to about 1/4 of infants delivered at 40-41 weeks of gestation, the group with the lowest cesarean rate.

Plurality and Medical Conditions--From 1996-2009, cesarean rates increased by 59% for single births, and by 38% for multiple births. In 2009, the cesarean rate for single births was 31.3, compared to a rate of 76.3 for multiple births. Cesarean rates also increased for women with diabetes, chronic hypertension, and pregnancy-associated hypertension.

State Variation--In 2009, cesarean rates varied considerably by State and region of the country (Table 2 and Figure 3). Although not all states fit the regional pattern, cesarean rates tended to be lowest in the upper Midwest (Minnesota, Wisconsin) and western mountain states (from Idaho to New Mexico), and highest in the southeastern states (from Texas to Florida). New Mexico (22.8), Utah (22.9), and Alaska (23.8) had the lowest cesarean rates, while Louisiana (39.6), New Jersey (39.4), Florida (38.1), and Mississippi (37.8) had the highest rates. The states with the lowest percentage increase from 1996-2009 were South Dakota (26%), New Mexico (33%) and Arkansas (37%) (Table 2 and Figure 4). In contrast, for 7 states (Connecticut, Colorado, Florida, Nevada, Oregon, Rhode Island, and Washington) cesarean rates increased by 74-85% from 1996-2009.

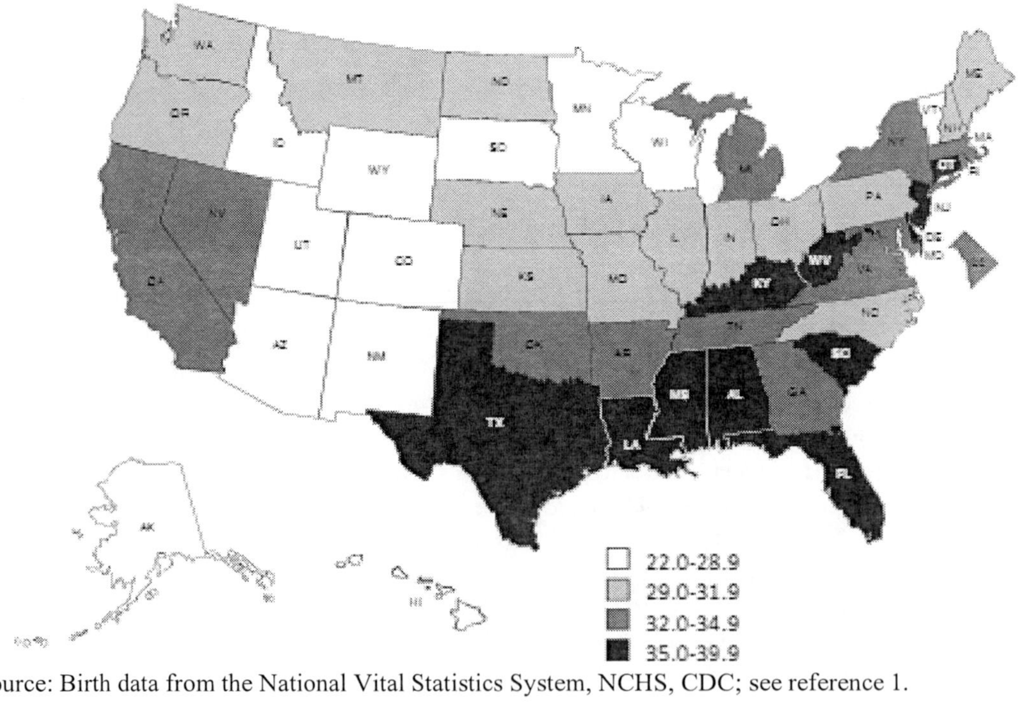

Source: Birth data from the National Vital Statistics System, NCHS, CDC; see reference 1.

Figure 3. Cesarean Rates by State: United States, 2009.

Table 2. Cesarean rates by state, 1996 and 2009, and percent change in cesarean rates 1996-2009

	1996	2009	Percent change 1996-2009
Alabama	23.3	34.9	53
Alaska	16.7	22.6	43
Arizona	16.1	27.1	70
Arkansas	25.3	34.6	37
California	20.6	32.6	60
Colorado	15.1	25.9	75
Connecticut	19.8	35.1	80
Delaware	21.0	33.2	70
District of Columbia	21.3	31.4	50
Florida	21.6	37.6	76
Georgia	20.9	32.9	61
Hawaii	17.5	26.8	54
Idaho	16.0	24.4	53
Illinois	19.3	30.9	63
Indiana	20.3	30.0	50
Iowa	18.6	29.3	63
Kansas	19.2	30.1	57
Kentucky	21.3	35.0	69
Louisiana	26.4	38.0	50
Maine	20.8	30.4	42
Maryland	21.6	33.1	55
Massachusetts	19.8	34.1	69
Michigan	20.2	31.5	59
Minnesota	16.9	26.4	62
Mississippi	26.6	37.1	42
Missouri	20.4	31.1	55
Montana	19.1	29.2	55
Nebraska	19.8	31.0	60
Nevada	19.3	33.7	75
New Hampshire	20.3	31.9	52
New Jersey	24.0	38.7	64
New Mexico	17.2	22.9	33
New York	22.9	34.5	52
North Carolina	21.1	30.8	48
North Dakota	18.9	28.1	55
Ohio	19.0	30.6	64
Oklahoma	22.5	34.2	54
Oregon	16.9	28.9	74
Pennsylvania	19.4	30.9	64
Rhode Island	17.7	33.3	85

Table 2. (Continued)

	1996	2009	Percent change 1996-2009
South Carolina	22.6	34.2	56
South Dakota	20.8	26.6	26
Tennessee	21.7	33.8	56
Texas	23.1	34.5	53
Utah	15.9	22.0	44
Vermont	16.5	27.2	68
Virginia	21.1	34.0	63
Washington	16.8	29.4	74
West Virginia	22.8	35.5	58
Wisconsin	15.6	25.2	65
Wyoming	18.3	27.0	54

Source: Birth data from the National Vital Statistics System, CDC, NCHS; see references 1 and 7.

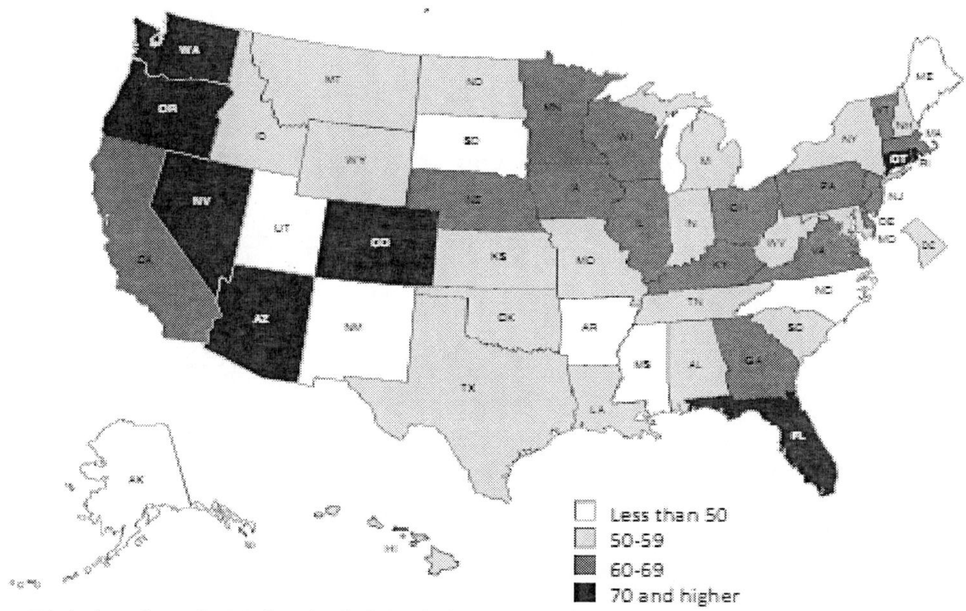

Source: Birth data from the National Vital Statistics System, NCHS, CDC.

Figure 4. Percent increase in cesarean rates by State: United States, 1996-2009.

Recent Studies Shed Light on the Reasons for the Increasing Trend

This section provides a brief review of the recent epidemiological literature to explore broader questions surrounding the recent increase in cesarean delivery, including possible changes in the medical risk profile of births and in indications for cesarean delivery, information on mother's opinions and preferences, and studies on cesarean delivery outcomes for the mother and neonate.

Trends in the Medical Risk Profile of Births and in Indications for Cesarean Delivery

Studies examining changes in the medical risk profile of births over time have found little evidence to suggest that the rising cesarean rates are due to such changes. [14-17] Declercq et al used birth certificate data to examine the medical risk profiles of women over time with regards to age, race/ethnicity, parity, gestational age, birthweight, and for a wide variety of medical risk factors and complications of labor and/or delivery. [10] They found that changing primary cesarean rates were not related to general shifts in mothers' medical risk profiles. Rather, cesarean rates associated with virtually every demographic or medical risk factor reported on birth certificates shifted in the same pattern as with the overall cesarean rates. They concluded that "changes in obstetrical practices were the major influence on the shifting pattern of primary cesarean rates." [15] A related study used multivariate logistic regression analysis to examine changes in primary cesarean rates over time for low risk women and found that the odds of having a primary cesarean in 2001 were 50% higher than the odds in 1996, after controlling for parity, birthweight, and maternal ethnicity, age and education. [14] Similarly, Rhodes et al found that excess weight gain during pregnancy and macrosomia did not explain the increase in cesarean delivery as cesarean rates increased in all weight gain categories, and the incidence of macrosomia actually declined from 1990 to 2000. [16] Donahue et al also found that recent increases in the cesarean rate were not related to increases in infant birthweight, as the mean birthweight of singleton term births in the US actually declined from1990 to 2005. [18]

Recent studies have also suggested that pre-pregnancy obesity (a measure not currently available from national birth certificate data) is related to higher primary cesarean rates. [19-20] However, rates of obesity among US women in all age groups increased during the 1990s, [21] while cesarean rates fell from 1991-96, and then increased from 1996-2000. Conversely, obesity rates did not increase from 1999-2008 among US women of reproductive age, [22-23] while the cesarean rate continued to climb; thus changes in obesity do not appear to be the primary driving force behind the increase in the cesarean rate.

These findings are consistent with a recent study by Barber et al which found that most of the increase in cesarean rates from 2003-2009 was due to more subjective and ill-defined indications such as nonreassuring fetal status and arrest of dilation, whereas cesarean rates associated with more objective indications such as malpresentation, cord prolapse, and placenta previa did not increase. [24] Similarly, Zhang et al found that many cesareans for dystocia were performed before 6cm of cervical dilation when many women may not yet be in the active phase of labor, suggesting that "clinical impatience may play a role in decision making." [25-26] A related group of studies examined trends in cesarean deliveries for women with no reported medical indications based on birth certificate data, hospital discharge data, or a combination of both. [14, 27-31] Although there are differences among studies in the definition of low risk, and questions about the completeness of reporting of various risk factors on birth certificates, all available studies, including those based on combined birth certificate and hospital discharge data, documented a recent increase in cesarean delivery among low-risk women with no reported medical indications for cesarean delivery. [14, 27-31]

Maternal Opinions Regarding Cesarean Delivery

The concept of 'maternal request cesarean' has been variously defined in the medical literature. In some cases, it has simply been defined as primary cesarean delivery in the absence of a medical or obstetric indication. [32-33] However, this definition does not take into account the complex and nuanced interaction between the obstetric care provider and the patient in decision making for cesarean section. [34] Some researchers have suggested a more precise definition as cesarean without a medical indication that was requested by the mother before labor. [34-35]

Few US studies have directly asked pregnant women about their preferences for delivery method. Although not a random sample, Listening to Mothers II was a national survey of 1,573 US women aged 18-45 who gave birth in a hospital to a singleton, still living infant in 2005, with results weighted to reflect the national population. [35] Of the 252 mothers with a primary cesarean in the survey, 3 indicated there was no medical indication for the cesarean and of these only one responded that she had made the decision to have a cesarean herself prior to beginning labor. [35] A recent NIH-funded study on Mode of First Delivery and Subsequent Childbearing interviewed 3,006 Pennsylvania women from 2009-early 2011 and found similar results. [36]

Results from the first Listening to Mothers Survey, conducted in 2002, found little interest in a future cesarean for non-medical reasons with just 6% of primiparous mothers interested in that option in the future. [37] A British national survey of mothers also found the phenomenon of maternal request cesareans to be extremely rare. [38]

Research from other countries with high cesarean rates, most notably Brazil [39] and Chile, [40] has found that rather than the cesarean rate being driven primarily by maternal demands, it is the interaction between mothers and their providers that leads to the decision to perform a cesarean without a clear medical indication. For example in Potter's study in Brazil, [39] more than 80% of primiparous mothers in the study anticipated a vaginal birth one month prior to their due date, yet almost half of these mothers (66% in private hospitals) ended up with a cesarean. Thus, although true maternal request cesareans doubtless occur, direct surveys of women seem to indicate that they are not numerous enough to account for the recent increase in the US cesarean rate.

Neonatal and Maternal Outcomes by Method of Delivery

Several recent review articles have examined the risks and benefits of cesarean without a medical reason vs. vaginal delivery for the mother and infant. [41-47] Several of these reviews were an outcome of the March 2006 National Institutes of Health (NIH) State-of-the-Science Conference on "Cesarean Delivery on Maternal Request". [44-47] The NIH panel, after a systematic review of the literature, noted the lack of well-controlled studies for many outcomes of interest; [47] however, four findings were supported by at least a moderate level of evidence. Cesarean without a medical reason (when compared to the combination of planned vaginal and unplanned cesarean delivery) was associated with: 1) a decreased risk of maternal hemorrhage; 2) an increased risk of respiratory problems for infants; 3) greater complications in subsequent pregnancies including uterine rupture and placental implantation problems, and 4) longer maternal hospital stays. [47] Several recent studies have further corroborated these findings. [31, 48-52] The NIH panel further noted that studies on neonatal and maternal mortality lacked statistical power and consistent methodologies to reliably assess the effect of delivery route. [47] As maternal and neonatal mortality are rare events for low-risk women in developed countries, very large sample sizes are often needed to detect statistically significant differences.

Several studies published since the NIH conference review may have the potential to shed further light on these issues. MacDorman et al examined neonatal mortality using linked birth and infant death certificate data for 1999-2002 from 5.7 million births with no reported risk for cesarean delivery, using an "intention-to-treat" methodology, and obtained an adjusted odds ratio of 1.69 (1.35-2.11) for cesarean without labor, compared to "planned vaginal delivery" (a category that included unplanned cesareans). [53] Villar et al, in a Latin American study found, for infants in cephalic presentations, an odds ratio of neonatal mortality for cesarean delivery of 1.9 (1.6-2.3), compared to vaginal delivery. [54] Betran et al, in a global study of the relationship between method of delivery and maternal and neonatal mortality, found that for countries with national cesarean rates above 15% "higher cesarean rates are predominantly correlated with higher maternal mortality. A similar pattern is found for infant and neonatal mortality." [55] These findings were corroborated by Villar for Latin America. [56] However, a more recent study of data from 193 countries found no relationship between cesarean rates above 15% and maternal or infant mortality rates. [57] Other recent studies have found increased risks of maternal mortality for low risk women delivered by cesarean, [58-59] while another study found substantial serious maternal morbidity associated with cesarean section, but no significant difference in maternal mortality. [52]

A related line of research has focused on the effect of multiple cesareans on maternal and neonatal morbidity and mortality. Repeat cesarean deliveries are associated with significantly higher maternal and neonatal morbidity and mortality, when compared to either cesarean or vaginal deliveries for women without a prior cesarean. [49-50, 60-61] The risk of poor outcome for both the mother and infant increases with the number of prior cesareans. [47] For example, Silver et al found that, compared to women having a first cesarean, the odds ratio (95% confidence interval) for life-threatening placenta accreta was 1.3 (0.7-2.3) for the second cesarean, 2.4 (1.3-4.3) for the third cesarean, and 9.0 (4.8-16.7) for the fourth cesarean. [60-61] In the Silver study, 27% of women were having their third or higher cesarean, although this figure may not be representative of the US population as a whole. [60] For this reason, the American College of Obstetricians and Gynecologists recommend avoiding a primary cesarean without a medical reason for women desiring several children. [61] In 2008, 32% of first births had a cesarean delivery, and more than 90% of these women will have a repeat cesarean delivery in their subsequent births. This creates a large population of women who are at elevated risk for maternal and neonatal morbidity and mortality.

Another way that cesarean section can impact neonatal and infant mortality is through its potential effect on the gestational age at delivery. Although ACOG recommends that cesareans without a medical indication not be performed before 39 weeks of gestation unless there is documentation of fetal lung maturity, studies indicate that this guideline is not always followed. [61-62] For example, Tita et al in a study of 13,000 repeat cesareans without a medical indication at 19 US academic centers found that 36% occurred before 39 weeks of gestation. [62] Several recent studies found a link between increases in cesarean section and/or induction of labor and increases in the preterm birth rate. [63-65] For example, MacDorman et al found that only half of singleton preterm births in 2006 were spontaneous vaginal deliveries, compared with 69% in 1991, and that obstetrical intervention (i.e. cesarean section and/or induction of labor) affected the gestational age at delivery for a large proportion (42%) of US infants in 2006. [63]

Discussion

Cesarean rates in the United States fell between 1991 and 1996 and then began to rise rapidly. In 2009, 1/3 of US births were cesarean deliveries. Over the past decade, cesarean rates increased sharply for women of all ages, all race/ethnic groups, all periods of gestation and in all States. Cesarean rates were highest for women aged 35 and over, for non-Hispanic black women, and for preterm births. About 58% of the increase in the cesarean rate from 1996 to 2003 was due to increases in the primary cesarean rate. Based on the trend in the repeat cesarean rate, a first cesarean delivery now virtually guarantees that subsequent deliveries will be cesarean deliveries. Multiple repeat cesarean deliveries are associated with significantly higher maternal and neonatal morbidity and mortality, when compared to either cesarean or vaginal deliveries for women without a prior cesarean. [49-51, 60-61]

Primary cesarean rates have also increased rapidly for low risk women and for women with no known medical reason for cesarean delivery. [14, 27-31] Although different studies used different methodologies which may limit comparisons, there appears to be a larger body of evidence now than at the time of the 2006 NIH conference for an increased risk of maternal and neonatal mortality and morbidity for cesareans without a medical reason compared to vaginal births. [49-56] In addition, the increase in the primary cesarean rate appears to be mainly due to changes in obstetric practice, and not to changes in the medical risk profile of births, or to increases in "maternal request". [14-15,35-40]

Discussions of the reasons for the growth in primary cesareans have centered on changing attitudes concerning cesareans among physicians and mothers. [66-69] Leitch and Walker related the rise in the cesarean rate to a change in medical practice; and concluded that although indications for cesarean did not change much over time "there has been a lowering in the overall threshold concerning the decision to carry out a caesarean section." [69] This, combined with the increase in cesareans without a medical indication, may account for much of the increase in the cesarean rate over the past decade. A more detailed examination is needed of mother, insurer, hospital and provider attitudes toward cesareans without a medical indication and of the nature of the interaction between mothers and their obstetric care providers in decision-making about the method of delivery. Research on the economic implications of the rising cesarean rate for hospitals, providers, insurers and parents is also essential.

Strengths of the birth certificate data to track trends in cesarean delivery include the comprehensive population-based nature of these data, which include all births in the United States for a given year. Most demographic items and some medical items (including maternal age, parity and method of delivery) are considered to be very well reported. [70-72] Limitations include incomplete reporting or absence of data on specific medical risk factors or complications. [70-72] Another limitation is the lack of comparable national data for repeat cesarean and VBAC delivery after 2003. Due to the staggered implementation of the 2003 revision of the birth certificate among US states, both revisions are currently in use in different states, thus it is not possible to construct national estimates for these measures. [9]

Interestingly, there are markedly different practice recommendations regarding cesarean delivery from the American and International obstetrical groups. In discussing the ethics of cesareans without a medical indication, the American College of Obstetricians and Gynecologists (ACOG) states that:

> If the physician believes that cesarean delivery promotes the overall health and welfare of the woman and her fetus more than vaginal delivery, he or she is ethically justified in performing a cesarean delivery. [67]

In contrast, the International Federation of Gynecology and Obstetrics (FIGO) states that:

> At present, because hard evidence of net benefit does not exist, performing Caesarean section for non-medical reasons is ethically not justified. [73]

Queenan noted that the underlying "question is not the ethics of patient choice, but lack of scientific proof of risks and benefits." [74] It is hoped that with an increasing body of research on the harms and benefits of cesarean vs. vaginal delivery, decision-making regarding these options will be increasingly evidence-based.

Disclaimer

The findings and conclusions in this article are those of the authors and do not necessarily represent the views of the Centers for Disease Control and Prevention.

References

[1] Martin JA, Hamilton BE, Ventura SJ, Osterman MJK, Kirmeyer S, Mathews TJ, Wilson EC. Births: Final data for 2009. *National vital statistics reports;* vol 60 no 1. Hyattsville, MD: National Center for Health Statistics. 2011. In press.

[2] Hall MJ, DeFrances CJ, Williams SN, et al. National hospital discharge survey: 2007 summary. *National health statistics reports* no. 29. Hyattsville (MD): National Center for Health Statistics; 2010.

[3] Organization for Economic Cooperation and Development. *OECD health data* 2010. Available at: http://www.ecosante.org. Accessed September 29, 2011.

[4] MacDorman MF, Declercq E, Menacker F. Recent Trends and Patterns in Cesarean and Vaginal Birth After Cesarean (VBAC) Deliveries in the United States. *Clin. Perinatol.* 2011; 38: 179–192.

[5] Taffel SM, Placek PJ, Moien M et al. 1989 U.S. cesarean section rate steadies-VBAC rate rises to nearly one in five. *Birth* 1991;18:73-7.

[6] MacDorman MF, Menacker F, Declercq E. Cesarean birth in the United States: Epidemiology, trends and outcomes. *Clin. Perinatol.* 2008;35:293-307.

[7] Menacker F, Hamilton BE. Recent trends in cesarean delivery in the United States. *NCHS Data Brief* no. 35. Hyattsville, Maryland: National Center for Health Statistics. 2010.

[8] Martin JA, Hamilton BE, Sutton PD et al. Births: Final Data for 2003. *National vital statistics reports*, vol 54 no 2. Hyattsville, MD: National Center for Health Statistics. 2005.

[9] Osterman MJK, Martin JA, Mathews TJ, Hamilton BE. Expanded data from the new birth certificate, 2008. *National vital statistics reports*, vol 59 no 7. Hyattsville, MD: National Center for Health Statistics. 2011.

[10] National Center for Health Statistics. *VitalStats - Birth* data, selected years. Available at: http://www.cdc.gov/nchs/data_access/vitalstats/ VitalStats_Births.htm. Accessed September 28, 2011.

[11] Martin JA, Hamilton BE, Sutton PD et al. Births: Final data for 2006. *National vital statistics reports* vol 57 no 7. Hyattsville, MD: National Center for Health Statistics. 2009.

[12] Declercq E, Young R, Cabral H, Ecker J. Is a rising cesarean delivery rate inevitable? *Trends in industrialized countries*, 1987 to 2007. Birth 2011;38:99-104.

[13] Ecker JL, Chen KT, Cohen AP, Riley LE, Lieberman ES. Increased risk of cesarean delivery with advancing maternal age: indications and associated factors in nulliparous women. *Am. J. Obstet. Gynecol.* 2001;185:883-7.

[14] Declercq E, Menacker F, MacDorman MF. Rise in "no indicated risk" primary cesareans in the United States, 1991-2001.*BMJ* 2005;330:71-72.

[15] Declercq E, Menacker F, MacDorman, MF. Maternal risk profiles and the primary cesarean rate in the United States, 1991-2002: *Am. J. Public Health* 2006;96:867-872.

[16] Rhodes JC, Schoendorf KC, Parker JD. Contribution of excess weight gain during pregnancy and macrosomia to the cesarean delivery rate, 1990-2000. *Pediatrics* 2003;111:1181-6.

[17] Reddy UM, Spong CY. Introduction. *Semin. Perinatol.* 2006;30:233-234.

[18] Donahue SMA, Kleinman KP, Gillman MW, Oken E. Trends in birth weight and gestational length among singleton term births in the United States 1990-2005. *Obstet. Gynecol.* 2010;115:357-64.

[19] Lu GC, Rouse DJ, DuBard M et al. The effect of the increasing prevalence of maternal obesity on perinatal morbidity. *Am. J. Obstet. Gynecol.* 2001;185:845-9.

[20] Kaiser PS, Kirby RS. Obesity as a risk factor for cesarean in a low risk population. *Obstet. Gynecol.* 2001;97:39-43.

[21] Flegal KM, Carroll MD, Ogden CL, Johnson DL. Prevalence and trends in obesity among US adults, 1999-2000. *JAMA* 2002;288:1723-7.

[22] Ogden CL, Carroll MD, Curtin LF et al. Prevalence of overweight and obesity in the United States, 1999-2004. *JAMA* 2006;295:1549-55.

[23] Flegal KM, Carroll MD, Ogden CL, Curtin LR. Prevalence and trends in obesity among US adults, 1999-2008. *JAMA* 2010;303:235-41.

[24] Barber EL, Lundsberg LS, Belanger K, et al. Indications contributing to the increasing cesarean delivery rate. *Obstetrics and Gynecolo*gy 2011;118:29-38.

[25] Zhang J, Troendle J, Reddy UM et al. Contemporary cesarean delivery practice in the United States. *Am. J. Obstet. Gynecol.* 2010;203(4): 326.e1-326.e10.

[26] Zhang J, Troendle J, Mikolajczyk R et al. The natural history of the normal first stage of labor. *Obstet. Gynecol.* 2010; 115:705-10.

[27] Menacker F, Declercq E, MacDorman MF. Cesarean delivery: Background, trends and epidemiology. *Semin. Perinatol.* 2006;30:235-41.

[28] Bailit JL, Love TE, Mercer B. Rising Cesarean Rates: Are Patients Sicker? *Am. J. Obstet. Gynecol.* 2004;191:800-1.

[29] Gregory, KD, Korst LM, Gornbein JA, et al: Using administrative data to identify indications for elective cesarean delivery. *Health Serv. Res.* 2002;37:1387-1401.

[30] Healthgrades. Healthgrades third annual report on "patient-choice" *Cesarean section rates in the United States*. September 2005. Available at: http://www.healthgrades.com

[31] Declercq E, Barger M, Cabral HJ et al. Maternal outcomes associated with planned primary cesarean births compared with planned vaginal births. *Obstet. Gynecol.* 2007;109:669-77.

[32] Wax, JR, Cartin A, Pinette MG, Blackstone J. Patient choice cesarean: An evidence-based review. *Obstetrical and Gynecological Survey* 2004;59:601-616.

[33] Gossman GL, Joesch JM, Tanfer K. Trends in maternal request cesarean delivery from 1991 to 2004. *Obstet. Gynecol.* 2006;108:1506-16.

[34] Gamble J, Creedy DK, McCourt C et al. A critique of the literature on women's request for cesarean section. *Birth* 2007;34:331-340.

[35] Declercq ER, Sakala C, Corry MP, Applebaum S. Listening to mothers II – *Report of the second national U.S. survey of women's childbearing experiences.* New York: Childbirth Connection, October 2006. Available at: http://www.childbirthconnection.org/article.asp?ck=10401.

[36] Kjerulff K, Velott D, Zhu J, Weisman DS, Hillemeier MM. *Maternal request cesarean section: How often does this occur?* Paper presented at the American Public Health Association annual meeting, Oct 29-Nov 2, 2011. Washington, DC.

[37] Declercq, ER, Sakala C, Corry MP, et al: Listening to Mothers: *Report of the First National U.S. Survey of Women's Childbearing Experiences.* New York. Maternity Center Association, October, 2002. Available at: http://www.childbirthconnection.org/pdfs/LtMreport.pdf.

[38] Redshaw M, Rowe R, Hockley C, Brocklehurst P. *Recorded Delivery: a national survey of women's experience with maternity care*, 2006. Oxford: National Perinatal Epidemiology Unit. 2007.

[39] Potter JE, Berquó E, Perpétuo I H O, et al: Unwanted caesarean sections among public and private patients in Brazil: prospective study. *BMJ* 2001;323:1155-1158.

[40] Murray S F. Relation between private health insurance and high rates of caesarean section in Chile: qualitative and quantitative study. BMJ 2000;321:1501-1505.

[41] Visco AG, Viswanathan M, Lohr K et al. Cesarean delivery on maternal request – Maternal and neonatal outcomes. *Obstet. Gyncol.* 2006;108:1517-29.

[42] Doherty EG, Eichenwald EC. Cesarean Delivery: Emphasis on the neonate. *Clinical Obstetrics and Gynecology* 2004: 47:332-41.

[43] Lavender T, Hofmeyr GJ, Neilson JP et al. Caesarean section for non-medical reasons at term (Review). *Cochrane Database of Systematic Reviews* 2006, Issue 3.

[44] Signore D, Hemachandra A, Klebanoff M. Neonatal mortality and morbidity after elective cesarean delivery versus routine expectant management: A decision analysis. *Semin. Perinatol.* 2006;30:288-295.

[45] Wax JR. Maternal request cesarean versus planned spontaneous vaginal delivery: Maternal morbidity and short term outcomes. *Semin. Perinatol.* 30:247-252. 2006.

[46] Vadnais M Sachs B. Maternal mortality with cesarean delivery: A literature review. *Semin. Perinatol.* 2006;30:242-246.

[47] NIH State-of-the-Science Conference Statement on Cesarean Delivery on Maternal Request. *NIH Consensus Science Statements.* 2006;23(1):1-29. Available at: http://consensus.nih.gov/2006/2006CesareanSOS027 main.htm.

[48] Kolas T, Saugstad OD, Daltveit AK et al. Planned cesarean versus planned vaginal delivery at term: Comparison of newborn infant outcomes. *Am. J. Obstet. Gynecol.* 2006;195:1538-43.

[49] Yang Q, Wen SW, Oppenheimer L et al. Association of caesarean delivery for first birth with placenta praevia and placental abruption in second pregnancy. *BJOG* 2007;114:609-613.

[50] Kennare R, Tucker G, Heard A, Chan A. Risks of adverse outcomes in the next birth after a first cesarean delivery. *Obstet. Gynecol.* 2007;109:270-6.

[51] Spong DY, Landon MB, Gilbert S et al. Risk of uterine repution and adverse perinatal outcome at term after cesarean delivery. *Obstet. Gynecol.* 2007;110:801-807.

[52] Liu S, Liston RM, Joseph KS et al. Maternal mortality and severe morbidity associated with low-risk planned cesarean delivery versus planned vaginal delivery at term. *CMAJ* 2007;176:455-460.

[53] MacDorman MF, Declercq E, Menacker F, Malloy MH. Neonatal mortality for primary cesarean and vaginal births to low-risk women: Application of an "intention-to-treat" model. *Birth* 2008;35:3-8.

[54] Villar J, Carroli G, Zavaleta N et al. Maternal and neonatal individual risks and benefits associated with caesarean delivery: Multicenter prospective study. *BMJ* 2007; 1025-1035. (published online first).

[55] Betran AP, Merialdi M, Lauer JA, et al. Rates of caesarean section: Analysis of global, regional and national estimates. *Paediatr. Perinat. Epidemiol.* 2007;21:98-113.

[56] Villar J, VAlladares E, Wojdyla D et al. Caesarean delivery rates and pregnancy outcomes: The 2005 WHO global survey on maternal and perinatal health in Latin America. *Lancet* 2006; 367:1819-29.

[57] Volpe FM. Correlation of cesarean rates to maternal and infant mortality rates: an ecological study of official international data. *Rev. Panam. Salud. Publica* 2011;29:303-8.

[58] Deneux-Tharaux C, Carmona E, Bouvier-Colle MH Breart G. Postpartum maternal mortality and cesarean delivery. *Obstet. Gynecol.* 2006;108:541-8.

[59] Schutte JM, Steegers EAP, Santema JG et al. Maternal deaths after elective cesarean section for breech presentation in the Netherlands. *Acta Obstetricia et Gynecologica.* 2007; 86:240-243.

[60] Silver RM, Landon MG, Rouse DJ et al. Maternal morbidity associated with multiple repeat cesarean deliveries. *Obstet. Gynecol.* 2006;107:1226-32.

[61] ACOG. Cesarean delivery on maternal request. ACOG Committee Opinion no. 394. *Obstet. Gynecol.* 2007;110:1501-4.

[62] Tita AT, Lai Y, Landon MB et al. Timing of elective repeat cesarean delivery at term and maternal perioperative outcomes. *Obstet. Gynecol.* 2011 177(2 pt 1):280-6.

[63] MacDorman MF, Declercq E, Zhang J. Obstetrical intervention and the singleton preterm birth rate in the United States from 1991-2006. *Am. J. Public Health.* 2010;100:2241-7.

[64] Bettegawda VR, Idas T, Davidoff MJ, et al. The relationship between cesaeran delivery and gestational age among US singleton births. *Clin. Perinatol.* 2008;35(2):309-324.

[65] Davidoff MJ, Dias T, Damus K et al. Changes in the gestational age distribution among US singleton births: Impact of rates of late preterm birth 1992 to 2002. *Semin. Perinatol.* 2006;30(1): 8-15.

[66] Minkoff H, Powderly KR, Chervenak F, et al: Ethical dimensions of elective primary cesarean delivery. *Obstet. Gynecol.* 2004;103:387-392.

[67] American College of Obstetricians and Gynecologists. Surgery and patient choice. *ACOG Committee Opinion* No. 395. Washington DC: American College of Obstetricians and Gynecologists. 2008.

[68] Hale RW, Harer WB. Elective prophylactic cesarean delivery. Editorial. *ACOG Clinical Review* 10(2):1 and 15, 2005.

[69] Leitch CR Walker JJ. The rise in caesarean section rate: the same indications but a lower threshold. *BJOG* 1998;105:621-6.

[70] Roohan, PJ, Josberger RE, Acar J, et al: Validation of birth certificate data in New York State. *J. Community Health* 2003;28:335-346.

[71] DiGiuseppe DL, Aron DC, Ranbom L, et al: Reliability of birth certificate data: A multi-hospital comparison to medical records information. *Matern. Child Health J.* 2002;6:169-179.

[72] Lydon-Rochelle MT, Holt VL, Cardenas V, et al: The reporting of pre-existing maternal medical conditions and complications of pregnancy on birth certificates and in hospital discharge data. *Am. J. Obstet. Gynecol.* 2005;193:125-134.

[73] International Federation of Gynecology and Obstetrics (FIGO). *Ethical Issues in Obstetrics and Gynecology.* FIGO: London, England. 2009.

[74] Queenan, JT. Elective Cesarean Delivery. *Obstet. Gynecol.* 2004;103:1135-1136.

In: Cesarean Section: Procedures, Complications and Recovery ISBN: 978-1-62081-214-3
Editor: Eyal Sheiner

Chapter IV

INDICATIONS FOR CESAREAN SECTIONS

Ciro Comparetto[1] and Franco Borruto[2]
[1]Division of Obstetrics and Gynecology, City Hospital, Prato, Italy
[2]Division of Obstetrics and Gynecology, Princesse Grace Hospital, Principality of Monaco

INTRODUCTION

Cesarean section (CS) has been practiced for ages, although originally as a universally postmortem procedure. [1,2] During the last 15 years, the CS rate was increased despite of the recommendations of the World Health Organization (WHO) to keep it below 10-15% (Figure 1). The concept of CS rate limitation has become obsolete. The increase in the CS rate is mainly justified by the decrease in maternal mortality and morbidity following elective CS: surgery-related risks have decreased and the confusion that was made between the risks of vaginal delivery and those of trial of labor (TOL) has to be clarified to show that maternal mortality and morbidity are not increased by elective CS. However, instrumental delivery and CS during labor remain two situations at high-risk both for the mother and her fetus. There is also an association between the increase in the CS rate and the decrease in PNM and morbidity, but this effect would only become clinically significant after a dramatic increase in the CS rate: this is the preventile principle of "marginal death". Numerous articles have been published reporting on the effects of vaginal delivery for the pelvic floor: urinary incontinence, pelvic organ prolapse, and especially fecal incontinence. All these publications concluded that CS has a protective effect. The rising duty to provide information to patients in high-risk obstetrical situations such as a history of CS also contributes to the overall increase in CS rate mainly through the elective CS rate. Indeed, when faced with the alternative choices of potentially severe complications either for themselves or their child, women are likely to choose what appears to be the safest mode of delivery for their child and thus to opt for a CS. Finally, widespread delivery of information to the patients about TOL itself and the risks of vaginal delivery is the first step towards a "principle of preference", which consists in giving an important place to the patient's choice in the decision-making process, and thus to recognize her right to ask for an elective CS [3,4].

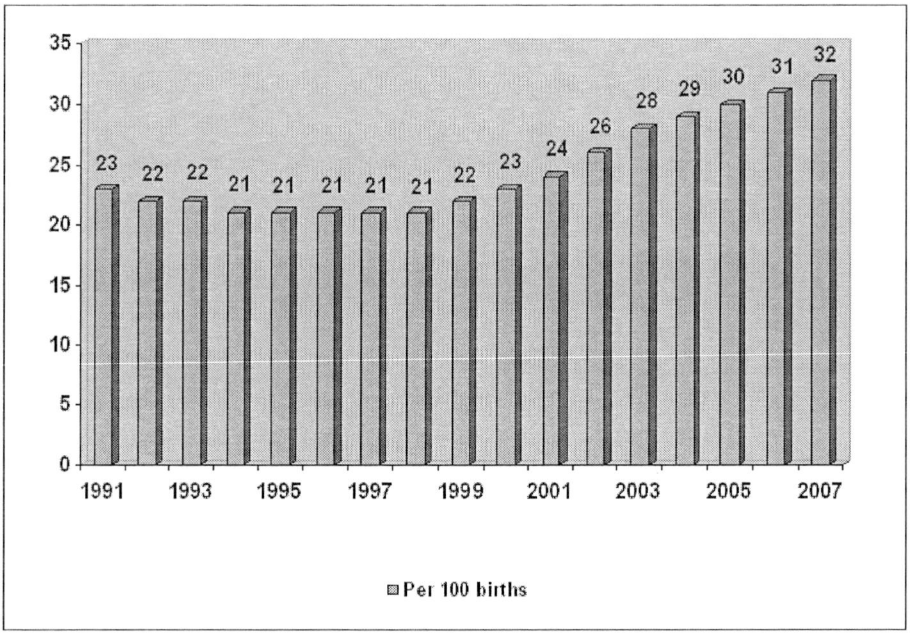

Figure 1. Cesarean section rates in the United States of America (modified from: Joy S. Cesarean delivery. http://emedicine.medscape.com/article/263424-overview, source: CDC/NCHS, National Vital Statistics System)

Indications

Although the CS rate has increased steadily for the past 40 years, further increase seems unlikely since the indications for performing the operation are already broadly defined (Tab. 1,2). Most of the earlier indications will remain unchanged (e.g. the presence of placenta previa and cephalo-pelvic disproportion). The trend toward vaginal delivery in perhaps 30% to 40% of breech births will probably have no material effect on the number of CS performed, and the present use of CS for multiple pregnancy will probably continue [5]. Decisions about the role of CS, forceps, and vacuum extraction (VE) in obstetrics continue to be a challenging part of daily obstetric practice, including the comparison of international rates of CS and vaginal births after CS (VBAC), the method of choice for the delivery of the low-birth weight (LBW) fetus presenting as vertex, the advantages of a prelabor CS for a fetus diagnosed with meningomyelocele, and the appropriate role for the midforceps delivery in the 1990s [6]. Spontaneous vaginal delivery without obstetric intervention remains the goal for most pregnant women. Midwives and obstetricians aim to support women in achieving this result, which is associated with the lowest risk of morbidity for both mother and baby. Despite the best efforts of the laboring woman and her carergivers, some women will fail to progress in the second stage of labor, and obstetric intervention will be required [7].

Table 1. Possible clinical indications, documented and undocumented, to cesarean section

Documented indications
Abnormal presentation or position
Human Immunodeficiency Virus infection
Fetal anomalies
Invasive cervical cancer
Vaginal obstructing mass
Multiple gestation, first twin non-vertex
Disorders of the pelvis
Placenta previa and severe abruptio placentae
Previous 2 cesarean sections
Umbilical cord prolapse
Threat of uterine rupture
Not always documented indications
Fetal heart rate alterations/overestimation of cardiotocography
Feto-pelvic disproportion
Non-progression of the presenting part
Fetal distress
Very low birth weight
Macrosomia and macrocephaly
Maternal pathology

Adapted from Nappi C, Guida M: Complicanze, errori e problematiche medico-legali in Ostetricia e Ginecologia. Rome: CIC Edizioni Internazionali; 2004.

Table 2. Non-clinical indications to cesarean section

Older maternal age
Mother's preference ("self-determination"), fear of pain
Insufficient cooperation of the pregnant woman
Absence of a support person during labor
Psychological pressure (pregnant-family)
Elimination of perineal damage
Pregnancy after infertility/sterility
Medium-high socio-economic conditions
Inadequate preparation of the delivery room staff
Unavailability and/or emotional status of the physician during labor
Fear of the physician not to avoid or to cause damage to the mother and/or the unborn child
Hostile legal climate ("defensive medicine")
Financial incentives (high value of the diagnosis-related group, higher income, insurance)
Fear of bad publicity by the physician

Adapted from Nappi C, Guida M: Complicanze, errori e problematiche medico-legali in Ostetricia e Ginecologia. Rome: CIC Edizioni Internazionali; 2004.

CS is indicated at any stage in the labor process in the presence of nonreassuring fetal status or when conservative measures fail in the setting of abnormal labor. In the absence of maternal or fetal indications for expedited delivery, CS is not indicated for latent phase disorders. When to intervene for protracted labor is arguable, but slow rates of labor progress are consistent with safe vaginal delivery. CS in the second stage should be avoided for at least 4 hours if there is progressive fetal descent [8]. CS for maternal reasons is needed for six main reasons: protracted labor, abruptio placentae, previous CS, eclampsia, placenta previa, and malpresentation [9].

The following chapter discusses the main obstetrical conditions which require or are associated with a higher incidence of CS, both in emergency and in non-emergency situations.

1) Emergency Cesarean Section

Obstetricians assume a dual role in the provision of health care for both mother and fetus during labor. Not only do they function as consultants for medical and surgical problems peculiar to labor, but they also assume a more broad-based role in the prevention of labor complications to achieve the best possible health maintenance for both patients. This includes the provision of continuous health care throughout pregnancy, delivery, and postpartum management [10]. The care of the pregnant patient presenting to the emergency department with labor or delivery complications requires an understanding of signs and symptoms of disease for the maternal and fetal patient [11]. Among all the emergency situations which may arise across the field of obstetrics, there are a small number which call for urgent practical steps to be taken in order to safeguard the life of the mother or the baby or both. These complications share several common characteristics in that they are rare difficult to predict, and can result in significant morbidity and mortality, so they require prompt action by well-trained staff and may involve the active and efficient co-operation of a range of different health care professionals. It is critically important that staff are fully aware of the procedures to be followed and the chain of command which will ensure that they are followed as efficiently and successfully as possible [12,13].

The obstetric patient poses exceptional challenges in the intensive care unit. Knowledge of the physiologic changes of pregnancy and specific pregnancy-related disorders is necessary for optimal management. The management of mechanical ventilation is based on principles of avoiding lung injury, and hypercapnia may be tolerated even during the pregnancy. When the clinician is faced with the extraordinary instance of cardiopulmonary arrest, perimortem CS must be considered to improve the potential for maternal and fetal survival [14]. The emergency department is a suboptimal location for delivery, and the greater prevalence of complicated presentations and emergency deliveries results in higher morbidity and mortality. Any woman greater than 20 weeks' gestation in labor is considered medically unstable and should be triaged quickly. Fetal viability occurs after 24 to 26 weeks' gestation. Placenta previa and abruptio placentae should be considered in a woman in labor with ongoing bleeding, and ultrasonographic (US) evaluation should be performed emergently. Continuous fetal monitoring is the best method to assess for fetal heart rate (FHR) variations, accelerations, or decelerations. After the fetus crowns, a finger sweep can exclude the presence of a cord prolapse. With a cord prolapse, the mother is instructed not to push, and the presenting part is elevated off of the cord. Perimortem CS is performed with gestational age greater than 24 to 26 weeks. The supine position can lead to aortocaval compression. Perimortem CS should be performed within 4 minutes of maternal cardiopulmonary arrest [15].

Acute abdominal pain in pregnancy challenges the diagnostic skills of the physician. With increasing traffic on our streets blunt trauma occurs and it might hurt pregnant women as well as their fetus. Even seat-belts can cause damage, if pelvic belts are used instead of shoulder belts. There is a variety of shock etiologies. Bleeding from the vagina is the most common complaint. Diagnosis does not allow any delay. It is always an emergency with hemorrhagic shock impending. The risk situation around even normal birth is well known. Emergencies will appear every time unannounced. There are post partum risks as well: they should not be underestimated when home-delivery is desired [16].

Among data on medical liability for obstetrical practice in labor ward, one of the claims concerns the decision-to-delivery interval during emergency CS, for which an optimal time is frequently advocated. A realistic review on this subject is needed. It mainly allows to note that:

1. unlike current opinion, neonatal prognosis is more dependent on the causal pathology than on decision-to-delivery interval;
2. the transfer time to the operating theater, which represents approximately half of this interval, should benefit an internal audit for each maternity as it is mainly dependent on organization and architectural specifications; and
3. the choice of mode of anesthesia in relation to the obstetrical context and the induction time has a strong incidence, which shows the importance of a good communication between the obstetrician and the anesthetist.

A detailed analysis of obstetrical context and of each sequence of the decision-to-delivery interval is more efficient and realistic for evaluation in medical liability cases than an optimal "gold standard". In addition, it allows a prophylactic reflexion for a risk management approach in each labor ward [17]. There are times when inter-departmental politics or indifference may sometimes spill onto service provision and threaten to affect patient care. There can be no doubt that an emergency CS cannot be delayed indefinitely. An unstable child who requires neonatal intensive care unit (NICU) or transfer can potentially occupy both Pediatric Senior House Officer (SHO) and Registrar for hours [18]. Lack of a standard definition and heterogeneity in patient selection criteria in the literature might have a role on the apparent inability to routinely begin an emergency CS in less than 30 minutes. Although there are some similarities in definitions and the criteria used for patient selection in multiple studies, the variability in the definitions could be responsible for some of the apparent timeliness performance deficiency in the literature [19,20].

a) Amniotic Fluid Embolism

Amniotic fluid embolism (AFE), also referred to as anaphylactoid syndrome of pregnancy, is a dramatic, rare, and frequently lethal complication of pregnancy which accounts for about 10% of all maternal deaths. The incidence ranges from 1:800 to 1:8,000. The mortality rate reaches 61-86%. Neonatal survival is reported at 70%. It must be suspected in all cases of sudden maternal collapse. For successful resuscitation, surgical delivery should be performed without delay [21-24]. AFE has a variable presentation, ranging from cardiac arrest and death through to mild degrees of organ system dysfunction with or without coagulopathy. The differential diagnosis includes pre-eclamptic toxemia/pregnancy-induced hypertension (PIH), anaphylaxis, and pulmonary embolism. AFE is believed to occur when the constituents of amniotic fluid enter the maternal circulation, leading to varying degrees of multiorgan compromise. There is no diagnostic test for AFE and the finding of fetal elements in the maternal circulation is non-specific. AFE was first described in 1926, gaining widespread recognition in 1941. Historically, AFE was thought to induce cardiovascular collapse by mechanical obstruction of the pulmonary circulation. It is now thought that a combination of left ventricular dysfunction and acute lung injury occur, with activation of several of the clotting factors. An immunological basis for these effects is postulated. There is no specific therapy and treatment is supportive. The mortality of the condition remains high [25,26].

b) Fetal Distress

Suspected fetal distress usually results in expedited delivery of a baby (often operatively). The potential harm to a mother and baby from operative delivery may not always be justified especially when fetal distress may be misdiagnosed. Even with a correct diagnosis, it is not clear whether an operative or conservative approach is better. There is no difference in PNM (relative risk [RR] 1.18, 95% confidence interval [CI] 0.56-2.48). There have been no contemporary trials of operative versus conservative management of suspected fetal distress. In settings without modern obstetric facilities, a policy of operative delivery in the event of meconium-stained liquor or FHR changes has not been shown to reduce PNM [27]. The technology of intrapartum surveillance made rapid strides from the 1960s through the 1980s but then stagnated as increasing resort to CS was made rather than improving measures of fetal condition and labor progress. However, despite CS rates commonly over 30%, medicolegally expensive mistakes continue to be made because it is difficult to teach clinicians to make reliable use of existing technology, e.g. cardiotocography (CTG) (Figure 2), US assessment of amniotic fluid index (AFI), biophysical profile (BPP), and blood flow patterns in fetal circulation detected by Doppler US [28-32].

Fetal blood sampling (FBS) with determination of pH and base excess (BE) is a valid supplement to continuous FHR monitoring. When used in conjunction with the conventional methods of FHR interpretation, FBS might slightly improve the accuracy of determination of the truly asphyxiated fetus, having a potentially ominous FHR pattern. Thus, its use may postpone or prevent the unnecessarily expeditious delivery of fetuses who are in fact not asphyxiated. Despite this usefulness, FBS has diffused poorly into the great majority of obstetric services in the United States of America (USA), primarily because of the minor, though real, technical inconveniences and analytic difficulties. Many defenders of FHR monitoring feel that its use without the availability of FBS is responsible for the overdiagnosis of fetal distress and the subsequent increase in CS rates. There are two possible ways out of this dilemma. First is the development of a simple method of continuously recording fetal tissue pH. Though there are such devices, they do not yet satisfy the necessary criteria of facility and simplicity, but improvements may be expected within several years. A second approach is to improve the accuracy of FHR interpretation, either by the application of available knowledge or by improvement in the understanding of FHR through further investigation. As to the application of presently available knowledge, avoidance of overcalling the presence of fetal distress could be facilitated by universal acceptance of the high prognostic accuracy of normal FHR variability to predict a vigorous fetus, even in the presence of other so-called ominous FHR patterns. Only a small number of fetuses have FHR patterns with absent or decreasing variability with periodic changes that cannot be ascribed to drugs or other nonasphyxial causes. Part of this small group may unnecessarily go to CS for fetal distress in the absence of FBS, but its influence on overall CS rates will be minor [33].

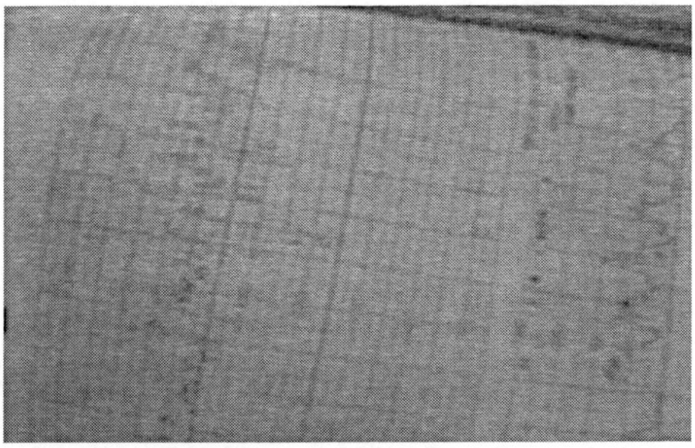

Figure 2. Cardiotocography (wanwordcommunications.com).

c) Perimortem Cesarean Section

Perimortem CS is a rare event often resulting in high mortality of mother and/or fetus. It represents a tragedy for the mother and the family and a crisis for the healthcare professionals managing such a case [34]. In previous centuries low infant survival rates led to negative opinions regarding the operation's usefulness.

A review of the past centuries' cases and a review of fetal physiology suggest that to obtain optimum infant survival, CS should be initiated within four minutes of maternal cardiac arrest. Legal liability from the operation is minimal [35]. The recommendation to perform a perimortem CS within four minutes of maternal cardiac arrest was introduced in 1986. This recommendation was based on the assumptions that cardiopulmonary resuscitation is ineffective in the third trimester because of aortocaval compression, and that fetal and perhaps maternal outcomes would be optimized by timely delivery. Published reports from 20 years support, but fall far from proving, that perimortem CS within 4 minutes of maternal cardiac arrest improves neonatal outcome [36]. Perimortem CS probably represents an underemphasized procedure on the skills list of the emergency physician. Although fraught with emotional and medico-legal overtones, the procedure can yield viable infants in at least 15% of cases and occasionally alters maternal hemodynamics so as to restore the pulse in a clinically dead woman [37].

d) Placenta Previa, Abruptio Placentae, and other Placental Abnormalities

Abnormal placentation is a serious complication of pregnancy. The disorder is also associated with significant maternal morbidity. Abnormal placentation, comprised of placenta previa, accreta, increta, and percreta, is a leading cause of post-partum hemorrhage (PPH) and indication for gravid hysterectomy [38]. The incidence of abnormal placental invasion has increased 10-fold in the past 50 years, reflecting the increased number of CS performed. Management relies on accurate early diagnosis with appropriate perioperative multidisciplinary planning to anticipate and avoid massive obstetric hemorrhage at delivery. Women at risk should plan to deliver at an institution with appropriate expertize and resources for managing this condition [39,40].

Placenta previa occurs in approximately one in 200 pregnancies. The cause is unknown, but endometrial damage due to prior pregnancy, CS, and other factors predispose to it. Diagnosis is usually made by transavaginal and transbdominal ultrasonography. False-positive diagnoses are common in the second trimester. Bleeding with placenta previa is usually associated with uterine contractions. Placenta accreta is common in the patient with one or more previous CS and placenta previa in the current pregnancy. Management of placenta previa depends on the gestational age and the status of the patient (amount of bleeding etc.); nevertheless it should involve avoidance of digital vaginal examination, delay of delivery until 36 weeks' gestation and/or documented fetal lung maturity, transfusion support to maintain maternal hematocrit greater than or equal to 30%, serial US, antepartum FHR monitoring, glucocorticoids, tocolytic therapy, and elective delivery by CS. Maternal mortality is rare with placenta previa. PNM is currently 4% to 8% primarily related to complications of prematurity [41].

Placenta accreta encompasses various types of abnormal placentation in which chorionic villi attach directly to or invade the myometrium. Placenta accreta is a significant cause of maternal morbidity and mortality and is now the most common reason for emergent postpartum hysterectomy. Its prevalence has risen tenfold in the USA over the past 50 years, primarily due to the increasing percentage of pregnant patients undergoing primary and repeat CS. Placenta previa and previous CS are the two most important known risk factors for placenta accreta. Accurate prenatal identification of affected pregnancies allows optimal obstetric management. U.S. remains the diagnostic standard, and routine U.S. examination at 18-20 weeks gestation affords an ideal opportunity to screen for the disorder. Placental lacunae and abnormal color Doppler imaging patterns are the most helpful U.S. markers for placenta accreta. In recent years, there has been an increased interest in magnetic resonance imaging (MRI) for the evaluation of placenta accreta, since it can provide information on depth of invasion and more clearly depict posterior placentas. The most reliable MRI findings are uterine bulging, heterogeneous placenta, and placental bands. Focal interruptions in the hypointense myometrial border may also be helpful. Placenta accreta is a clinical and diagnostic challenge that is being encountered with increasing frequency. Clinicians should be aware of the clinical issues, risk factors, and imaging findings associated with placenta accreta to facilitate optimal case management [42,43]. There is a paucity of information about the management of placenta previa accreta. A multidisciplinary team approach is essential to reduce neonatal and maternal morbidity and mortality. The mainstay of treatment is by demolitive CS, however in carefully selected cases, conservative options may be considered with caution [44].

Abruptio placentae is an important cause of vaginal bleeding in the latter half of pregnancy. The key factor in the pathophysiology is hemorrhage at the decidual-placental interface. Small episodes may escape clinical detection, but severe grades impact significantly on fetal and maternal morbidity and mortality, with the most frequent complications being fetal death, severe maternal shock, disseminated intravascular coagulopathy (DIC), and renal failure. Important risk factors for the development of abruptio placentae are previous abruptio, hypertensive diseases, abdominal trauma, intrauterine growth restriction (IUGR), and smoking. The diagnosis is essentially made on the clinical picture that includes vaginal bleeding (usually dark blood), abdominal pain, and uterine contractions. The essence of management is restoration of circulating volume followed by delivery of the fetus and placenta, most often by CS when the diagnosis is clear and the fetus alive and viable. Aggressive resuscitation and expeditious vaginal delivery are the goals when the fetus is dead [45,46].

e) Trauma

Trauma is not rare among pregnant patients. Various anatomic and physiologic changes of pregnancy may alter the type of injury experienced by pregnant women. These changes may also alter the manifestations of given injuries and the treatment required to re-establish maternal-fetal hemostasis. Fortunately, most traumas experienced by pregnant individuals is minor and is associated with good prognosis for both the mother and her fetus. Blunt trauma as a result of automobile collision is the most frequent form of serious injury involving pregnant women. However, several cases of penetrating abdominal wounds have also been reported. Both blunt and penetrating trauma may frequently injure the uterus. Fetal intracranial injury and fracture, as well as abruptio, often occur as a result of blunt trauma. Multiple direct fetal, placental, and cord injuries have been reported as a result of penetrating trauma. Both blunt and penetrating trauma frequently cause injury to other intra-abdominal organs, and blunt trauma is associated with an especially high incidence of pelvic fracture and retroperitoneal hemorrhage. Laparotomy is often required to treat such injuries. At the time of the laparotomy, difficult decisions are required in determining whether the fetus is best delivered or left in utero. Recent technologic advances for assessing fetal status may be helpful in these decisions. Rarely, a mother may expire with her living fetus undelivered, and a rapid postmortem CS may save the fetal life. During the last several years, the prognosis for both trauma victims and gravid women with complicated pregnancies and their fetuses has improved markedly. Hopefully, during the next several years, the knowledge and therapeutic modalities developed to treat each group will be combined to provide optimal care for the pregnant trauma victim and her fetus [47]. Trauma during pregnancy has presented very unique challenges over the centuries. From the first report of Ambrose Pare of a gunshot wound to the uterus in the 1600s to the present, there have existed controversies and inconsistencies in diagnosis, management, prognostics, and outcome. Anxiety is heightened by the addition of another, smaller patient. Trauma affects 7% of all pregnancies and requires admission in 4 of 1000 pregnancies. The incidence increases with advancing gestational age. Just over half of trauma during pregnancy occurs in the third trimester. Motor vehicle crashes comprise 50% of these traumas, and falls and assaults account for 22% each. These data were considered to be underestimates because many injured pregnant patients are not seen at trauma centers. Trauma during pregnancy is the leading cause of nonobstetric death and has an overall 6% to 7% maternal mortality. Fetal mortality has been quoted as high as 61% in major trauma and 80% if maternal shock is present. The anatomy and physiology of pregnancy make diagnosis and treatment difficult [48].

f) Umbilical Cord Prolapse

Umbilical cord prolapse with fetal distress is a serious obstetrical complication unfamiliar to many emergency physicians although it represents an acute emergency with high mortality. Appropriate prehospital, emergency department, and obstetrical suite care is needed including a bladder-filling technique and in rare cases even tocolysis that can buy valuable time by temporarily relieving pressure on the cord [49]. The frequency of cord prolapse is 0.21% over a 10-year period. Neonatal mortality is 20/1000. Predisposing factors are breech presentation, prematurity, twin pregnancy, and multiparity. Despite much progress in obstetrics, the frequency of cord prolapse has not changed over time. The consequences are not as lethal as in the past, because of progress in diagnosis and neonatal resuscitation. Fetal prognosis might be however severe [50,51].

2) Non-Emergency Cesarean Section

a) Fetal and Adnexal Causes

1. Abnormal Fetal Presentations

Abnormal presentation and position are encountered infrequently during labor. Breech and transverse presentations should be converted to cephalic presentations by external cephalic version (ECV) or delivered by CS. Face, brow, and compound presentations are usually managed expectantly. Occipito-posterior positions can be delivered as such or rotated to occipito-anterior positions. As with any position or presentation, an obstetrician should not hesitate to abandon any rotational or operative vaginal procedure and proceed to CS if rotation or descent does not occur with relative ease [52]. Current trends in the obstetrical management of abnormal fetal presentations have contributed to the sharp rise in the overall use of CS for delivery. Recent literature questions this need. Many investigators are re-evaluating this shift from more traditional approaches [53].

Breech Presentation

Breech presentation might place the fetus at an increased risk. In the management of the selected mature breech presentation, a policy of selected vaginal delivery will result in 4 perinatal deaths for every 1000 patients delivered. A similar probability of neurologic handicap, at least until discharge from hospital, can also be attributed to this method of delivery. These unfavorable outcomes were reported less frequently in more recent reports covering the years since 1974. In these cases, the probability of fetal death due to a trial of vaginal delivery is approximately 2 in 1000. CS rates have risen, however, and 18-40% of TOL for breech presentation now result in emergency CS. Decision analysis has demonstrated that a policy of elective CS for all cases would not necessarily increase maternal mortality and morbidity. Thus, the greater dangers of emergency compared with non-elective surgery may abolish the advantages of attempting a vaginal delivery. Depending on the relative dangers of elective and emergency CS, planned delivery becomes the safer option when 16-30% of trials of vaginal breech delivery are unsuccessful [54]. In light of recent studies that further clarify the long-term risks of vaginal breech delivery, the American College of Obstetricians and Gynecologists (ACOG) recommends that the decision regarding mode of delivery should depend on the experience of the health care provider. CS will be the preferred mode for most physicians because of the diminishing expertise in vaginal breech delivery. Planned vaginal delivery of a term singleton breech fetus may be reasonable under hospital-specific protocol guidelines for both eligibility and labor management. Before a vaginal breech delivery is planned, women should be informed that the risk of perinatal or neonatal mortality or short-term serious neonatal morbidity may be higher than if a CS is planned, and the patient's informed consent should be documented [55].

Vaginal breech birth can be associated with a higher risk of PNM and short-term neonatal morbidity than elective CS. Careful case selection and labor management in a modern obstetrical setting may achieve a level of safety similar to elective CS. Planned vaginal delivery is reasonable in selected women with a term singleton breech fetus. With careful case selection and labor management, PNM occurs in approximately 2 per 1000 births and serious short-term neonatal morbidity in approximately 2% of breech infants. Many recent retrospective and prospective reports of vaginal breech delivery that follow specific protocols have noted excellent neonatal outcomes. Long-term neurological infant outcomes do not differ by planned mode of delivery even in the presence of serious short-term neonatal morbidity. For a woman with suspected breech presentation, pre- or early labor US might be performed to assess type of breech presentation, fetal growth and estimated weight, and attitude of fetal head. Contraindications to labor include:

1. cord presentation;
2. IUGR or macrosomia;
3. any presentation other than a frank or complete breech with a flexed or neutral head attitude;
4. clinically inadequate maternal pelvis; and
5. fetal anomaly incompatible with vaginal delivery.

Vaginal breech delivery can be offered when the estimated fetal weight is between 2500 g and 4000 g. Clinical pelvic examination should be performed to rule out pathological pelvic contraction. Radiologic pelvimetry is not necessary for a safe TOL: good progress in labor is the best indicator of adequate fetal-pelvic proportions. Continuous electronic FHR monitoring is preferable in the first stage and mandatory in the second stage of labor. When membranes rupture, immediate vaginal examination is recommended to rule out prolapsed cord. In the absence of adequate progress in labor, CS is advised. Induction of labor is not recommended for breech presentation. Oxytocin augmentation is acceptable in the presence of uterine dystocia. A passive second stage without active pushing may last up to 90 minutes, allowing the breech to descend well into the pelvis. Once active pushing commences, if delivery is not imminent after 60 minutes, CS should be considered. The active second stage of labor should take place in or near an operating room with equipment and personnel available to perform a timely CS if necessary. A health care professional skilled in neonatal resuscitation should be in attendance at the time of delivery. The health care provider for a planned vaginal breech delivery needs to possess the requisite skills and experience. An experienced obstetrician-gynecologist comfortable in the performance of vaginal breech delivery should be present at the delivery to supervise other health care providers, including a trainee. The requirements for emergency CS, including availability of the hospital operating room team and the approximate 30-minute timeline to commence a laparotomy, must be in accordance with the recommendations of the Society of Obstetricians and Gynecologists of Canada (SOGC) Policy Statement, "Attendance at Labor and Delivery" (Clinical Practice Guidelines [CPG] No. 89, update 2009). The health care provider should have rehearsed a plan of action and should be prepared to act promptly in the rare circumstance of a trapped after-coming head or irreducible nuchal arms: symphysiotomy or emergency abdominal rescue can be life saving. Total breech extraction is inappropriate for term singleton breech delivery. Effective maternal pushing efforts are essential to safe delivery and should be encouraged. At the time of delivery of the after-coming head, an assistant should be present to apply suprapubic pressure to favor flexion and engagement of the fetal head. Spontaneous or assisted breech delivery is acceptable. Fetal traction should be avoided, and fetal manipulation should be applied only after spontaneous delivery to the level of the umbilicus. The fetal head may deliver spontaneously, with the assistance of suprapubic pressure, by Mauriceau-Smellie-Veit maneuver, or with the assistance of Piper forceps. In the absence of a contraindication to vaginal delivery, a woman with a breech presentation should be informed of the risks and benefits of a TOL and elective CS, and informed consent should be obtained. A woman's choice of delivery mode should be respected. The consent discussion and chosen plan should be well documented and communicated to labor-room staff. Hospitals offering a TOL should have a written protocol for eligibility and intrapartum management. Women with a contraindication to a TOL should be advised to have a CS [56-58].

ECV, the transabdominal manipulation of a breech-presenting fetus into a head-down position before birth, is common in traditional ethno-obstetric systems as well as in the modern scientific obstetrics. It is suggested that ECV may constitute an attractive conservative management strategy for breech presentation in scientific obstetric systems as well as in those developing countries where the skill to do versions is part of the traditional inventory of midwifery skills [59].

2. Fetal Anomalies

Conflicting data exist regarding optimal mode of delivery for many fetal conditions. CS may improve neonatal outcome for fetuses with isolated meningomyelocele, hydrocephalus with concomitant macrocephaly, anterior wall defects with extracorporeal liver, sacrococcygeal teratomas, hydrops, and alloimmune thrombocytopenia with low platelet count at term. Hydrocephalus without macrocephaly, anterior wall defects without an extracorporeal liver, ovarian cysts, skeletal dysplasias, fetuses whose mothers have immune thrombocytopenic purpura, and fetuses with alloimmune thrombocytopenia with acceptable platelet counts may safely be delivered vaginally [60]. Our ability to diagnose fetuses with congenital anomalies has dramatically increased over the past two decades and with improved surgical treatment for some defects, more women may choose to continue their pregnancies. Babies with neural tube defects (NTD) presenting by the breech benefit from CS but there is no clear evidence that CS improves outcome in those with a vertex presentation. When the size of the sac exceeds 6 cm, CS may be justified to decrease the risk of disruption. For sacrococcygeal teratoma, the current approach is based on the size of the tumor. In a fetus with a tumor of less than 5 cm, vaginal delivery may be attempted. About ventral wall defects, there is no conclusive evidence that CS is beneficial for fetuses with omphalocele. Because of the heterogeneity of the studies, it is difficult to assess the net impact of mode of delivery in cases of gastroschisis. There is no evidence of significant differences in outcome among fetuses delivered by the vaginal versus the abdominal route. Trauma to the abdominal viscera can occur during either route, and careful delivery is thus mandated [61].

Unique studies using modern US techniques describe the evolution of spina bifida and the subsequent varying development of hydrocephalus. In addition, the dilated fetal stomach is shown to be an ominous sign of complications in cases of gastroschisis. Such complications can be decreased by prenatal supervision using CTG, which detects signs of fetal distress. Recent studies confirm previous findings that CS does not improve the outcome in cases of fetal gastroschisis or spina bifida. Recent research has demonstrated the development of severe fetal malformations. New studies have shown the positive effects of fetal supervision in cases of gastroschisis. Furthermore, CS is not beneficial compared with vaginal delivery in such cases. Fetal surgery is still undergoing rapid development and has the potential to improve outcome [62]. The literature on CS for anomalous infants reports insufficient information on comorbid neonatal conditions. In a minority of cases, a CS is reasonable to prevent dystocia or optimize outcome. Areas for future investigation include prospective, randomized controlled trials (RCT) of prelabor CS compared with vaginal deliveries for myelomeningocele and anterior abdominal wall defects. The rarity of other lesions likely precludes RCT [63].

b) Maternal and Pregnancy-Associated Causes

1. Dystocia

The diagnosis of dystocia is currently a leading indication for CS. Efforts to identify abnormal labor and correct abnormal contraction patterns, fetal malposition, and inadequate expulsive efforts may help eliminate many CS without compromising the outcome for either the mother or the fetus. CS for dystocia should not be performed in the latent phase of labor or in the active phase of labor unless adequate uterine activity has been achieved. CS in the second stage of labor may be reduced if, after re-evaluation of the fetus and pelvis, there is potential for correction of uterine forces with oxytocin, correction of malposition, operative vaginal delivery, or safe continued observation. Use of either a low-dose or high-dose oxytocin regimen is appropriate for augmentation of labor. [64] Early oxytocin augmentation was defined as immediate oxytocin administration when dystocia was identified. Early oxytocin was associated with an increase in the probability of spontaneous vaginal delivery (RR 1.09, 95% CI 1.03-1.17). For every 20 patients treated with early oxytocin augmentation, one additional spontaneous vaginal delivery is expected. Although the point estimate for the effect on CS (RR 0.87, 95% CI 0.71-1.06) and on operative vaginal delivery (RR 0.84, 95% CI 0.70-1.00) showed modest protective effects, the CI for both estimates included the null effect. A decrease in antibiotic use (RR 0.45, 95% CI 0.21-0.99) was observed with early intervention. Early oxytocin was associated with an increased risk of hyperstimulation (RR 2.90, 95% CI 1.21-6.94) without evidence of adverse neonatal effects. Early oxytocin for augmentation in labor is associated with an increase in spontaneous vaginal delivery [65,66].

2. Infections

There are a limited number of infections in a pregnant woman that warrant CS to prevent perinatal transmission. Pregnant women with active genital herpes lesions or with known Herpes Simplex Virus (HSV) infection and a prodromal illness consistent with recurrence at the time of presentation in labor should undergo CS. Pregnant women who are Human Immunodeficiency Virus (HIV) infected and have detectable viremia (> 1000 copies/ml) should be counseled regarding the potential benefits of CS as an adjunct to antiretroviral (ARV) therapy. Hepatitis C Virus (HCV) can be transmitted intrapartum, but prevention of HCV transmission by CS has not been proved effective and is not generally indicated. A limited number of other infectious agents can be transmitted through the birth canal but do not constitute an indication for CS [67].

Hepatitis C Virus

HCV vertical transmission is considered the main route of HCV infection in children. Some authors have stated that CS can reduce perinatal HCV transmission. However, the findings are heterogeneous and high-quality studies are lacking. Aggregation of study results did not show a significant decrease in HCV vertical transmission among study (mothers who underwent CS) versus control (mothers who gave birth vaginally) patients (pooled odds ratio

[OR] 1.1, 95% CI 0.45-2.67). The p value was 0.35 for the test of heterogeneity. Thus it seems that CS does not decrease perinatal HCV transmission from HCV-ribonucleic acid (RNA)+/HIV- mothers to infants [68,69].

Herpes Simplex Virus

Genital herpes is the leading cause of genital ulcer disease worldwide and it is one of the most common sexually transmitted infections (STI). Genital HSV infection during pregnancy poses significant risks, predominantly vertical transmission of infection with resulting neonatal disease. While uncommon, neonatal infection has a high mortality rate and significant long-term morbidity [70]. The type 2 HSV (HSV-2) is mainly localized in the genital region and is transmitted by sexual intercourse. A distinction must be made between primary and recurrent infection. During pregnancy, infection of the generative tract with HSV-2 can be expected in 0.1% of cases, depending on the patient's social status. Fifty percent of all infections in pregnancy are asymptomatic. Miscarriages are common before the 20th week of pregnancy (33%), while later there is a slight increase in premature confinement. Where HSV-2 infection exists at the time of birth, CS is the method of choice for delivery. If rupture of the amnion has occurred over 4 hours, surgical delivery to prevent infection is no longer justified [71].

Human Immunodeficiency Virus

HIV infection during pregnancy is a condition that requires multidisciplinary care. Care must be rendered that is appropriate for both the mother and the fetus. Prevention of mother-to-child transmission of HIV is of paramount concern. To prevent transmission, universal testing for HIV infection in pregnant women is ideal. In the USA and other developed countries, great strides have been made toward decreasing the risk of HIV transmission to infants to < 2% with use of a combination of highly active ARV therapy (HAART) during the antepartum period and during labor and delivery, scheduled CS when appropriate, avoidance of breast-feeding, and 6 weeks of zidovudine (ZDV) prophylaxis for infants. The continuation of ARV therapy after delivery depends on the needs of the mother with regard to treatment of her own health. In resource-limited countries, where simplified and shortened courses of ARV regimens have been used, reduction in mother-to-child transmission has also been shown, although not as effectively as that with HAART. In these settings, exclusive breast-feeding for 6 months is recommended to reduce the risk of postnatal transmission [72]. Management of infection with HIV dramatically improved during the 1990s. The advent of high-performance quantitative HIV assays and HAART were important developments in HIV medicine. As a result, HIV mortality and morbidity have significantly reduced. This improvement in life quality and expectancy through the use of HAART has led to an increase in the number of HIV-infected patients wishing to have children. The mother-to-child transmission which was of major concern previously can now be significantly reduced by newer management strategies [73]. Both the WHO and the USA Department of Health and Human Services (HHS) have recently substantially revised perinatal HIV treatment guidelines based on emerging data, much of it from the developing world. Management of HIV infection in pregnancy and delivery is complicated by concerns for maternal and fetal drug toxicity, acquisition of ARV resistance, prior therapy, co-infections with other viruses, as well as incident opportunistic infections. Intrapartum and peripartum obstetric management, including the role of CS, continue to evolve in the setting of maternal HIV infection. Finally, new data have expanded the role of antiviral therapy in allowing safer infant feeding choices for HIV-infected mothers in resource-limited settings [74-77]. This topic is discussed in chapter 18.

Human Papillomavirus

Recurrent respiratory papillomatosis (RRP) was first described in the 1800s, but it was not until the 1980s when it was convincingly attributed to Human Papilloma Virus (HPV). RRP is categorized into juvenile onset and adult onset depending on presentation before or after the age of 12 years, respectively. The prevalence of this disease is likely variable depending on the age of presentation, country, and socioeconomic status of the population being studied, but is generally accepted to be between 1 and 4 per 100000. Despite the low prevalence, the economic burden of RRP is high given the multiple procedures required by patients. Multiple studies have shown that the most likely route of transmission of HPV in RRP is from mother to child during labor. Exceptions to this may include patients with congenital RRP who have been exposed in utero and adult patients who may have been exposed during sexual contact. Although CS may prevent the exposure of children to the HPV virus during childbirth, its effectiveness in preventing RRP is debatable and the procedure itself carries an increased risk of complications. The quadrivalent HPV vaccine holds the most promise for the prevention of RRP by eliminating the maternal reservoir for HPV [78].

3. Maternal Request and Refusal of Cesarean Section

CS on maternal request is defined as a primary CS at maternal request in the absence of any medical or obstetric indication. Potential risks of CS on maternal request include a longer maternal hospital stay, an increased risk of respiratory problems for the baby, and greater complications in subsequent pregnancies, including uterine rupture and placental implantation problems. CS on maternal request should not be performed before gestational age of 39 weeks has been accurately determined unless there is documentation of lung maturity. CS on maternal request is not recommended for women desiring several children, given that the risks of placenta previa, placenta accreta, and the need for gravid hysterectomy increase with each CS [79]. The literature is nearly unanimous in recommending elective CS at 39 weeks of gestation because of the lower rates of neonatal respiratory complications compared to 38 weeks. However, elective CS at 39 weeks or more may have maternal and other fetal consequences compared to delivery at 38 weeks, which are not always addressed in these studies. Between 38 and 39 weeks of gestation, approximately 10-14% of women go into spontaneous labor, meaning that a considerable number of women scheduled for an elective CS at 39 weeks will deliver earlier in an unscheduled, frequently emergency, CS. The incidence of maternal morbidity and mortality is higher among women undergoing non-elective CS than among those undergoing elective ones. Complications may be greater among women after numerous repeat CS and among older women. Other than reducing the frequency of non-elective CS, bringing forward the timing of elective CS to 38 weeks, may occasionally prevent intrauterine fetal demise which has been shown to increase with increasing gestational age and to avoid other fetal consequences related to the emergency delivery. All these considerations need to be weighed against the medical and the economic impact of the increase in neonatal morbidity resulting from births at 38 weeks compared to 39 weeks. Until prospective RCT are conducted, we are unlikely to be able to precisely answer all risk/benefit questions as to the best timing of scheduled elective CS. It is reasonable to inform pregnant women of the risk of each of the above options and to respect her autonomy and decision-making [80].

The requirements for a legal assessment of the CS on request can be deduced from the general criteria for the legitimacy of medical treatment: indication of treatment, adequacy of treatment (quality), and informed consent. The problem of indication is of particular relevance under the aspect of criminal law. Even if one takes the view that a CS on request is an operation without indication, this does not automatically amount to unconscionability, as defined by Criminal Code, since such an operation may be justified by the consent of the woman. This leads to the problem of comprehensive information on the risks of such an operation. Moreover, it appears to be questionable to reject the indication of a CS on request. The information requirements with reference to liability law can only be formulated with the background of the general information requirements for methods of delivery. The general principle that the greater the risk of operation and the more difficult the decision to be taken are, the more intensive should be the information provided, results in comprehensive duties of information in the case of the CS on request. At present, court rulings establish natural birth to be the first choice of treatment. However, if the risk/benefit assessment should lead to new results due to new medical findings in the future, this will require some discourse within the profession and possibly a new establishment of the medical standard. With regard to the professional aspect, the doctor in charge is entitled to refuse a CS on request [81]. Litigation in obstetric and gynecologic practice has arisen as an important issue. The four most common clinical causes of medical litigation in obstetrics and gynecology are cases involving fetal distress, uterine rupture after a vaginal birth in a woman with a previous CS, shoulder dystocia, and misdiagnosis of breast cancer. Litigation raised in most of the cases is driven by bad outcomes and not by malpractice. Additionally, both juries and the public often expect perfection as the natural result of pregnancy and any deviation from this expectation has to be the result of someone's negligence. For this reason, it has become mandatory for doctors in hospitals and private practices to acquire a sufficient knowledge relating to modern management, to document carefully in writing their procedural and management plans, and to become familiar with the legal aspects of medical practice. Adequate communication and a written patient's consent form are of paramount importance. Maintenance of high standards in daily practice with continuous training, clear communication, and a signed patient's informed consent form along with the appropriate documentation of any procedure carried out, may provide professional safety to practicing obstetricians and gynecologists in case of medical litigation [82].

The issue of CS in the absence of any specific medical indication has sparked intense conversation, as it raises questions about the nature of autonomy in birth. Whereas mainstream bioethical discourse is used to associating autonomy with having a large array of choices, this conception of autonomy does not seem adequate to capture concerns and intuitions that have a strong grip outside this discourse. An empirical and conceptual exploration of how delivery decisions ought to be negotiated must be guided by a rich understanding of women's agency and its placement within a complicated set of cultural meanings and pressures surrounding birth. It is too early to be "for" or "against" women's access to CS in the absence of traditional medical indications, and indeed, a simple pro- or con- position is never going to do justice to the subtlety of the issue. The right question is not whether women ought to be allowed to choose their delivery approach but, rather, taking the value of women's autonomy in decision-making around birth as a given, what sorts of guidelines, practices, and social conditions will best promote and protect women's full inclusion in a safe and positive birth process [83]. Primary and repeat CS rates have reached their highest levels both nationally and internationally, with 30.3% of live births in the USA being CS. Some cite the increase in CS on maternal request as a contributing factor, although data have yet to confirm this. Concern about the rising number of CS performed, and the lack of clear knowledge about health outcomes for both mother and neonate as a result of this trend prompted the National Institute of Child Health and Human Development (NICHD) and the Office of Medical Applications of Research (OMAR) of the National Institutes of Health (NIH) to convene a State-of-the-Science Conference on the topic of CS on maternal request from March 27 to 29, 2006. Before this conference, a study was conducted by the ACOG to assess practice patterns and opinions related to CS on maternal request among obstetricians-gynecologists. It was found that most obstetricians-gynecologists recognized an increased demand for CS on maternal request in their practices [84-86].

Recent position statements by the American Academy of Pediatrics (AAP) and the ACOG and the emergence of legal and ethical analyses on the nature of compelled CS have instigated much discussion on how the primary care physician should respond when a pregnant woman refuses to consent to surgery [87]. In fact, a contemporary ethico-legal dilemma concerns the circumstances, if any, in which a pregnant woman's refusal of medical treatment may be judicially overridden either in her interests or those of the unborn child. On the one hand, the obstetrician will be concerned about the interests of both his patients in potentially life-threatening situations when they can be protected by what might be regarded as relatively straightforward procedures and where to fail to take those steps might expose the practitioner to allegations of negligence. On the other hand, the imposition of treatment in these circumstances will necessarily interfere with the woman's rights of autonomy and self-determination. In such cases also, the conduct of medical procedures in the face of an express prohibition by the woman may give rise to liability for battery. At the heart of an analysis of this issue is the status of the fetus as it is the fact of the woman patient's pregnancy. In regard to this aspect, the approach of the courts in various jurisdictions has arguably been confused and contradictory. Medical treatment of a pregnant woman is lawful in the absence or refusal of consent. This issue is of practical importance to physicians and raises ethico-legal issues about the relative and competing rights of a pregnant woman and the fetus. These rulings have centered on the status of the fetus and have, therefore, suffered from confusion. They have also suffered from hasty decisions made in perceived emergency situations. In the USA, maternal rights are outweighing fetal rights. It has been concluded that courts should not compel pregnant women to submit to medical treatment and any judicial authority in these matters should arise from legislation [88]. This topic is thoroughly discussed in chapter 20.

4. Multiple Gestation

Multi-fetal gestations are associated with increased frequency of maternal, fetal, and neonatal complications. Specific management for multi-fetal pregnancies include early diagnosis, meticulous follow-up, early decrease of maternal activity, midwives at home, psychological care, delivery by CS, and a neonatologist for each baby at the time of delivery [89]. The assessment of optimal delivery for twin gestations is complex due to the relatively high frequency of obstetrical complications and to the heterogeneity of delivery management in these conditions. There is limited role for TOL after CS in twin gestation with a policy of active management [90]. Compared to CS, large retrospective population-based studies demonstrated increased neonatal morbidity and mortality of the second twin associated with vaginal delivery. Some then suggested that systematic planned CS could protect second twins from increased neonatal mortality and morbidity. These results have not been confirmed in retrospective studies in which candidates for vaginal delivery were carefully selected, and second twin delivery actively managed, with internal version when the fetal head is above a 0 station in case of cephalic presentation and with systematic immediate total breech extraction in case of non cephalic presentation. Taking into account the poor external validity of the population-based studies, and the reassuring results of the hospital retrospective studies, attempted vaginal delivery after 34 weeks, when the first twin is in cephalic presentation, still appears as a safe option in low-risk populations. Progress in the assessment of the risks associated with the mode of delivery could result from a large nationwide observational prospective study, a RCT being, even more than in the breech delivery issue, an inappropriate method for evaluating these risks [91,92].

5. Previous Cesarean Delivery

Provided there are no contraindications, a woman with one previous transverse lower uterine segment (LUS) CS should be offered a TOL with appropriate discussion of maternal and perinatal risks and benefits. The process of informed consent with appropriate documentation should be an important part of the birth plan in a woman with a previous CS. The intention of a woman undergoing a TOL after CS should be clearly stated, and documentation of the previous uterine scar should be clearly marked on the prenatal record. For a safe labor after CS, a woman should deliver in a hospital where a timely CS is available. The woman and her health care provider must be aware of the hospital resources and the availability of obstetric, anesthetic, pediatric, and operating-room staff. Each hospital should have a written policy in place regarding the notification and/or consultation for the physicians responsible for a possible timely CS. In the case of a TOL after CS, an approximate time frame of 30 min should be considered adequate in the set-up of an urgent laparotomy. Continuous electronic fetal monitoring of women attempting a TOL after CS is recommended. Suspected uterine rupture requires urgent attention and expedited laparotomy to attempt to decrease maternal and perinatal morbidity and mortality. Oxytocin augmentation is not contraindicated in women undergoing a TOL after CS. Medical induction of labor with oxytocin may be associated with an increased risk of uterine rupture and should be used carefully after appropriate counseling. Medical induction of labor with prostaglandin (PG) E2 (dinoprostone) is possibly associated with an increased risk of uterine rupture and should only be used in rare circumstances and after appropriate counseling. PGE1 (misoprostol) is possibly associated with a high-risk of uterine rupture and is not recommended as a routine part of a TOL after CS. A Foley catheter may be safely used to ripen the cervix in a woman planning a TOL after CS. The available data suggest that a TOL in women with more than one previous CS is likely to be successful but is associated with a higher risk of uterine rupture. Multiple gestation is not a contraindication to TOL after CS. Diabetes mellitus and macrosomia are not contraindications to TOL after CS. Women delivering within 18 months of a CS should be counseled about an increased risk of uterine rupture in labor. Postdatism is not a contraindication to a TOL after CS. Every effort should be made to obtain the previous CS operative report to determine the type of uterine incision used. In situations where the scar is unknown, information concerning the circumstances of the previous delivery is helpful in determining the likelihood of a low transverse incision. If the likelihood of a lower transverse incision is high, a TOL after CS can be offered [93-95].

Trial of VBAC is considered acceptable after one CS, however, women wishing to have trial after two CS are generally not allowed or counseled appropriately of efficacy and complications. Vaginal birth after two CS (VBAC-2) success rate is considered 71.1%, uterine rupture rate 1.36%, hysterectomy rate 0.55%, blood transfusion 2.01%, neonatal unit admission rate 7.78%, and perinatal asphyxial injury/death 0.09%. While maternal morbidity increases with increased number of cesarean sections, when compared with their term counterparts, late pre-term infants face increased morbidity. Establishing the optimal time of delivery for both mother and child is a major challenge faced by clinicians [96-103] (Figure 3).

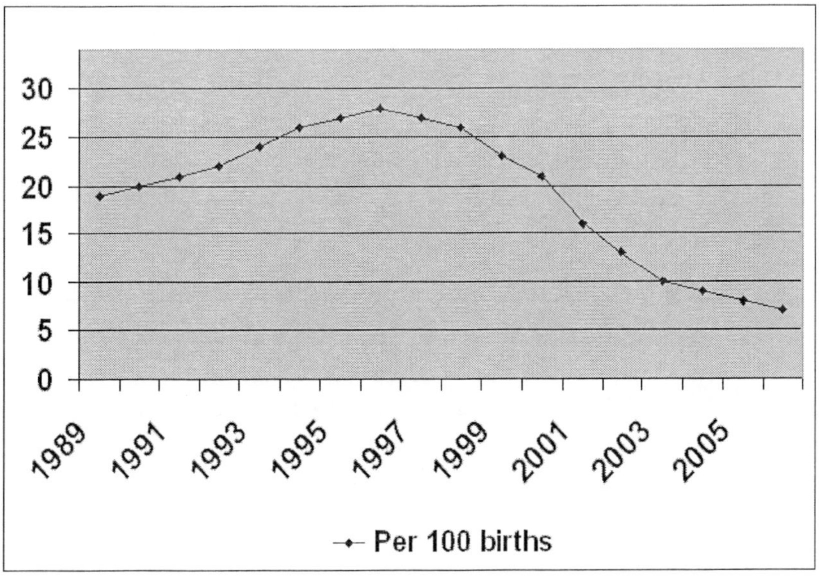

Figure 3. Vaginal births after cesarean rates, Unites States, 1989-2006 (modified from: Viniker DA. Cesarean section rate. http://www.2womenshealth.com/Cesarean-Section-Rate.htm, source: U.S. National Center for Health Statistics).

Cesarean Section Rate Reduction

Between 1965 and 1986, the USA CS rate increased from 4.5% to 24.1%. Various programs and policies have been proposed or implemented to reduce CS rates. In recent decades, many other nations have also experienced a sharply escalating CS rate. It is reasonable to conclude that a largely uncontrolled international pandemic of medically unnecessary CS is occurring. The level of political, analytic, and programmatic activity that has occurred in the USA regarding medically unnecessary surgical births does not seem to be paralleled in other nations with sharply escalating rates [104]. The rate of CS in Great Britain (GB) and the USA, ascertained from a survey, is higher than warranted by the known and agreed obstetric indications for this operation, which suggest a rate of 10-15% would be adequate. It is argued that the fall in PNM which has occurred over the period during which the CS rate has risen is not the main reason for this fall. The training of obstetricians to deal with anxiety, provision of primary maternity care by appropriately trained midwives and general or family practitioners, and changes in management protocols could cut the CS rate. In studies of midwifery care the CS rate is even lower and it is possible that labor proceeds more efficiently if the woman knows her caregivers and labors at home, as in The Netherlands. Although CS is much safer than in the past, it is still has significant morbidity for the woman and economic costs for society [105].

Although infant mortality has declined during the same period, there is little evidence that more frequent CS is the cause. CS benefit health in certain circumstances, but the incidence of those indications has not increased. CS also has risks, the most significant for the infant being iatrogenic prematurity or respiratory disease. Maternal mortality is 2-4 times higher and morbidity is 5-10 times higher after a CS compared to vaginal birth. The four indications responsible for most of the rise in CS rates (previous CS, dystocia, breech presentation, and fetal distress) are those conferring the least clear-cut benefit. Demographically, women who are most likely to experience pregnancy complications, LBW births, or infant mortality are least likely to have a CS. Social, economic, and other factors seem to have a greater influence on the decision to perform a CS than does expected medical benefit. The development of neonatal intensive care, expanded access to prenatal care, and greater availability of abortion and family planning have contributed more to falling infant mortality. It has been estimated that approximately half the CS currently performed in the USA are medically unnecessary, resulting in considerable avoidable maternal mortality and morbidity, and a cost of over $1 billion each year [106]. In studies using matched or adjusted cohorts, USA women beginning labor with midwives and/or in out-of-hospital settings have attained CS rates that are considerably lower than similar women using prevailing forms of care, i.e. physicians in hospitals. This CS reduction involved no compromise in mortality and morbidity outcome measures. Moreover, groups of women at elevated risk for adverse perinatal outcomes have attained excellent outcomes and CS rates well below the general population rate with these care arrangements. The midwives' understanding of and approaches to major medical indications for CS contrast strikingly with prevailing medical knowledge and practice. Cohort studies documenting such a reduction, studies showing other benefits of such forms of care, and the increasing reluctance of physicians to provide obstetrical services, suggests that childbearing families would realize many benefits from greatly expanded use of midwives and out-of-hospital birth settings [107].

Examination of processes and standards of care in light of findings and theory in the areas of gender and psychosocial development leads to the conclusion that the present model of obstetric services is consistent with a masculine style, and offers far less than optimal care for women. In fact, the gender-inappropriate elements of the model itself probably contribute to the excessive rates of interventions in labor. Social, political, and historical factors are seen to support the obstetric model as is, leading to some pessimism about the possibility that the model could be modified sufficiently without major social change [108, 109].

Non-clinical interventions, those applied independent of patient care in a clinical encounter, may have a role in reducing unnecessary CS. Two RCT were shown to be effective in reducing CS rates: a nurse-led relaxation training programme for women with a fear or anxiety of childbirth and birth preparation sessions. However, both RCT were small in size and targeted younger mothers with their first pregnancies. There is insufficient evidence that prenatal education and support programmes, computer patient decision-aids, decision-aid booklets, and intensive group therapy are effective. A cluster-RCT of guideline implementation with mandatory second opinion resulted in a small, statistically significant reduction in total CS rates (adjusted RD -1.9, 95% CI -3.8 to -0.1). This reduction was predominately in intrapartum sections. A study of mandatory second opinion and peer review feedback at department meetings found statistically significant results at 48 months for reducing repeat CS rates (change in level was -6.4%, 95% CI -9.7% to -3.1%, and change in slope -1.14%, 95% CI -1.9% to -0.3%) but not for total CS rates. A cluster-RCT of guideline implementation with support from local opinion leaders increased the proportion of women with a previous CS being offered a TOL (absolute difference 16.8%) and the number who had a vaginal birth (VBAC rates) (absolute difference 13.5%). There was insufficient evidence that audit and feedback, training of public health nurses, insurance reform, external peer review, and legislative changes are effective. Implementation of guidelines with mandatory second opinion can lead to a small reduction in CS rates, predominately in intrapartum sections. Peer review, including pre-CS consultation, mandatory secondary opinion, and post-CS surveillance can lead to a reduction in repeat CS rates. Guidelines disseminated with endorsement and support from local opinion leaders may increase the proportion of women with previous CS being offered a TOL in certain settings. Nurse-led relaxation classes and birth preparation classes may reduce CS rates in low-risk pregnancies [110].

Conclusion

CS is now advocated by many as a routine technique with major advantages over vaginal delivery. In fact, it has been suggested that labor and vaginal delivery are no longer the desired consequence of pregnancy, a conclusion that reflects perceived medical advantages and patient and physician convenience [111]. The indications of CS are increasing. The need to respect maternal desire in the decision making has been supported by law and ethics. Some of the other contributors to the increasing CS rate are breech with failed ECV, decreasing rate of trial of scar, increasing induction rate and electronic FHR monitoring, and changing demography. Despite the adverse effects of CS, the incidence of severe morbidity and mortality is low. The strategies put forward to reduce the CS rate have not been effective and in no country or province, the CS rate has come down. CS rate should not be looked at in isolation or as high or low. It is the product of changing obstetric practice and societal norms and demographics. CS rates do not reflect the performance of a maternity unit [112].

The reported benefits of planned CS include greater safety for the baby, less pelvic floor trauma for the mother, avoidance of labor pain, and convenience. The potential disadvantages, from observational studies, include increased risk of major morbidity or mortality for the mother, and problems in subsequent pregnancies, including uterine scar rupture and greater risk of stillbirth and neonatal morbidity. An unbiased assessment of advantages and disadvantages would assist discussion of what has become a contentious issue in modern obstetrics. There is no evidence from RCT, upon which to base any practice recommendations regarding planned CS for non-medical reasons at term. In the absence of trial data, there is an urgent need for a systematic review of observational studies and a synthesis of qualitative data to better assess the short- and long-term effects of CS and vaginal birth [113]. For some CS remains a major surgical procedure with a corresponding level of risk, which must only be employed in the presence of specific complications and in conjunction with a clearly defined set of indications. Others consider CS quite simply to be the most efficient and straightforward means to deliver as well as the one attended by the least amount of risk. Opinion among those most immediately affected is likewise divided: for many women, the experience of vaginal birth is among the most fulfilling of their entire life (comparable only to sexuality-related moments of ecstasy), while other women come to regard birth as the worst thing that ever happened to them an experience attended by pain and fear [114].

REFERENCES

[1] Lurie S. The changing motives of cesarean section: from the ancient world to the twenty-first century. *Arch. Gynecol. Obstet.* 2005;271:281-5.

[2] Todman D. Childbirth in ancient Rome: from traditional folklore to obstetrics. *Aust. N. Z. J. Obstet. Gynaecol.* 2007;47:82-5.

[3] Rozenberg P. Evaluation of cesarean rate: a necessary progress in modern obstetrics. *J. Gynecol. Obstet. Biol. Reprod.* (Paris). 2004;33:279-89.

[4] Turner MJ. The use of quality control performance charts to analyze cesarean delivery rates nationally. *Int. J. Gynaecol. Obstet.* 2011;113:175-7.

[5] Danforth DN. Cesarean section. *JAMA.* 1985;253:811-8.

[6] Robertson P. Operative and assisted delivery. *Curr. Opin. Obstet. Gynecol.* 1991;3:769-72.

[7] Murphy DJ. Failure to progress in the second stage of labour. *Curr. Opin. Obstet. Gynecol.* 2001;13:557-61.

[8] Mancuso MS, Rouse DJ. Cesarean delivery for abnormal labor. *Clin. Perinatol.* 2008;35:479-90.

[9] Dumont A, de Bernis L, Bouvier-Colle MH, Bréart G; MOMA study group. Caesarean section rate for maternal indication in sub-Saharan Africa: a systematic review. *Lancet.* 2001;358:1328-33.

[10] Weinstein D, Ezra Y, Elchalal U. Management of labor and labor complications. *Curr. Opin. Obstet. Gynecol.* 1995;7:437-41.

[11] Gianopoulos JG. Emergency complications of labor and delivery. *Emerg. Med. Clin. North Am.* 1994;12:201-17.

[12] Calder AA. Emergencies in operative obstetrics. *Baillieres Best Pract. Res. Clin. Obstet. Gynaecol.* 2000;14:43-55.

[13] Kochenour NK. Intrapartum obstetric emergencies. *Crit. Care Clin.* 1991;7:851-64.

[14] Shapiro JM. Critical care of the obstetric patient. *J. Intensive Care Med.* 2006;21:278-86.

[15] Stallard TC, Burns B. Emergency delivery and perimortem C-section. *Emerg. Med. Clin. North Am.* 2003;21:679-93.

[16] Ludwig H. Emergencies in obstetrics. *Ther. Umsch.* 1996;53:477-96.

[17] Pierre F, Rudigoz RC. Emergency caesarean delivery: is there an ideal decision-to-delivery interval? *J. Gynecol. Obstet. Biol. Reprod.* (Paris). 2008;37:41-7.

[18] Papanikitas AN. Obstetrician vs. paediatrician: does inter-professional indifference compromise emergency caesarean safety? *Int. J. Surg.* 2008;6:5-6.

[19] Schauberger CW, Chauhan SP. Emergency cesarean section and the 30-minute rule: definitions. *Am. J. Perinatol.* 2009;26:221-6.

[20] Munnur U, Bandi V, Guntupalli KK. Management principles of the critically ill obstetric patient. *Clin. Chest Med.* 2011;32:53-60.

[21] Ratten GJ. Amniotic fluid embolism – 2 case reports and a review of maternal deaths from this cause in Australia. *Aust. N. Z. J. Obstet. Gynaecol.* 1988;28:33-5.

[22] Davies MG, Harrison JC. Amniotic fluid embolism: maternal mortality revisited. *Br. J. Hosp. Med.* 1992;47:775-6.

[23] D'Addato F, Repinto A, Angeli G. Amniotic fluid embolism in trial of labor. A case report. *Minerva Ginecol.* 1997;49:217-20.

[24] Peitsidou A, Peitsidis P, Tsekoura V, Spathi A, Tzaneti A, Samanta E, Siampalioti G, Kioses E. Amniotic fluid embolism managed with success during labour: report of a severe clinical case and review of literature. *Arch. Gynecol. Obstet.* 2008;277:271-5. Epub 2007 Nov 20.

[25] Fletcher SJ, Parr MJ. Amniotic fluid embolism: a case report and review. *Resuscitation.* 2000;43:141-6.

[26] Mato J. Suspected amniotic fluid embolism following amniotomy: a case report. *AANA J.* 2008;76:53-9.

[27] Hofmeyr GJ, Kulier R. Operative versus conservative management for "fetal distress" in labour. *Cochrane Database Syst. Rev.* 2000;(2):CD001065.

[28] Steer PJ. Surveillance during labour. *J Perinat Med. 2009*;37:451-6.

[29] Pattison N, McCowan L. WITHDRAWN. Cardiotocography for antepartum fetal assessment. *Cochrane Database Syst. Rev.* 2010;1:CD001068.

[30] Khunpradit S, Lumbiganon P, Laopaiboon M. Admission tests other than cardiotocography for fetal assessment during labour. *Cochrane Database Syst. Rev.* 2011;6:CD008410.

[31] Alfirevic Z, Stampalija T, Gyte GM. Fetal and umbilical Doppler ultrasound in high-risk pregnancies. *Cochrane Database Syst. Rev.* 2010;1:CD007529.

[32] Molina FS, Nicolaides KH. Ultrasound in labor and delivery. *Fetal Diagn Ther.* 2010;27:61-7.

[33] Parer JT. The current role of intrapartum fetal blood sampling. *Clin Obstet. Gynecol.* 1980;23:565-82.

[34] Warraich Q, Esen U. Perimortem caesarean section. *J. Obstet. Gynaecol.* 2009;29:690-3.

[35] Katz VL, Dotters DJ, Droegemueller W. Perimortem cesarean delivery. *Obstet. Gynecol.*. 1986;68:571-6.

[36] Katz V, Balderston K, DeFreest M. Perimortem cesarean delivery: were our assumptions correct? *Am. J. Obstet. Gynecol.* 2005;192:1916-20.

[37] Strong TH Jr, Lowe RA. Perimortem cesarean section. *Am. J. Emerg. Med.* 1989;7:489-94.

[38] Kazandi M. Conservative and surgical treatment of abnormal placentation: report of five cases and review of the literature. *Clin. Exp. Obstet. Gynecol.* 2010;37:310-2.

[39] Ophir E, Singer-Jordan J, Odeh M, Hirch Y, Maksimovsky O, Shaider O, Yvry S, Solt I, Bornstein J. Abnormal placental invasion – A novel approach to treatment case report and review. *Obstet. Gynecol. Surv.* 2009;64:811-22.
[40] Rudra A, Chatterjee S, Sengupta S, Wankhede R, Nandi B, Maitra G, Mitra J. Management of obstetric hemorrhage. *Middle East J. Anesthesiol.* 2010;20:499-507.
[41] Mabie WC. Placenta previa. *Clin. Perinatol.* 1992;19:425-35.
[42] Baughman WC, Corteville JE, Shah RR. Placenta accreta: spectrum of US and MR imaging findings. *Radiographics*. 2008;28:1905-16.
[43] Comstock CH. The antenatal diagnosis of placental attachment disorders. *Curr. Opin. Obstet. Gynecol.* 2011;23:117-22.
[44] Allahdin S, Voigt S, Htwe TT. Management of placenta praevia and accreta. *J. Obstet. Gynaecol.* 2011;31:1-6.
[45] Hall DR. Abruptio placentae and disseminated intravascular coagulopathy. *Semin. Perinatol.* 2009;33:189-95.
[46] Doumouchtsis SK, Arulkumaran S. The morbidly adherent placenta: an overview of management options. *Acta Obstet. Gynecol. Scand.* 2010;89:1126-33.
[47] Lavin JP Jr, Polsky SS. Abdominal trauma during pregnancy. *Clin. Perinatol.* 1983;10:423-38.
[48] Barraco RD, Chiu WC, Clancy TV, Como JJ, Ebert JB, Hess LW, Hoff WS, Holevar MR, Quirk JG, Simon BJ, Weiss PM; EAST Practice Management Guidelines Work Group. Practice management guidelines for the diagnosis and management of injury in the pregnant patient: the EAST Practice Management Guidelines Work Group. *J. Trauma.* 2010;69:211-4.
[49] Barnett WM. Umbilical cord prolapse: a true obstetrical emergency. *J. Emerg. Med.* 1989;7:149-52.
[50] Dufour P, Vinatier D, Bennani S, Tordjeman N, Fondras C, Monnier JC, Codaccioni X, Lequien P, Puech F. Cord prolapse. Review of the literature. A series of 50 cases. *J. Gynecol. Obstet. Biol. Reprod.* (Paris). 1996;25:841-5.
[51] Lin MG. Umbilical cord prolapse. *Obstet. Gynecol. Surv.* 2006;61:269-77.
[52] Stitely ML, Gherman RB. Labor with abnormal presentation and position. *Obstet. Gynecol. Clin. North Am.* 2005;32:165-79.
[53] Gimovsky M, Hennigan C. Abnormal fetal presentations. *Curr. Opin. Obstet. Gynecol.* 1995;7:482-5.
[54] Bingham P, Lilford RJ. Management of the selected term breech presentation: assessment of the risks of selected vaginal delivery versus cesarean section for all cases. *Obstet. Gynecol.*. 1987;69:965-78.
[55] ACOG Committee on Obstetric Practice. ACOG Committee Opinion No. 340. Mode of term singleton breech delivery. *Obstet. Gynecol.*. 2006;108:235-7.
[56] Kotaska A, Menticoglou S, Gagnon R, Farine D, Basso M, Bos H, Delisle MF, Grabowska K, Hudon L, Mundle W, Murphy-Kaulbeck L, Ouellet A, Pressey T, Roggensack A; Maternal Fetal Medicine Committee; Society of Obstetricians and Gynaecologists of Canada. Vaginal delivery of breech presentation. *J. Obstet. Gynaecol. Can.* 2009;31:557-66, 567-78.

[57] Kotaska A, Menticoglou S, Gagnon R, Farine D, Basso M, Bos H, Delisle MF, Grabowska K, Hudon L, Mundle W, Murphy-Kaulbeck L, Ouellet A, Pressey T, Roggensack A; Society of Obstetricians and Gynaecologists of Canada. SOGC clinical practice guideline: Vaginal delivery of breech presentation: no. 226, June 2009. *Int. J. Gynaecol. Obstet.* 2009;107:169-76.

[58] Kok M, Cnossen J, Gravendeel L, Van Der Post JA, Mol BW. Ultrasound factors to predict the outcome of external cephalic version: a meta-analysis. *Ultrasound Obstet. Gynecol.*. 2009;33:76-84.

[59] Jordan B. External cephalic version as an alternative to breech delivery and cesarean section. *Soc. Sci. Med.* 1984;18:637-51.

[60] Kuller JA, Katz VL, Wells SR, Wright LN, McMahon MJ. Cesarean delivery for fetal malformations. *Obstet. Gynecol. Surv.* 1996;51:371-5.

[61] Anteby EY, Yagel S. Route of delivery of fetuses with structural anomalies. *Eur J. Obstet.. Gynecol. Reprod Biol.* 2003;106:5-9.

[62] Lingman G. Management of pregnancy and labour in cases diagnosed with major fetal malformation. *Curr. Opin. Obstet. Gynecol.* 2005;17:143-6.

[63] Hamrick SE. Cesarean delivery and its impact on the anomalous infant. *Clin. Perinatol.* 2008;35:395-406.

[64] ACOG technical bulletin. Dystocia and the augmentation of labor. Number 218 – December 1995 (replaces no. 137, December 1989, and no. 157, July 1991). American College of Obstetricians and Gynecologists. *Int. J. Gynaecol. Obstet.* 1996;53:73-80.

[65] Wei SQ, Luo ZC, Xu H, Fraser WD. The effect of early oxytocin augmentation in labor: a meta-analysis. *Obstet. Gynecol.*. 2009;114:641-9.

[66] Wei SQ, Luo ZC, Qi HP, Xu H, Fraser WD. High-dose vs low-dose oxytocin for labor augmentation: a systematic review. *Am. J. Obstet. Gynecol.*. 2010;203:296-304.

[67] Sharma D, Spearman P. The impact of cesarean delivery on transmission of infectious agents to the neonate. *Clin. Perinatol.* 2008;35:407-20.

[68] Ghamar Chehreh ME, Tabatabaei SV, Khazanehdari S, Alavian SM. Effect of cesarean section on the risk of perinatal transmission of hepatitis C virus from HCV-RNA+/HIV- mothers: a meta-analysis. *Arch. Gynecol. Obstet.* 2011;283:255-60..

[69] Indolfi G, Resti M. Perinatal transmission of hepatitis C virus infection. *J. Med. Virol.* 2009;81:836-43.

[70] Aga IE, Hollier LM. Managing genital herpes infections in pregnancy. *Womens Health* (Lond Engl). 2009;5:165-72.

[71] Koenig UD. The importance of herpes simplex virus type 2 (HSV-2) infection pregnancy and the period following birth. *Z. Geburtshilfe Perinatol.* 1977;181:380-9.

[72] Anderson BL, Cu-Uvin S. Pregnancy and optimal care of HIV-infected patients. *Clin. Infect. Dis.* 2009;48:449-55.

[73] Reshi P, Lone IM. Human immunodeficiency virus and pregnancy. *Arch. Gynecol. Obstet.* 2010;281:781-92.

[74] Vogler MA, Singh H, Wright R. Complex decisions in managing HIV infection during pregnancy. *Curr. HIV/AIDS Rep.* 2011;8:122-31.

[75] Mepham SO, Bland RM, Newell ML. Prevention of mother-to-child transmission of HIV in resource-rich and -poor settings. *BJOG.* 2011;118:202-18.

[76] Legardy-Williams JK, Jamieson DJ, Read JS. Prevention of mother-to-child transmission of HIV-1: the role of cesarean delivery. *Clin. Perinatol.* 2010;37:777-85.

[77] Van Dyke RB. Mother-to-child transmission of HIV-1 in the era prior to the availability of combination antiretroviral therapy: the role of drugs of abuse. *Life Sci.* 2011;88:922-5.

[78] Larson DA, Derkay CS. Epidemiology of recurrent respiratory papillomatosis. *APMIS.* 2010;118:450-4.

[79] American College of Obstetricians and Gynecologists. ACOG Committee Opinion No. 394, December 2007. Cesarean delivery on maternal request. *Obstet. Gynecol.*. 2007;110:1501.

[80] Salim R, Shalev E. Health implications resulting from the timing of elective cesarean delivery. *Reprod. Biol. Endocrinol.* 2010;8:68.

[81] Becker-Schwarze K. Legal problems in an elective cesarean section. *Zentralbl. Gynakol.* 2001;123:111-6.

[82] Mavroforou A, Koumantakis E, Michalodimitrakis E. Physicians' liability in obstetric and gynecology practice. *Med. Law.* 2005;24:1-9.

[83] Obstetrics and Gynecology Risk Research Group, Kukla R, Kuppermann M, Little M, Lyerly AD, Mitchell LM, Armstrong EM, Harris L. Finding autonomy in birth. *Bioethics.* 2009;23:1-8.

[84] Coleman VH, Lawrence H, Schulkin J. Rising cesarean delivery rates: the impact of cesarean delivery on maternal request. *Obstet. Gynecol.* Surv. 2009;64:115-9.

[85] Michaluk CA. Cesarean delivery by maternal request: what neonatal nurses need to know. *Neonatal. Netw.* 2009;28:145-50.

[86] Mazzoni A, Althabe F, Liu NH, Bonotti AM, Gibbons L, Sánchez AJ, Belizán JM. Women's preference for caesarean section: a systematic review and meta-analysis of observational studies. *BJOG.* 2011;118:391-9.

[87] Doukas DJ, Elkins TE. Compelled cesarean section. An ethical perspective. *Prim. Care.* 1993;20:721-8.

[88] Rossiter GP. Contemporary transatlantic developments concerning compelled medical treatment of pregnant women. *Aust. N. Z. J. Obstet. Gynaecol.* 1995;35:132-8.

[89] Pons JC, Frydman R. Quadruplet pregnancies: management and obstetric and pediatric outcome. *J. Gynecol. Obstet. Biol. Reprod.* (Paris). 1992;21:557-62.

[90] Sentilhes L, Bouhours AC, Biquard F, Gillard P, Descamps P, Kayem G. Delivery of twins. *Gynecol. Obstet. Fertil.* 2009;37:432-41.

[91] Schmitz T, Azria E, Cabrol D, Goffinet F. Is vaginal delivery in twin pregnancy still an option? An analysis of the literature data. *J. Gynecol. Obstet. Biol. Reprod.* (Paris). 2009;38:367-76.

[92] Rossi AC, Mullin PM, Chmait RH. Neonatal outcomes of twins according to birth order, presentation and mode of delivery: a systematic review and meta-analysis. *BJOG.* 2011;118:523-32.

[93] Martel MJ, MacKinnon CJ; Clinical Practice Obstetrics Committee of the Society of Obstetricians and Gynaecologiests of Canada. Guidelines for vaginal birth after previous Caesarean birth. *J. Obstet. Gynaecol. Can.* 2004;26:660-83.

[94] Martel MJ, MacKinnon CJ; Clinical Practice Obstetrics Committee, Society of Obstetricians and Gynaecologists of Canada. Guidelines for vaginal birth after previous Caesarean birth. *J. Obstet. Gynaecol. Can.* 2005;27:164-88.

[95] Society of Obstetricians and Gynaecologists of Canada. SOGC clinical practice guidelines. Guidelines for vaginal birth after previous caesarean birth. Number 155 (Replaces guideline Number 147), February 2005. *Int. J. Gynaecol. Obstet.* 2005;89:319-31.
[96] Tzur T, Weintraub AY, Sheiner E, Wiznitzer A, Mazor M, Holcberg G. Timing of elective repeat caesarean section: maternal and neonatal morbidity and mortality. *J Matern. Fetal. Neonatal. Med.* 2011;24:58-64.
[97] Gregory KD, Fridman M, Korst L. Trends and patterns of vaginal birth after cesarean availability in the United States. *Semin. Perinatol.* 2010;34:237-43.
[98] Lydon-Rochelle MT, Cahill AG, Spong CY. Birth after previous cesarean delivery: short-term maternal outcomes. *Semin. Perinatol.* 2010;34:249-57.
[99] Silver RM. Delivery after previous cesarean: long-term maternal outcomes. *Semin. Perinatol.* 2010;34:258-66.
[100] Landon MB. Predicting uterine rupture in women undergoing trial of labor after prior cesarean delivery. *Semin. Perinatol.* 2010;34:267-71.
[101] Patel RM, Jain L. Delivery after previous cesarean: short-term perinatal outcomes. *Semin. Perinatol.* 2010;34:272-80.
[102] O'Shea TM, Klebanoff MA, Signore C. Delivery after previous cesarean: long-term outcomes in the child. *Semin. Perinatol.* 2010;34:281-92.
[103] Kaimal AJ, Kuppermann M. Understanding risk, patient and provider preferences, and obstetrical decision making: approach to delivery after cesarean. *Semin. Perinatol.* 2010;34:331-6.
[104] Sakala C. Medically unnecessary cesarean section births: introduction to a symposium. *Soc. Sci. Med.* 1993;37:1177-98.
[105] Francome C, Savage W. Caesarean section in Britain and the United States 12% or 24%: is either the right rate? *Soc. Sci. Med.* 1993;37:1199-218.
[106] Shearer EL. Cesarean section: medical benefits and costs. *Soc. Sci. Med.* 1993;37:1223-31.
[107] Sakala C. Midwifery care and out-of-hospital birth settings: how do they reduce unnecessary cesarean section births? *Soc. Sci. Med.* 1993;37:1233-50.
[108] LoCicero AK. Explaining excessive rates of cesareans and other childbirth interventions: contributions from contemporary theories of gender and psychosocial development. *Soc. Sci. Med.* 1993;37:1261-9.
[109] Mutryn CS. Psychosocial impact of cesarean section on the family: a literature review. *Soc. Sci. Med.* 1993;37:1271-81.
[110] Khunpradit S, Tavender E, Lumbiganon P, Laopaiboon M, Wasiak J, Gruen RL. Non-clinical interventions for reducing unnecessary caesarean section. *Cochrane Database Syst. Rev.* 2011;6:CD005528.
[111] Singh R, Nath Trivedi A. Is the caesarean section rate a performance indicator of an obstetric unit? *J. Matern. Fetal. Neonatal. Med.* 2011;24:204-7.
[112] Grisaru S, Samueloff A. Primary nonmedically indicated cesarean section ("section on request"): evidence based or modern vogue? *Clin. Perinatol.* 2004;31:409-30.
[113] Lavender T, Hofmeyr GJ, Neilson JP, Kingdon C, Gyte GM. Caesarean section for non-medical reasons at term. *Cochrane Database Syst. Rev.* 2006;3:CD004660.
[114] Husslein P. Elective caesarean section versus vaginal delivery. Whither the end of traditional obstetrics? *Arch. Gynecol. Obstet.* 2001;265:169-74.

In: Cesarean Section: Procedures, Complications and Recovery ISBN: 978-1-62081-214-3
Editor: Eyal Sheiner

Chapter V

BREECH DELIVERY: EPIDEMIOLOGY AND CESAREAN DELIVERY

***Henry Chong Lee**[*,1] **and Jeffrey B. Gould**[2]*
[1]Pediatrics, University of California, San Francisco,
Department of Pediatrics, Division of Neonatology, San Francisco, CA, US
Pediatrics, Department of Pediatrics, Division of Neonatal and
[2]Developmental Medicine, Director, Perinatal Epidemiology and Health Outcomes
Research Unit, Stanford University School of Medicine, Stanford, CA, US

INTRODUCTION

Breech presentation, in which the fetus's bottom presents downward toward the cervix, was described as early as about 400 – 600 A.D. in the Moschion manuscript with figures of the fetus, which were adopted by obstetric texts of the 16 to 18th centuries. [1,2] Leonardo di Vinci described a fetus in complete breech presentation in his notebook. [1] There are three types of breech presentation: frank breech which is the most common in which hips are flexed and knees extended with buttocks presenting and feet near the head, complete breech when hips and knees are flexed with buttocks and feet presenting in a cross-legged position, and footling or incomplete breech, when one or both feet present first.

INCIDENCE

A precise incidence of breech presentation at birth is difficult to ascertain. The reported incidence of breech is usually 3-4%, ranging from 2.7% to 5.2%. [3-7] This variability may be due to demographic differences in the composition of the population under study and in the operational definition of breech delivery. When considering the reported rates of breech

* Corresponding author: Henry Chong Lee, MD, MS, University of California, San Francisco, 533 Parnassus Avenue, Room U503, San Francisco, CA 94143-0734, (415) 476-1888 (phone), (415) 476-9976 (fax), email: LeeHC@peds.ucsf.edu.

presentation, one should note the inclusion criteria, as incidence can be significantly influenced by the composition of the population under study. For example, preterm infants and multiple gestation births are more likely to have higher incidence of breech as are infants with congenital anomalies. When reporting rates, it should be noted whether these groups were excluded from analysis.

For example, using the Netherlands Perinatal Registry which included more than 1.3 million singleton births, the breech incidence in an 8 year period was 5.2% for all singletons, but only 3% for term singletons. [8] However these may be higher estimates then what might be expected in a general population in that the Netherlands registry captures data at higher proportions (95-99%) for births at higher risk centers than at low risk hospitals (90%). Because data is biased towards centers where breech presentation would be expected to be higher, the rate reported could be an overestimate of actual country-wide incidence.

A second difficulty in estimating the incidence of breech is ascertainment. The best estimate of the true incidence of breech would presumably be from data collection from a large population. When using administrative datasets, it is important to see how variables are defined and recorded. Large population data such as a country's vital records dataset may not differentiate between breech presentation and other malpresentations. In our study of United States birth certificate data, we found a breech incidence in the whole U.S. population of 3.8% over a 7 year period, which included more than 28 million births. [6] The coding for U.S. birth certificate data has included "malpresentation" as part of the breech variable. Therefore, the validity of this measure, while commonly used as an estimate of breech presentation rates, is dependent on the diagnosis of other malpresentations. In our analysis, we also saw a variation of breech incidence by state ranging from an incidence of 1.5 to 4.1%. While the ascertainment of breech or transverse lie should be uniform, it is possible that there may be variability in the diagnosis of other malpresentations.

Etiology / Associations, Congenital Malformations

In some infants, breech presentation may occur as a result of disorders in which there is decreased movement in utero. Infants with congenital malformations and / or neuromuscular disorders have been found with higher incidence of breech than expected and conversely, breech infants have been found with higher rates of malformations. [4,9,10] A study of cases from dysmorphology clinics found that the proportion of breech presentation for various congenital disorders, such as Trisomy 18 and Zelleweger syndrome, was higher than expected. [11] Breech incidence was as high as 50% for Prader-Willi syndrome, a well known cause of hypotonia. Fetal alcohol syndrome and Smith-Lemli-Opitz syndrome had breech incidence of 40%. When considering studies of developmental outcome in breech infants, it would be important to consider the potential impact of these associations.

Prematurity and Size

The incidence of breech declines as a function of increasing gestational age, as more fetuses engage in the vertex position as pregnancy ensues. In a study of the Netherlands

Perinatal Registry, the incidence of breech decreased linearly with gestation from 40% at 24 weeks to 3% at term. In our analysis of the United States birth certificates, we found a similar decline for singletons, however starting at 25% incidence at 24 weeks and declining to 3% at 39 weeks and 2% at 40 weeks (figure 1).

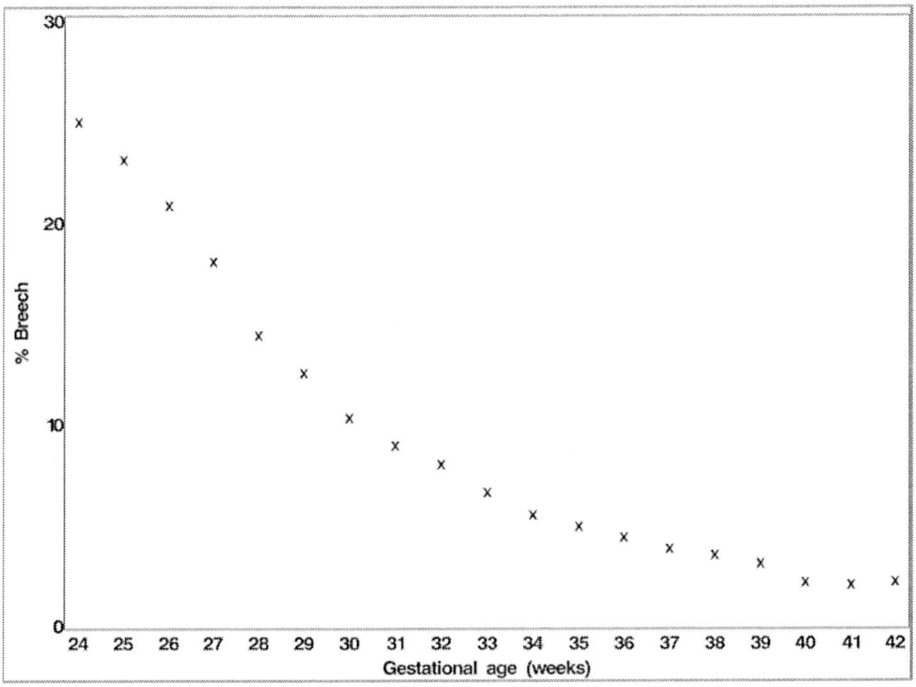

Figure 1. Incidence of breech presentation at birth by gestational age. Data source: National Center for Health Statistics.

Another study of singletons born in Washington State reported similar rates – 20.6% at 25 – 26 weeks gestation, declining to 2.6% at 40 weeks. [12] These differences at earlier gestations between the U.S. data and the Netherlands may be due to differences in reporting or management of preterm births. The steeper drop from 39 to 40 weeks (which is seen at 37 weeks in the Netherlands Registry) may be due to elective cesarean deliveries occurring prior to those gestational age weeks.

Small size independent of gestational age has also been shown as a risk factor for breech presentation. After controlling for gestational age, parity, and maternal age, a 500 gram decrease in birth weight was associated with an increased risk of breech presentation in singletons (OR 1.32, 95% CI 1.26, 1.38). [10] In a similar study of Australian term newborns, small for gestational age (< 10th percentile for birth weight) was associated with breech presentation (OR 1.33, 95% CI 1.28, 1.38). [13]

Gender

In a study of the Netherlands Perinatal Registry, for infants born after 32 weeks gestation, there were significantly more singleton girls than boys in breech position at delivery. [8] The study included more than 70,000 breech births. At 40 weeks, 43.4% of breech infants were boys, with 3.6% of girls and 2.8% of boys being born in breech position. This difference in breech presentation with females having higher incidence has also been shown in other cohorts. [3,13,14] In our investigation of the United States birth certificate dataset from 2003, we also found a higher incidence of breech in singleton females (3.3%) than males (3.0%). [15] The reason for this gender difference may be due to the smaller size of girls or differences in body proportion.

Multiple Births

Breech presentation is more common in multiple births. In twin pregnancies, the incidence of breech in the first presenting or lower twin has been reported to be 17.7% to 27.0%. [16] For the second presenting twin, the incidence was higher, from 30.7% to 40.8%. [16] The incidence of breech in higher order multiples has been less well reported, although it would presumably be higher than for singletons. In a series of 41 triplet pregnancies, the incidence of breech in the first presenting triplet was 17.6%, the second triplet 28.5%, and the third triplet 29.1%. [17] It is notable that almost all of those pregnancies were preterm, which is also associated with breech presentation.

Developmental Dysplasia of the Hip

Breech presentation has been noted as a risk factor for developmental dysplasia of the hip (DDH). The etiology of DDH is multi-factorial including genetic predisposition and hormonal. However, intra-uterine mechanical factors would likely play an important role in the forces which cause hip instability and dysplasia, and would explain the higher risk of DDH seen in breech born infants. The risk of DDH from breech presentation is probably a result of some period of time spent in that position, and has been shown to remain higher for infants who were in breech position at 36 weeks, but then subsequently delivered in vertex position after version. [18]

The incidence of DDH is difficult to pinpoint for several reasons: the condition encompasses a spectrum of hip instability from subluxation to dislocation, there is no gold standard for diagnosis, and the condition may be present or absent at varying times in an infant's life. [19] Earlier studies describing risk factors for DDH were based on registries of patients with that condition. As the incidence of breech is relatively stable across populations, knowing the proportion of breech in a cohort of DDH can give an idea of the increased risk conferred by the abnormal position in utero. Reported incidence of breech in such studies ranges from 11% to 25% in patients with DDH. [20-22]

A population based approach may allow for a clearer indication of the risk of a breech infant for DDH. In an Australian cohort, breech presentation was found to be the most significant factor associated with DDH. [23] Vaginally delivered breech infants (OR 17.2, 95% CI 12.8, 23.0) and cesarean delivered breech infants (OR 10.0, 95% CI 8.6 11.7) were more likely to have DDH compared to non-breech presentation.

In a population based study of the Norwegian birth registry of more than 1 million births, the breech rate of neonatal hip instability was 4.4% compared to the overall prevalence of 0.9%. [24] In that study, neonatal hip instability was defined as positive Ortolani sign or congenital dislocation of the hip. There was a slight increase in prevalence for vaginally delivered breech infants (4.54%) compared to cesarean born breech infants (4.25%).

Mortality and Morbidity

The process of labor and delivery present several risks to the fetus presenting in breech position, including cord prolapse, head entrapment, and other birth traumas. [25-27] Other associated morbidities include potential brain injury, spinal cord injury, brachial plexus injury, skull fracture, fracture of long bones or clavicle, and genital injury; such injuries may be more prevalent in vaginal breech births. [28-36]

Determining the risk contribution of breech presentation to various morbidities is not always straightforward. The presence of various obstetric conditions and injuries may partly be a result of the factors which led to breech presentation, and not the breech presentation per se. Breech presentation would also influence the mode of delivery, which could potentially contribute to or attenuate certain morbidities. For example, cord prolapse is more common in preterm infants and the preterm state could have contributed to the prolapse as well as breech presentation.

Cord prolapse is a rare obstetric complication which often requires emergent cesarean delivery, with an incidence of 0.1% to 0.6% in the general population, and ensuing cord compression can lead to asphyxia and encephalopathy. [27] The reported incidence of cord prolapse is 2% to 6% in breech presentation with a decreasing trend in more recent reports. [27] This may be partly due to the increase in elective cesarean delivery for breech infants. In a large case-control study examining risk factors of cord prolapse, breech presentation conferred a significantly higher risk of prolapse (OR 2.5, 95% CI 1.7, 3.9) after controlling for other factors. [37]

Infants born in breech position are at generally higher risk of asphyxia and encephalopathy, conferring a 4 to 20-fold risk compared to vertex births. [38-42] This risk is present for both preterm and term infants, but is more of a factor for term births. [39]

Neonatal mortality is higher for infants born in breech position, this risk likely related to the above morbidities, conferring a 1.5 to 2-fold risk compared to vertex births. [29,43-45] When considering mortality, there is the possibility of risk factors for breech presentation also being risks for mortality. During a 9 year period in California amongst term births, there were 0.6 deaths per 1,000 breech deliveries compared to 0.3 per 1000 vertex deliveries. [29] Neonatal mortality was higher for breech babies born vaginally (1.8 per 1000).

Version

External version of breech fetuses can be attempted in order to reduce the potential for complications and cesarean delivery. The procedure has been shown to reduce the incidence of breech presentation at term. [46,47] At 36 weeks gestation, the success rate is about 65%.

[25] Complications such as placental separation or umbilical cord compression can lead to the need for emergent cesarean delivery. However, the current literature has not shown a significantly high rate of ultimate adverse outcomes for infant or mother. [48] Although cesarean delivery may be necessary due to a complication or failure of version, the overall cesarean rate could be reduced by attempts at version. [25,46]

Cesarean and Breech

The suggestion that cesarean delivery may be of routine benefit for breech presentation surfaced in the 1950's. [25,49,50] Prior to that time, vaginal breech delivery was the standard. The cesarean rate for breech steadily increased in the United States in the 1970's. At one university center in the 1970's, the cesarean rate for singleton breech infants with birth weight greater than 2,500 grams increased from 13% to 54%, and from 5% to 55% in smaller infants. [51]

Retrospective Studies

Most past studies on the potential benefit of cesarean delivery for term infants have been retrospective cohort studies and have had relatively low power to detect significant differences in both neonatal and maternal outcomes. [52-54] Some investigators have found no significant impact from the mode of delivery when considering other factors, both short and long term. [55-58] Others have found reduction in mortality and morbidity. [5,7,29,59] Conclusions from such studies have been difficult to make due to their retrospective nature and issues of selection bias and confounding. The framework for when to have a trial of labor for certain patients have not been uniform, nor the reasons for switching to cesarean delivery.

Larger population-based studies have also been performed which have tended to show some benefit to cesarean in regard to mortality. In a study of 3,447 term breech births in the North West Thames region, there was a relative risk of 20 (95% CI, 2.5, 163) of mortality for vaginal vs. cesarean delivery. However, this study did not incorporate potential confounders in the analysis. A study of term breech births (n = 100,667) in California from 1991 to 1999 found higher mortality (OR 9.2, 95% CI 3.3, 25.6) for singleton breech vaginal vs. cesarean delivery, but no difference in mortality by mode of delivery when the mother had a prior vaginal delivery. [29] However, morbidities such as asphyxia and brachial plexus injury were increased for vaginal delivery in both nulliparous mothers and those with prior vaginal delivery.

Other large observational studies have also shown that cesarean delivery for breech presentation is associated with lower incidence of acidemia, low Apgar score, birth trauma, and neurologic injury. [7,60-62] Although such studies may have power to detect differences in outcome, they often have less clinical detail, particularly regarding the decisions surrounding the mode of delivery. This limits the practical application of these studies, due to the potential that the factors which influenced the mode of delivery could ultimately have impacted outcome, more so than the mode of delivery itself. In an era where the benefit of cesarean is at least contemplated by many obstetricians, could there have been extenuating circumstances which led to a vaginal delivery, which could have been the cause of the adverse outcome, and not the mode of delivery per se? Presumably, a study with more clinical details could be beneficial in answering such questions. However, with more detail, one generally compromises on sample size and power.

Randomized Trials

There have been three randomized trials examining this question. Two were published more than 20 years ago and had relatively small sample size. In a randomized trial of 208 term frank breech infants, the ultimate decision for vaginal delivery was based on x-ray pelvimetry. Of 112 women assigned to the vaginal group, 52 had inadequate pelvic measurements and were scheduled for cesarean delivery. Of the 60 planned vaginal deliveries, 49 had successful vaginal births and 11 ultimately underwent cesarean delivery for difficulties during labor. Their conclusion was that in selected cases, vaginal delivery could be performed in term frank breech presentation. [63] A randomized trial of 105 term nonfrank breech infants also found that 59% of those assigned to the planned vaginal group had inadequate dimensions on x-ray pelvimetry. [64] Although they concluded that selective vaginal delivery was a potential option, their numbers were small, with 31 patients ultimately delivering vaginally, one of which ended in neonatal death due to "inadequate resuscitation".

The largest randomized trial conducted by Hannah et al., the Term Breech Trial, was a multicenter trial involving 2083 women in 121 hospitals in 26 countries. [65] The initial results were published in October 2000 and demonstrated improved outcome for selective cesarean delivery. [65] They found a lower rate of neonatal mortality and serious morbidity in the planned cesarean group (1.6% vs. 5.0%) without significant maternal morbidity or mortality. However, follow-up data from this trial did not demonstrate improvement in outcomes for cesarean delivery neither for infants at 2 years, nor for mothers, although there was also no harm seen for mothers. [66,67] The number of patients followed up to 2 years was reduced from the original group to 923 children.

Several studies have found increased morbidity for mothers undergoing cesarean compared to vaginal delivery. [7,58,68] However, the Term Breech Trial found similar outcomes and no significant increase in morbidity for mothers in the planned cesarean group compared to selective delivery. [66]

If there is a select group of singleton breech infants that can be delivered safely by skilled practitioners, the potential for training and maintaining the skill level of obstetricians may be limited. Even in Sweden, where breech vaginal deliveries were relatively high, the average number of estimated vaginal deliveries by each obstetrician would be less than one per year. [7]

Recent Trends

Largely in response to the Term Breech Trial, the American College of Obstetricians and Gynecologists Committee on Obstetric Practice published an opinion statement in 2001 which recommended cesarean delivery for singleton term breech presentation. [69] The opinion statement was modified in 2006 to allow for the possibility of vaginal delivery in specific situations with skilled physicians and appropriate counseling of mothers. [70] Although there has been some controversy surrounding the implications of the Term Breech Trial, it appears to have had implications for practice as seen by increased cesarean rates in various countries.

In Sweden, the cesarean section rate for term breech infants increased from 75.3% to 86.0% from 1999 to 2001. [71] In the Netherlands, the cesarean section rate increased from 50% to 80% within two months after publication of the Term Breech Trial. [72] In France, the cesarean rate for term breech presentation increased from 14.5% in 1972 to 42.6% in 1995/1998 to 74.5% in 2003. [73] In the United States, cesarean rates had already been high at 83.8% in 1997. There was a modest increase up to 85.1% in 2003 after the recommendations surrounding the Term Breech Trial. [6]

It is worth noting that there is somewhat wide variability of cesarean delivery rates for breech across different states, ranging from 62 to 96% within the same year. [6] We found that those states having higher reporting of breech incidence tended to have lower rates of cesarean delivery for breech (figure 2).

It is possible that lowered rates in those states may be secondary to an overestimate of breech incidence rather than a true decrease in cesarean delivery for breech presentation due to inclusion of infants who were in "malpresentation" and not truly in breech presentation. This would be the case if cases labeled as "malpresentation" represented relatively benign situations in which cesarean delivery would not usually be required.

There still remain researchers in the obstetric community who believe that in the care of a skilled provider and in selected circumstances, delivery of a breech infant by vaginal route can be a safe practice. [68,74,75]

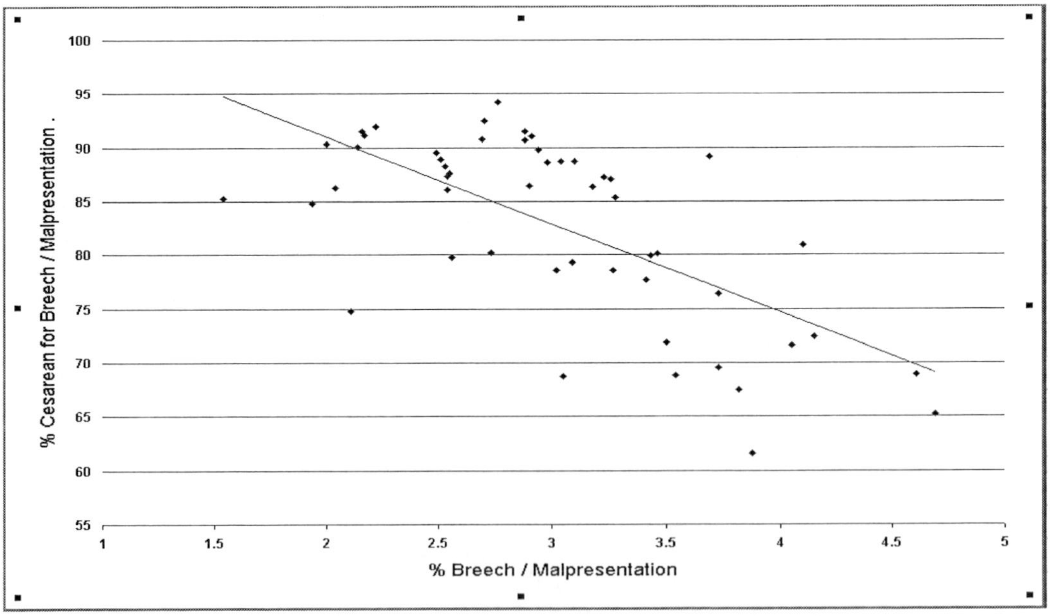

Figure 2. Cesarean rates for breech presentation by breech incidence for individual states. Data source: National Center for Health Statistics.

Preterm Breech and Cesarean

The potential benefit of cesarean delivery for preterm breech infants has also been debated. Although there have been a few randomized trials attempted for preterm breech and mode of delivery, they have suffered from poor enrollment, possibly due to both a lack of enthusiasm in both practitioners and patients. [76-78] One study which involved 26 centers was only able to recruit 13 patients from 6 of those centers over a period of 17 months, despite many more patients having been eligible for the study. [77] The largest study was able to recruit 38 patients over a five year period. [78] Although there was a trend toward higher Apgar scores in the immediate cesarean group, there were not enough numbers to draw conclusions about the optimal mode of delivery in this population.

There have been multiple retrospective studies on preterm breech mode of delivery. These have shown a potential benefit of cesarean compared to vaginal delivery in regard to mortality. [45,79-81] Other outcomes such as intraventricular hemorrhage, chronic lung disease, retinopathy of prematurity, and adverse neurologic sequelae have been associated with vaginal delivery compared to cesarean delivery in breech infants with birth weights 750 to 1,500 grams or gestational age < 32 weeks. [82-85] However, the conclusions of such studies are limited due to their retrospective design. The decisions regarding mode of delivery would be influenced by the circumstances surrounding viability of preterm infants and the mother's health. It is also possible that the medical management of an infant could also be influenced by the mode of delivery, with a stronger push for survival after a mother has undergone a surgical delivery.

Despite this uncertainty, the majority of preterm infants are delivered by cesarean, with greater than 80% cesarean rates for most gestational age groups and often exceeding 90% in the US. [86]

Conclusion

Breech presentation occurs at approximately 3-4% at birth. Although the majority of infants born in breech position will be healthy "well babies", there is increased risk of adverse outcome, which may in part be due to the "cause" of breech presentation, and in some situations, the circumstances of the breech delivery. There has been an increasing trend in cesarean delivery of breech due to various studies which have shown an advantage to planned cesarean delivery, most notably the Term Breech Trial. [65] However, there is still debate about the necessity of cesarean delivery for all breech births. [87,88] As another randomized clinical trial of large magnitude seems unlikely, epidemiologic studies may continue to play an important role in furthering this debate.

References

[1] Confino E, Gleicher N, Elrad H, Ismajovich B, David MP. The breech dilemma. A review. *Obstet. Gynecol. Surv.* Jun 1985;40(6):330-337.

[2] Barbour AHF. Early Contributions of Anatomy to Obstetrics. *Edinburgh Medical Journal.* 1888;34(4):328-335.
[3] Hall MH, Carr-Hill R. Impact of sex ratio on onset and management of labour. *Br. Med. J. (Clin Res Ed).* Aug 7 1982;285(6339):401-403.
[4] Ho NK. Neonatal outcome of breech babies in Toa Payoh Hospital 1984-1989. *Singapore Med. J.* Aug 1992;33(4):333-336.
[5] Thorpe-Beeston JG, Banfield PJ, Saunders NJ. Outcome of breech delivery at term. *Bmj.* Sep 26 1992;305(6856):746-747.
[6] Lee HC, El-Sayed YY, Gould JB. Population trends in cesarean delivery for breech presentation in the United States, 1997-2003. *Am. J. Obstet. Gynecol..* Jul 2008;199(1):59 e51-58.
[7] Roman J, Bakos O, Cnattingius S. Pregnancy outcomes by mode of delivery among term breech births: Swedish experience 1987-1993. *Obstet. Gynecol..* Dec 1998;92(6):945-950.
[8] Rietberg CC, Elferink-Stinkens PM, Visser GH. *Term breech delivery in The Netherlands*, Utrecht University; 2006.
[9] Axelrod FB, Leistner HL, Porges RF. Breech presentation among infants with familial dysautonomia. *J. Pediatr.* Jan 1974;84(1):107-109.
[10] Rayl J, Gibson PJ, Hickok DE. A population-based case-control study of risk factors for breech presentation. *Am. J. Obstet. Gynecol..* Jan 1996;174(1 Pt 1):28-32.
[11] Braun FH, Jones KL, Smith DW. Breech presentation as an indicator of fetal abnormality. *J. Pediatr.* Mar 1975;86(3):419-421.
[12] Hickok DE, Gordon DC, Milberg JA, Williams MA, Daling JR. The frequency of breech presentation by gestational age at birth: a large population-based study. *Am. J. Obstet. Gynecol.* Mar 1992;166(3):851-852.
[13] Roberts CL, Algert CS, Peat B, Henderson-Smart D. Small fetal size: a risk factor for breech birth at term. *Int. J. Gynaecol. Obstet.* Oct 1999;67(1):1-8.
[14] Jonas O, Roder D. Breech presentation in South Australia, 1987-1989. *Aust. N. Z. J. Obstet. Gynaecol.* Feb 1993;33(1):17-21.
[15] *2003 Natality public-use tape and CD-ROM.* Hyattsville, MD: National Center for Health Statistics.
[16] Sekulic SR, Petrovic DS, Runic R, Williams M, Vejnovic TR. Does a probability of breech presentation of more than 50% exist among diseases and medical conditions? *Twin Res. Hum. Genet.* Aug 2007;10(4):649-654.
[17] Ziadeh SM. Perinatal outcome in 41 sets of triplets in Jordan. *Birth.* Sep 2000;27(3):185-188.
[18] Andersson JE, Oden A. The breech presentation and the vertex presentation following an external version represent risk factors for neonatal hip instability. *Acta Paediatr.* Aug 2001;90(8):895-898.
[19] Clinical practice guideline: early detection of developmental dysplasia of the hip. Committee on Quality Improvement, Subcommittee on Developmental Dysplasia of the Hip. American Academy of Pediatrics. *Pediatrics.* Apr 2000;105(4 Pt 1):896-905.
[20] Woolf CM, Koehn JH, Coleman SS. Congenital hip disease in Utah: the influence of genetic and nongenetic factors. *Am. J. Hum. Genet.* Sep 1968;20(5):430-439.
[21] Carter CO, Wilkinson JA. Genetic and environmental factors in the etiology of congenital dislocation of the hip. *Clin. Orthop. Relat. Res.* Mar-Apr 1964;33:119-128.

[22] Record RG, Edwards JH. Environmental influences related to the aetiology of congenital dislocation of the hip. *Br. J. Prev. Soc. Med.* Jan 1958;12(1):8-22.

[23] Chan A, McCaul KA, Cundy PJ, Haan EA, Byron-Scott R. Perinatal risk factors for developmental dysplasia of the hip. *Arch. Dis. Child Fetal. Neonatal. Ed.* Mar 1997;76(2):F94-100.

[24] Hinderaker T, Daltveit AK, Irgens LM, Uden A, Reikeras O. The impact of intra-uterine factors on neonatal hip instability. An analysis of 1,059,479 children in Norway. *Acta Orthop. Scand.* Jun 1994;65(3):239-242.

[25] Bowes Jr. WA, Thorp Jr. JM. Clinical Aspects of Normal and Abnormal Labor. In: Creasy RK, Resnik R, eds. *Maternal-Fetal Medicine.* 5th ed. Philadelphia: Saunders; 2004:671-706.

[26] Dilbaz B, Ozturkoglu E, Dilbaz S, Ozturk N, Sivaslioglu AA, Haberal A. Risk factors and perinatal outcomes associated with umbilical cord prolapse. *Arch. Gynecol. Obstet.* May 2006;274(2):104-107.

[27] Lin MG. Umbilical cord prolapse. *Obstet. Gynecol. Surv.* Apr 2006;61(4):269-277.

[28] Bassaw B, Rampersad N, Roopnarinesingh S, Sirjusingh A. Correlation of fetal outcome with mode of delivery for breech presentation. *J. Obstet. Gynaecol.* Apr 2004;24(3):254-258.

[29] Gilbert WM, Hicks SM, Boe NM, Danielsen B. Vaginal versus cesarean delivery for breech presentation in California: a population-based study. *Obstet. Gynecol..* Nov 2003;102(5 Pt 1):911-917.

[30] Tiwary CM. Testicular injury in breech delivery: possible implications. *Urology.* Oct 1989;34(4):210-212.

[31] Erkaya S, Tuncer RA, Kutlar I, Onat N, Ercakmak S. Outcome of 1040 consecutive breech deliveries: clinical experience of a maternity hospital in Turkey. *Int. J. Gynaecol. Obstet.* Nov 1997;59(2):115-118.

[32] Nadas S, Gudinchet F, Capasso P, Reinberg O. Predisposing factors in obstetrical fractures. *Skeletal Radiol.* 1993;22(3):195-198.

[33] Vialle R, Pietin-Vialle C, Ilharreborde B, Dauger S, Vinchon M, Glorion C. Spinal cord injuries at birth: a multicenter review of nine cases. *J. Matern Fetal. Neonatal. Med.* Jun 2007;20(6):435-440.

[34] Franken EA, Jr. Spinal cord injury in the newborn infant. *Pediatr Radiol.* Mar 20 1975;3(2):101-104.

[35] van Ouwerkerk WJ, van der Sluijs JA, Nollet F, Barkhof F, Slooff AC. Management of obstetric brachial plexus lesions: state of the art and future developments. *Childs Nerv. Syst.* Nov 2000;16(10-11):638-644.

[36] Geutjens G, Gilbert A, Helsen K. Obstetric brachial plexus palsy associated with breech delivery. A different pattern of injury. *J. Bone Joint Surg. Br.* Mar 1996;78(2):303-306.

[37] Critchlow CW, Leet TL, Benedetti TJ, Daling JR. Risk factors and infant outcomes associated with umbilical cord prolapse: a population-based case-control study among births in Washington State. *Am. J. Obstet. Gynecol..* Feb 1994;170(2):613-618.

[38] Lindstrom K, Hallberg B, Blennow M, Wolff K, Fernell E, Westgren M. Moderate neonatal encephalopathy: pre- and perinatal risk factors and long-term outcome. *Acta Obstet. Gynecol. Scand.* 2008;87(5):503-509.

[39] MacDonald HM, Mulligan JC, Allen AC, Taylor PM. Neonatal asphyxia. I. Relationship of obstetric and neonatal complications to neonatal mortality in 38,405 consecutive deliveries. *J. Pediatr.* May 1980;96(5):898-902.

[40] Milsom I, Ladfors L, Thiringer K, Niklasson A, Odeback A, Thornberg E. Influence of maternal, obstetric and fetal risk factors on the prevalence of birth asphyxia at term in a Swedish urban population. *Acta Obstet. Gynecol. Scand.* Oct 2002;81(10):909-917.

[41] Mbweza E. Risk factors for perinatal asphyxia at Queen Elizabeth Central Hospital, Malawi. *Clin. Excell Nurse Pract.* May 2000;4(3):158-162.

[42] Chandra S, Ramji S, Thirupuram S. Perinatal asphyxia: multivariate analysis of risk factors in hospital births. *Indian Pediatr.* Mar 1997;34(3):206-212.

[43] Kambarami RA. Levels and risk factors for mortality in infants with birth weights between 500 and 1,800 grams in a developing country: a hospital based study. *Cent Afr. J. Med.* Nov-Dec 2002;48(11-12):133-136.

[44] Evans N, Hutchinson J, Simpson JM, Donoghue D, Darlow B, Henderson-Smart D. Prenatal predictors of mortality in very preterm infants cared for in the Australian and New Zealand Neonatal Network. *Arch. Dis. Child Fetal Neonatal Ed.* Jan 2007;92(1):F34-40.

[45] Demol S, Bashiri A, Furman B, Maymon E, Shoham-Vardi I, Mazor M. Breech presentation is a risk factor for intrapartum and neonatal death in preterm delivery. *Eu.r J. Obstet. Gynecol. Reprod. Biol.* Nov 2000;93(1):47-51.

[46] Hofmeyr GJ, Kulier R. External cephalic version for breech presentation at term. *Cochrane Database Syst. Rev.* 2000(2):CD000083.

[47] Zhang J, Bowes WA, Jr., Fortney JA. Efficacy of external cephalic version: a review. *Obstet. Gynecol.* Aug 1993;82(2):306-312.

[48] Nassar N, Roberts CL, Barratt A, Bell JC, Olive EC, Peat B. Systematic review of adverse outcomes of external cephalic version and persisting breech presentation at term. *Paediatr Perinat Epidemiol.* Mar 2006;20(2):163-171.

[49] Goethals TR. Cesarean section as the method of choice in management of breech delivery. *Am. J. Obstet. Gynecol.* Mar 1956;71(3):536-552.

[50] Wright RC. Reduction of perinatal mortality and morbidity in breech delivery through routine use of cesarean section. *Obstet. Gynecol.* Dec 1959;14:758-763.

[51] Bowes WA, Jr., Taylor ES, O'Brien M, Bowes C. Breech delivery: evaluation of the method of delivery on perinatal results and maternal morbidity. *Am. J. Obstet. Gynecol.* Dec 1 1979;135(7):965-973.

[52] Bingham P, Hird V, Lilford RJ. Management of the mature selected breech presentation: an analysis based on the intended method of delivery. *Br. J. Obstet. Gynaecol.* Aug 1987;94(8):746-752.

[53] Cheng M, Hannah M. Breech delivery at term: a critical review of the literature. *Obstet. Gynecol..* Oct 1993;82(4 Pt 1):605-618.

[54] Hannah M, Hannah W. Caesarean section or vaginal birth for breech presentation at term. *Bmj.* Jun 8 1996;312(7044):1433-1434.

[55] Munstedt K, von Georgi R, Reucher S, Zygmunt M, Lang U. Term breech and long-term morbidity -- cesarean section versus vaginal breech delivery. *Eur. J. Obstet. Gynecol. Reprod. Biol.* Jun 2001;96(2):163-167.

[56] Danielian PJ, Wang J, Hall MH. Long-term outcome by method of delivery of fetuses in breech presentation at term: population based follow up. *Bmj.* Jun 8 1996;312(7044):1451-1453.
[57] McBride WG, Black BP, Brown CJ, Dolby RM, Murray AD, Thomas DB. Method of delivery and developmental outcome at five years of age. *Med J Aust.* Apr 21 1979;1(8):301-304.
[58] Sanchez-Ramos L, Wells TL, Adair CD, Arcelin G, Kaunitz AM, Wells DS. Route of breech delivery and maternal and neonatal outcomes. *Int. J. Gynaecol. Obstet.* Apr 2001;73(1):7-14.
[59] Golfier F, Vaudoyer F, Ecochard R, Champion F, Audra P, Raudrant D. Planned vaginal delivery versus elective caesarean section in singleton term breech presentation: a study of 1116 cases. *Eur. J. Obstet. Gynecol. Reprod Biol.* Oct 2001;98(2):186-192.
[60] Herbst A, Thorngren-Jerneck K. Mode of delivery in breech presentation at term: increased neonatal morbidity with vaginal delivery. *Acta Obstet. Gynecol. Scand.* Aug 2001;80(8):731-737.
[61] Ulander VM, Gissler M, Nuutila M, Ylikorkala O. Are health expectations of term breech infants unrealistically high? *Acta Obstet. Gynecol. Scand.* Feb 2004;83(2):180-186.
[62] Rietberg CC, Elferink-Stinkens PM, Brand R, van Loon AJ, Van Hemel OJ, Visser GH. Term breech presentation in The Netherlands from 1995 to 1999: mortality and morbidity in relation to the mode of delivery of 33824 infants. *BJOG.* Jun 2003;110(6):604-609.
[63] Collea JV, Chein C, Quilligan EJ. The randomized management of term frank breech presentation: a study of 208 cases. *Am. J. Obstet. Gynecol.* May 15 1980;137(2):235-244.
[64] Gimovsky ML, Wallace RL, Schifrin BS, Paul RH. Randomized management of the nonfrank breech presentation at term: a preliminary report. *Am. J. Obstet. Gynecol.* May 1 1983;146(1):34-40.
[65] Hannah ME, Hannah WJ, Hewson SA, Hodnett ED, Saigal S, Willan AR. Planned caesarean section versus planned vaginal birth for breech presentation at term: a randomised multicentre trial. Term Breech Trial Collaborative Group. *Lancet.* Oct 21 2000;356(9239):1375-1383.
[66] Hannah ME, Whyte H, Hannah WJ, et al. Maternal outcomes at 2 years after planned cesarean section versus planned vaginal birth for breech presentation at term: the international randomized Term Breech Trial. *Am. J. Obstet. Gynecol.* Sep 2004;191(3):917-927.
[67] Whyte H, Hannah ME, Saigal S, et al. Outcomes of children at 2 years after planned cesarean birth versus planned vaginal birth for breech presentation at term: the International Randomized Term Breech Trial. *Am. J. Obstet. Gynecol.* Sep 2004;191(3):864-871.
[68] Irion O, Hirsbrunner Almagbaly P, Morabia A. Planned vaginal delivery versus elective caesarean section: a study of 705 singleton term breech presentations. *Br. J. Obstet. Gynaecol.* Jul 1998;105(7):710-717.
[69] ACOG committee opinion: number 265, December 2001. Mode of term single breech delivery. *Obstet. Gynecol..* Dec 2001;98(6):1189-1190.

[70] ACOG Committee Opinion No. 340. Mode of term singleton breech delivery. *Obstet. Gynecol.* Jul 2006;108(1):235-237.

[71] Alexandersson O, Bixo M, Hogberg U. Evidence-based changes in term breech delivery practice in Sweden. *Acta Obstet. Gynecol. Scand.* Jun 2005;84(6):584-587.

[72] Rietberg CC, Elferink-Stinkens PM, Visser GH. The effect of the Term Breech Trial on Medical Intervention Behavior and Neonatal Outcome in The Netherlands: An Analysis of 35,453 Term Breech Infants. *Obstet. Gynecol. Surv.* May 2005;60(5):289-290.

[73] Carayol M, Blondel B, Zeitlin J, Breart G, Goffinet F. Changes in the rates of caesarean delivery before labour for breech presentation at term in France: 1972-2003. *Eur. J. Obstet.. Gynecol. Reprod. Biol.* May 2007;132(1):20-26.

[74] Kayem G, Goffinet F, Clement D, Hessabi M, Cabrol D. Breech presentation at term: morbidity and mortality according to the type of delivery at Port Royal Maternity hospital from 1993 through 1999. *Eur J. Obstet. Gynecol. Reprod. Biol.* May 10 2002;102(2):137-142.

[75] Hauth JC, Cunningham FG. Vaginal breech delivery is still justified. *Obstet. Gynecol..* Jun 2002;99(6):1115-1116.

[76] Lumley J, Lester A, Renou P, Wood C. A failed RCT to determine the best method of delivery for very low birth weight infants. *Control Clin Trials.* Jun 1985;6(2):120-127.

[77] Penn ZJ, Steer PJ, Grant A. A multicentre randomised controlled trial comparing elective and selective caesarean section for the delivery of the preterm breech infant. *Br. J. Obstet. Gynaecol.* Jul 1996;103(7):684-689.

[78] Zlatnik FJ. The Iowa premature breech trial. *Am. J. Perinatol.* Jan 1993;10(1):60-63.

[79] Lee KS, Khoshnood B, Sriram S, Hsieh HL, Singh J, Mittendorf R. Relationship of cesarean delivery to lower birth weight-specific neonatal mortality in singleton breech infants in the United States. *Obstet. Gynecol..* Nov 1998;92(5):769-774.

[80] Main DM, Main EK, Maurer MM. Cesarean section versus vaginal delivery for the breech fetus weighing less than 1,500 grams. *Am. J. Obstet. Gynecol..* Jul 1 1983;146(5):580-584.

[81] Ananth CV, Vintzileos AM. Trends in cesarean delivery at preterm gestation and association with perinatal mortality. *Am. J. Obstet. Gynecol..* Jun 2011;204(6):505 e501-508.

[82] Gorbe E, Chasen S, Harmath A, Patkos P, Papp Z. Very-low-birthweight breech infants: short-term outcome by method of delivery. *J. Matern Fetal. Med.* May-Jun 1997;6(3):155-158.

[83] Granati B, Rondinelli M, Capoti C, Carnielli V, Bottos M, Rubaltelli FF. The premature breech presentation: outcome of newborn infants born by vaginal or abdominal delivery. *Am. J. Perinatol.* Jan 1984;1(2):145-147.

[84] Weissman A, Blazer S, Zimmer EZ, Jakobi P, Paldi E. Low birthweight breech infant: short-term and long-term outcome by method of delivery. *Am. J. Perinatol.* Jul 1988;5(3):289-292.

[85] Lodha A, Zhu Q, Lee SK, Shah PS. Neonatal outcomes of preterm infants in breech presentation according to mode of birth in Canadian NICUs. *Postgraduate medical journal.* Mar 2011;87(1025):175-179.

[86] Lee HC, El-Sayed YY, Gould JB. Delivery mode by race for breech presentation in the US. *J Perinatol.* Mar 2007;27(3):147-153.

[87] Yamamura Y, Ramin KD, Ramin SM. Trial of vaginal breech delivery: current role. *Clin. Obstet. Gynecol.* Jun 2007;50(2):526-536.
[88] Turner MJ. The Term Breech Trial: are the clinical guidelines justified by the evidence? *J. Obstet. Gynaecol.* Aug 2006;26(6):491-494.

In: Cesarean Section: Procedures, Complications and Recovery ISBN: 978-1-62081-214-3
Editor: Eyal Sheiner

Chapter VI

CESAREAN SECTION PROCEDURES

Avi Harlev* and Eyal Sheiner
Department of Obstetrics and Gynecology,
Soroka University Medical Center,
Faculty of Health Sciences,
Ben-Gurion University of the Negev,
Beer-Sheva, Israel

INTRODUCTION

Cesarean section (CS) is defined as a surgical birth of a fetus through the abdominal wall (laparotomy) and the uterine wall (hysterotomy).

The percentage of United States CS increased from 20.7% in 1996 to 31.1% in 2006 [1]. The rate of CS is steadily rising and in 2008, nearly one-third (32.3%) of US births were by CS. Cesarean section is the most common major surgical procedure for women in the United States, with 1.4 million surgeries annually [2].

Cesarean section as a surgical procedure confers an increased risk of wound complications, iatrogenic injury to bladder/bowel, anesthetic risk and venous thromboembolism [3].

Hence, it is mandatory to use the optimal surgical technique to minimize morbidity. Notwithstanding the traditional CS stages (Table 1), several surgical techniques and modifications are being used to perform this common surgical procedure. This chapter reviews the evidence base of some of the procedures used in a CS.

---

* Address all correspondence to: Avi Harlev, M.D. Department of Obstetrics and Gynecology, Soroka University Medical Center, P.O. Box 151, Beer Sheva 84101, ISRAEL, Tel: +972-8-640-3762, Fax: +972-8-640-3057, e-mail harlev@bgu.ac.il.

Table 1. Cesarean section optional stages

1.	Patient positioning
2.	Skin preparation
3.	Sterile covers
4.	Skin incision
5.	Subcutaneous tissuesseparation
6.	Opening of the fascia
7.	Rectus musclesseparation
8.	Opening of the peritoneum
9.	Bladder flap formation
10.	Uterine incision and extension
11.	Delivery of the fetus
12.	Delivery of the placenta
13.	Exteriorizing the uterus
14.	Cervical dilatation
15.	Uterinecleansing
16.	Uterine closure
17.	Peritoneum closure
18.	Fascia closure
19.	Subcutaneous sutures
20.	Skin closure

Preoperative Issues

Urinary Catheterization

Most of the surgeons place a urinary indwelling catheter routinely before the CS. The major role of placing the catheter is to empty the urine bladder in order to maximize exposure of the lower uterine segment and to avoid bladder injury. Several studies compared CS results of patients with and without the catheter [4-7]. All studies concluded that in low risk patients, non-placement of indwelling urinary catheter during CS was more convenient to women with no increase in intraoperative complications and it reduced the risk of urinary infection. A recently published systemic review concluded that in hemodynamically stable patients, routine use of indwelling urinary catheters for CS is not necessary, and can be harmful [8]. If the patient is hemodynamically stable and can void before the operation, a catheter placement may be avoided. Others recommend single catheterization before starting the procedure [9]. In cases of urgent CS it's recommended to place an indwelling catheter.

Hair Removal

The preparation of the patient for surgery has traditionally included the routine removal of body hair from the intended surgical wound site. No studies were performed regarding hair removal for CS. A Cochrane systemic review concluded that there is no difference in wound infection among patients who have had hair removed prior to surgery and those who have not; there is no difference when patients are shaved or clipped one day before surgery or on the day of surgery [10].

Preparation of the Skin

In order to reduce surgical site infection, skin antiseptic cleansing is performed since the patient's skin is a major source of the pathogens. The agents that are traditionally used are Iodophores, such as iodine plus polyvinyl pyrolidine (povidone±iodine) and tincture of chlorhexidinegluconate (0.5%in 70% isopropyl alcohol) [9]. Darouiche et al. randomly assigned adults undergoing clean-contaminated surgery in six hospitals to preoperative skin preparation with either chlorhexidine-alcohol scrub or povidone-iodine scrub and paint. The primary outcome was any surgical-site infection within 30 days after surgery. Secondary outcomes included individual types of surgical-site infections. They concluded that preoperative cleansing of the patient's skin with chlorhexidine-alcohol is superior to cleansing with povidone-iodine for preventing surgical-site infection after clean-contaminated surgery [11].

Intraoperative Issues

Abdominal Skin Incision

The 2 major methods of the skin incision is either the transverse or the vertical incision.

The Vertical Incision

The vertical incision is performed in the midline, from 3 cm above the pubis to 3 cm beneath the umbilicus. In cases of severe intra-abdominal adhesion, the surgeon may elongate the incision cephalad (Figure 1).

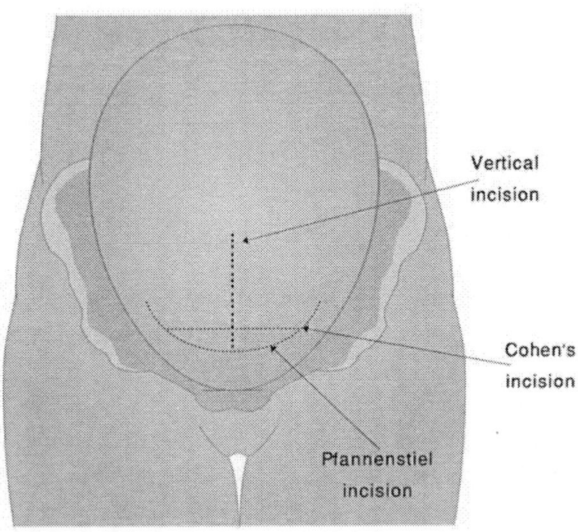

Position of various skin incisions.

Figure 1. Positions of various skin incisions.

The Transverse Incision

The transverse incision is more frequently used than the vertical incision due to less postoperative pain, greater wound strength, and better cosmetic results compared to the vertical midline incision [12]. The 2 most commonly used transverse incisions are the Pfannenstiel and the Joel Cohen's incision (Figure 1).

The Pfannenstiel incision is made at the level of the pubic hairline and is extended somewhat beyond the lateral borders of the rectus muscles. The skin and subcutaneous tissue are incised using a lower, transverse, slightly curvilinear incision [13]. The Joel Cohen's incision is a straight transverse incision through skin only, 3 cm below the level of the anterior-superior iliac spines. The subcutaneous tissues are opened only in the middle 3 cm [14].

While comparing the transverse incisions, Franchi et al. examined the results of 152 women who underwent the Joel-Cohen to 158 women who underwent the Pfannenstiel incision [15]. The total operative time was similar in both groups (Joel-Cohen 32 min (12-60) vs. Pfannenstiel 33 min (18-70)). The extraction time was shorter in the Joel-Cohen group. No difference was found between groups in terms of intraoperative and postoperative complications. In addition, no difference was found in the neonatal neurodevelopmental assessment at 6 months of age in relation to the abdominal incision performed. The authors concluded that the Joel-Cohen method of opening the abdomen at CS is faster than the Pfannenstiel technique at delivering the fetus. However, considering the absence of benefits to the mother and the fetus there is no clear indication for performing a Joel-Cohen incision [15].

In contrast to the previous study, other studies found the Joel-Cohen incision to be superior compared to the Pfannenstiel incision in several aspects. A study of 101 women compared Joel-Cohen to the Pfannenstiel incision [16]. The Joel–Cohen incision was associated with significantly shorter operating time, less post-operative discomfort indicated by fewer analgesic requirements, and lower febrile morbidity. A Cochrane review on the type of transverse incision concluded that the Joel-Cohen incision has advantages compared to the Pfannenstiel incision.

These are less fever, pain and analgesic requirements; less blood loss; shorter duration of surgery and hospital stay [17]. A recently published Cochrane review [18] found the Joel-Cohen incision compared with Pfannenstiel to be associated with less blood loss, shorter operating time, postoperatively reduced time to oral intake, less fever, shorter duration of postoperative pain, fewer analgesic injections and shorter time from skin incision to the birth of the baby.

On the contrary, a multi-center prospective study of 5123 cesarean sections, evaluated maternal nosocomial infection rates according to the incision technique used for caesarean delivery.

The overall nosocomial infection and endometritis rates were higher for the Joel-Cohen than Pfannenstiel incision (4.5% vs. 3.3%, 0.8% vs. 0.3%, respectively). The Joel-Cohen incision was found as an independent risk factor for endometritis. The authors concluded that the Joel-Cohen technique is faster than the Pfannenstiel technique but is associated with a higher incidence of endometritis.

Bladder Flap Formation

Bladder injuries during a CS occur in 0.27% in primary CS and 0.81% in repeated CS [19]. A common procedure aimed to reduce bladder injuries is performing a bladder flap. In this procedure, the vesicouterine serosa is picked up with smooth forceps and is incised in the midline with Metzenbaum scissors. The incision is carried out laterally in a curvilinear manner. The vesicouterine fold is then tented with forceps or a pair of hemostats, which allows direct visualization as the bladder flap is bluntly created using the index and middle fingers of the surgeon's hand. Sharp dissection may be necessary, particularly in repeat operations [20].

In order to estimate the necessity of bladder flap formation, a randomized trial [21] compared 49 women who underwent this procedure during a CS to 53 women who did not. Significant differences were observed in median skin incision-delivery interval (5 versus 7 minutes, $P < .001$), median total operating time (35 versus 40 minutes, $P = .004$), and median blood loss (Delta hemoglobin 0.5 versus 1 g/dL, $P = .009$) in favor of the study group. Postoperative microhematuria was reduced in the study group (21% versus 47%, $P < .01$). There was no difference in bowel function. The authors concluded that omission of the bladder flap provides short-term advantages such as reduction of operating time and incision-delivery interval, and reduced blood loss.

The effect of bladder flap formation during CS on the uterine scar was evaluated during a subsequent CS [22]. The investigators found that forming bladder flap during CS leads to an inflammatory and fibrotic reaction, resulting in inflammation reactive and regenerative processes, mesothelial hyperplasia and submesothelial fibrosis. CS without the procedure reduces the inflammatory processes and the subsequent intraperitoneal adhesions and adhesions between the bladder and uterus.

However, none of the studies regarding bladder flap formation was satisfactorily powered to detect differences in bladder injury which is infrequent. Furthermore, although the evidence we do have does not appear to support routine bladder flap formation, it is probable that many obstetricians will be adhere to this traditional surgical step [23].

Uterine Incision

The uterus may be entered by either a transverse or a vertical incision. The more commonly used is the low transverse section incision. This incision is favored since the lower uterine segment is less vascular than the body of the uterus, and the incision is easier to repair. This leads to a reduction in operative complications, especially hemorrhage, and also a reduction in morbidity [24]. Compared with a classical incision, it is located at a site least likely to rupture during a subsequent pregnancy [25], and does not promote adherence of bowel or omentum to the incisional line [13].

While opening the uterus in a CS, a small incision is performed in the middle of the lower uterine segment with a scalpel and then extended. This extension can be performed either with scalpel or scissors (sharp extension) or using the fingers (blunt extension). Comparing the blunt ($n = 139$) and sharp ($n = 147$) expansion groups, Rodriguez et al. [26] noted no difference in the incidence of unintended extension, postoperative endometritis, duration of surgery, or estimated blood loss. The frequency of unintended extension (1.4%, 15.5%, and

35.0% for no labor and first and second stages, respectively) correlated with the stage of labor.

Table 2. Indications for vertical uterine incision

- Poorly developed lower uterine segment (eg, extremely preterm breech presentation)
- Transvers fetal lie, back up
- Large leiomyoma in lower uterine segment
- Severe lower segment intra-abdominal adhesions
- Anterior placenta previa or accreta
- Postmortem delivery

Another randomized study intended to compare the incidence of intra-operative hemorrhage while using the sharp vs. blunt extension of the uterine incision [27]. Compared with the blunt group, the estimated blood loss (886 versus 843mL, P = 0.001), change in the mean hematocrit (6.1% versus 5.5%, P = 0.003), incidence of postpartum hemorrhage (13% versus 9%; relative risk = 1.23, 95% CI 1.03, 1.46) and need for a transfusion (2% versus 0.4%; relative risk = 1.65, 95% CI 1.25, 2.21) were significantly greater in the sharp extension group. Extensions of the uterine incision (defects occurring outside the line of the original incision) were reported by both trials, and in both cases they were more common in the sharp extension group. Nonetheless, combining these data in a meta-analysis gave a non-significant RR of 0.41 (95% CI 0.31 to 0.54) [24].

The vertical or the so-called classical incision is a vertical incision into the body of the uterus above the lower uterine segment and reaches the uterine fundus [13]. No randomized study compares transverse and vertical uterine incision. The vertical incision is reserved today for special cases only (table 2).

Delivery of the Newborn

In a cephalic presentation, the surgeon slips his hand into the uterine cavity between the symphysis and fetal head. The head is raised gently with the fingers and palm through the incision, aided by trans-abdominal fundal pressure[13]. When the fetal head is impacted (e.g. when operating in an advanced second stage of the labor), several methods may aid to deliver the baby. The fetal head may be pushed cephalad from the vagina ('push' method) or the fetal leg may be delivered first and reverse breech technique ('pull' method) may be carried out. Reviewing 3105 CS reports, Levy et al. noted the 'push' or 'pull' methods in 48 (1.5%) cases. Women that were delivered by the 'pull' method had significantly lower rate of postpartum fever (5% versus 46%; odds ratios, 0.06; 95% confidence intervals, 0.007-0.51) and extensions of the uterine incision (15% versus 50%; odds ratio, 0.17; 95% CI, 0.04-0.74) compared to those that were delivered by the 'push' method. Neonatal outcomes were good in all cases [28]. Moreover, another study found that patients in the 'push' group had statistically significant higher rates of maternal and fetal morbidity (longer operation time, more blood loss, extension of uterine incision, endometritis, longer hospital stay and higher hospital bills) than the pull method ($P<0.05$). They concluded that the 'pull' method of delivery of impacted fetal head at caesarean section for obstruction is safer and faster than the 'push' method [29].

An alternative technique to deliver the fetus in cases of impacted fetal head is an instrumental delivery using vacuum extraction or forceps. Compared in a small prospective study [30], the use of vacuum extraction did not demonstrate fewer extensions of the uterine incision or lesser amounts of blood loss as measured by serial hemoglobin determinations.

There was a trend for the forceps group to require a longer period of time for delivery. Women in the vacuum group reported significantly lower pain scores. There were no serious neonatal injuries in both groups.

Delivery of the Placenta

The placenta can be delivered by either manual shearing of the placenta or by controlled cord traction [9]. Several prospective and randomized trials compared the delivery of the placenta methods [31-35].

A Cochrane review addressing the issue [36] found that manual shearing of the placenta was associated with more endometritis, blood loss, lower hematocrit after delivery, greater hematocrit fall after delivery and longer duration of hospital stay. The authors concluded that delivery of the placenta with cord traction at caesarean section has more advantages compared to manual removal.

Cervical Dilatation

Routine cervical dilatation during the CS was considered a method to maximize uterine drainage. Uterine drainage will assumingly prevent fluid and blood stasis inside the uterine cavity and subsequently reduce metritis [37]. Correspondingly, by reducing potential uterine atony, cervical dilatation might lessen the incidence of postpartum hemorrhage [38].

In a retrospective study of 666 elective CS performed by our group [39], 348 underwent routine cervical dilatation. No significant differences were found between the cervical dilatation and the comparison group regarding postpartum febrile morbidity (5.1 and 3.1% respectively; $p=0.071$), hospitalization duration (4.1 ± 1.4 and 4.1 ± 2.0 days; $p=0.95$), wound infection (0.9% and 1.25%, $p=0.451$) or anemia rate (9.50 ± 0.73 and 9.54 ± 0.65, $p=0.91$). Nevertheless, among patients following a previous vaginal delivery, cervical dilatation was significantly associated with post-operative fever (OR=5.8; 95%CI 1.2-38.0; $P=0.021$).

The authors concluded that routine cervical dilatation during elective CS does not reduce post-operative morbidity. Moreover, among patients with a previous vaginal delivery cervical dilatation is a risk factor for febrile morbidity.

Uterine Closure

Immediately after delivering the placenta, the uterus should be massaged and oxytocin is administered in order to prevent hemorrhage. Closure of the uterus is extremely important to prevent future scar dehiscence. The question of whether to suture the uterus intra-abdominally versus extra-abdominally was addressed in a review that compared 6 randomized trials; there were no statistically significant differences between the groups in most of the outcomes identified, except for febrile morbidity and length of hospital stay. With extra-abdominal closure of the uterine incision, febrile morbidity was lower (relative risk 0.41, 95%, CI 0.17 to 0.97), and the hospital stay was longer (weighted mean difference 0.24 days, 95% CI 0.08 to 0.39) [40]. A more recent meta-anlysis [41] included 5 more randomized trials to compare the site of uterine suture. Combining all 11 trials, No significant differences in either postoperative or intraoperative complications were demonstrated between the extra-abdominal (n=1605) and intra-abdominal repair (n=1578) groups. Operative time, estimated blood loss, and hospital stay were all unaffected by repair technique. This study cannot exclude differences in rare complications, such as serious venous air embolism or maternal death. The authors concluded that both techniques are valid surgical options.

An important question regarding uterine closure is whether to perform a single or double layer suture. The potential advantages of a single layer include reduced operating time, less tissue disruption, and less introduction of foreign suture material into the wound. These potential advantages may translate into reduced operative and postoperative morbidity for women. On the other hand, a double layer closure may supply improved hemostasis and wound healing, and possibly a reduced risk of uterine rupture in a subsequent pregnancy. Comparing 11 trials [24], single layer closure of the uterine incision compared with double layer closure was associated with a statistically significant reduction in mean blood loss, duration of the operative procedure and the presence of post-operative pain. There were no statistically significant differences identified for morbidity (including endometritis), blood loss, postoperative anemia, or wound infection. Nevertheless, the authors concluded that while single layer closure of the uterine incision is associated with a reduction in blood loss and the duration of the procedure, there were other aspects of the intervention which could significantly impact on these findings [24]. In our institute a double layer uterine closure is mandatory, mainly due to the potential risk for uterine rupture.

Closure of the Peritoneum

Of all the CS procedures, the closure of the peritoneum is the most debatable, and hence, the most investigated procedure. During the CS, both the visceral and parietal peritoneum is incised. Both short and long term effects of peritoneal closure should be considered before making the decision.

A randomized trial of 200 women back in 1996 compared continuous double layer closure of uterine incision in addition to closure of visceral and parietal peritoneum to uterine incision sutured in one layer and the visceral and parietal peritoneum left open [42]. They found that non closure of the peritoneum reduced operative time and postoperative narcotic requirement, and had no adverse effect on postoperative recovery. They concluded that a double-layer closure of low uterine incision, re-approximation of bladder flap, and closure of parietal peritoneum, as in the standard technique, does not seem to be essential steps of CS.

The rising prevalence of repeated CS makes the association between closure of the peritoneum and adhesion formation an important consideration. This association was studied with conflicting results. A randomized trial of 45 women who underwent a subsequent CS concluded that closure of the peritoneum increases the operating time, but may decrease the risk of adhesions [43]. Alike, a systematic review [44] has demonstrated that according to current data in the literature, non-closure of the peritoneum after caesarean section is associated with more adhesion formation compared to closure. On the other hand, a randomized trial of 120 women demonstrated that surgical peritoneal closure resulted in more advanced adhesion formation and recommended not to close the peritoneum [45]. A recent randomized study [46] concluded that closure or non-closure of the peritoneum at CS did not lead to large differences in the adhesion rate.

Most previous studies on management of the visceral peritoneum have found non-closure to confer benefit as regards short-term febrile morbidity [23]. It seems that in order to minimize adhesions and their consequences, non-closure of the visceral but closure of the parietal peritoneal layers, would appear the most judicious CS technique. Yet, although studies have constantly established non-closure of the visceral layer to be advantageous, clinical equipoise over the benefits of parietal peritoneal closure persists [23].

Effects of visceral peritoneal closure on scar formation at CS were histologically evaluated at a subsequent CS, comparing women who underwent peritoneal closure at first CS to those who did not [47]. Closure of the visceral peritoneum at CS may produce an inflammatory reaction and adhesions, evidenced by reactive and regenerative mesothelial hyperplasia and submesothelial fibrosis.

While examining the association between upward bladder traction by visceral peritoneal closure during CS and the impact on postpartum urinary complaints, Shahin et al. reported [48] that compared to visceral peritoneal non-closure, CS with visceral closure is associated with significant postpartum frequency of urination and incontinence that disappear without treatment almost completely within 6 months.

Parietal peritoneal closure during CS is associated with a higher incidence of early and persistent postoperative pain. A high pain score on the 1st day is a predictor of persistent pain [49]. Interestingly, intra-peritoneal instillation of 200 mg of lidocaine decreased the incidence and scores of post-cesarean pain when the parietal peritoneum was sutured [50].

Skin Closure

The closure of the skin imposes 2 questions. The first is weather to perform subcutaneous approximation sutures; the second is whether to staple or use one of the skin suturing techniques. Reviewing seven studies involving 2056 women, Anderson et al. [51] found that the risk of hematoma or seroma was reduced with fat closure compared with non-closure (RR 0.52, 95%, CI 0.33 to 0.82). No difference in the risk of wound infection alone or other short-term outcomes was found. No long-term outcomes were reported. Moreover, a meta-analysis [52] of randomized trials comparing subcutaneous sutures in different abdominal wall thickness concluded that suture closure of subcutaneous fat during CS results in a 34% decrease in risk of wound disruption in women with fat thickness greater than 2 cm.

Data regarding the skin closure method is limited. A Cochrane review [53] in 2003 found only one randomized trial suitable for evaluation. The randomized trial [54] of 66 women found that skin incisions closed with subcuticular closure following CS result in less postoperative discomfort and are more cosmetically appealing at the six-week postoperative visit as compared to incisions closed with staples. Despite this, the Cochrane reviewers, after evaluating the results, concluded that there is no conclusive evidence about how the skin should be closed after caesarean section. Rousseau et al. [55] randomized 101 patients to either subcuticular sutures or staples. Pain at 6 weeks postoperatively was significantly less in the staple group (0.17 vs. 0.51; P = .04), operative time was shorter in that group (24.6 vs. 32.9 minutes; P < .0001) and no difference was noted in incision appearance and women's satisfaction. The conclusion was that staples are the method of choice for skin closure for elective term cesareans. A recent meta-analysis [56] reviewed five RCTs and one prospective cohort study. Staple closure (n=803) was associated with a twofold higher risk of wound infection or separation compared with subcuticular suture closure (n=684) (13.4% versus 6.6%, pooled OR 2.06, 95% confidence interval [CI] 1.43-2.98). Staple closure was associated with shorter duration of surgery, whereas the two techniques appeared equivalent overall with regard to pain, cosmetic result, and patient satisfaction. The conclusion was that staple closure is faster to perform but associated with a higher risk of wound complications.

REFERENCES

[1] MacDorman MF, Menacker F, Declercq E. Cesarean birth in the United States: epidemiology, trends, and outcomes. *Clin. Perinatol.* 2008;35(2):293-307, v.

[2] MacDorman M, Declercq E, Menacker F. Recent trends and patterns in cesarean and vaginal birth after cesarean (VBAC) deliveries in the United States. *Clin. Perinatol.* 2011;38(2):179-92.

[3] ACOG Committee Opinion No. 394, December 2007. Cesarean delivery on maternal request. *Obstet. Gynecol.* 2007;110(6):1501.

[4] Barnes JS. Is it better to avoid urethral catheterization at hysterectomy and caesarean section? *Aust. N. Z. J. Obstet. Gynaecol.* 1998;38(3):315-6.

[5] Ghoreishi J. Indwelling urinary catheters in cesarean delivery. *Int. J. Gynaecol. Obstet.* 2003;83(3):267-70.

[6] Senanayake H. Elective cesarean section without urethral catheterization. *J. Obstet. Gynaecol. Res.* 2005;31(1):32-7.

[7] Nasr AM, ElBigawy AF, Abdelamid AE, Al-Khulaidi S, Al-Inany HG, Sayed EH. Evaluation of the use vs nonuse of urinary catheterization during cesarean delivery: a prospective, multicenter, randomized controlled trial. *J. Perinatol.* 2009;29(6):416-21.

[8] Li L, Wen J, Wang L, Li YP, Li Y. Is routine indwelling catheterisation of the bladder for caesarean section necessary? A systematic review. *Bjog* 2011;118(4):400-9.

[9] Hema KR, Johanson R. Techniques for performing caesarean section. *Best Pract. Res. Clin. Obstet. Gynaecol.* 2001;15(1):17-47.

[10] Tanner J, Woodings D, Moncaster K. Preoperative hair removal to reduce surgical site infection. *Cochrane Database Syst. Rev.* 2006;3:CD004122.

[11] Darouiche RO, Wall MJ, Jr., Itani KM, et al. Chlorhexidine-Alcohol versus Povidone-Iodine for Surgical-Site Antisepsis. *N. Engl. J. Med.* 2010;362(1):18-26.

[12] Berghella V, Baxter JK, Chauhan SP. Evidence-based surgery for cesarean delivery. *Am. J. Obstet. Gynecol.* 2005;193(5):1607-17.

[13] Cunningham F.G LKJ, Bloom S.L, Hauth J.C, Rouse D.J, Spong C.Y. Williams Obstetrics, Twenty-Third Edition: McGraw-Hill Companies; 2010.

[14] Wallin G, Fall O. Modified Joel-Cohen technique for caesarean delivery. *Br. J. Obstet. Gynaecol.* 1999;106(3):221-6.
[15] Franchi M, Ghezzi F, Raio L, et al. Joel-Cohen or Pfannenstiel incision at cesarean delivery: does it make a difference? *Acta Obstet. Gynecol. Scand* 2002;81(11):1040-6.
[16] Mathai M, Ambersheth S, George A. Comparison of two transverse abdominal incisions for cesarean delivery. *Int. J. Gynaecol. Obstet.* 2002;78(1):47-9.
[17] Mathai M, Hofmeyr GJ. Abdominal surgical incisions for caesarean section. *Cochrane Database Syst. Rev.* 2007(1):CD004453.
[18] Hofmeyr GJ, Mathai M, Shah A, Novikova N. Techniques for caesarean section. *Cochrane Database Syst. Rev.* 2008(1):CD004662.
[19] Rahman MS, Gasem T, Al Suleiman SA, Al Jama FE, Burshaid S, Rahman J. Bladder injuries during cesarean section in a University Hospital: a 25-year review. *Arch. Gynecol. Obstet.* 2009;279(3):349-52.
[20] Gabbe SG NJ, Simpson JL. Gabbe: Obstetrics: Normal and Problem Pregnancies, 5th ed. Philadelphia: Chuchill Livingstone Elsevier; 2007.
[21] Hohlagschwandtner M, Ruecklinger E, Husslein P, Joura EA. Is the formation of a bladder flap at cesarean necessary? A randomized trial. *Obstet. Gynecol.* 2001;98(6):1089-92.
[22] Malvasi A, Tinelli A, Guido M, et al. Effect of avoiding bladder flap formation in caesarean section on repeat caesarean delivery. *Eur. J. Obstet. Gynecol. Reprod Biol* 2011.
[23] Walsh CA. Evidence-based cesarean technique. *Curr. Opin. Obstet. Gynecol.* 2010;22(2):110-5.
[24] Dodd JM, Anderson ER, Gates S. Surgical techniques for uterine incision and uterine closure at the time of caesarean section. *Cochrane Database Syst. Rev.* 2008(3):CD004732.
[25] Schutterman EB, Grimes DA. Comparative safety of the low transverse versus the low vertical uterine incision for cesarean delivery of breech infants. *Obstet. Gynecol.* 1983;61(5):593-7.
[26] Rodriguez AI, Porter KB, O'Brien WF. Blunt versus sharp expansion of the uterine incision in low-segment transverse cesarean section. *Am. J. Obstet. Gynecol.* 1994;171(4):1022-5.
[27] Magann EF, Chauhan SP, Bufkin L, Field K, Roberts WE, Martin JN, Jr. Intra-operative haemorrhage by blunt versus sharp expansion of the uterine incision at caesarean delivery: a randomised clinical trial. *Bjog* 2002;109(4):448-52.
[28] Levy R, Chernomoretz T, Appelman Z, Levin D, Or Y, Hagay ZJ. Head pushing versus reverse breech extraction in cases of impacted fetal head during Cesarean section. *Eur. J. Obstet. Gynecol. Reprod. Biol.* 2005;121(1):24-6.
[29] Fasubaa OB, Ezechi OC, Orji EO, et al. Delivery of the impacted head of the fetus at caesarean section after prolonged obstructed labour: a randomised comparative study of two methods. *J. Obstet. Gynaecol.* 2002;22(4):375-8.
[30] Bofill JA, Lencki SG, Barhan S, Ezenagu LC. Instrumental delivery of the fetal head at the time of elective repeat cesarean: a randomized pilot study. *Am. J. Perinatol.* 2000;17(5):265-9.

[31] McCurdy CM, Jr., Magann EF, McCurdy CJ, Saltzman AK. The effect of placental management at cesarean delivery on operative blood loss. *Am. J. Obstet. Gynecol.* 1992;167(5):1363-7.

[32] Magann EF, Dodson MK, Allbert JR, McCurdy CM, Jr., Martin RW, Morrison JC. Blood loss at time of cesarean section by method of placental removal and exteriorization versus in situ repair of the uterine incision. *Surg. Gynecol. Obstet.* 1993;177(4):389-92.

[33] Magann EF, Dodson MK, Harris RL, Floyd RC, Martin JN, Morrison JC. Does method of placental removal or site of uterine incision repair alter endometritis after cesarean delivery? *Infect. Dis. Obstet. Gynecol.* 1993;1(1):65-70.

[34] Lasley DS, Eblen A, Yancey MK, Duff P. The effect of placental removal method on the incidence of postcesarean infections. *Am. J. Obstet. Gynecol.* 1997;176(6):1250-4.

[35] Merchavy S, Levy A, Holcberg G, Freedman EN, Sheiner E. Method of placental removal during cesarean delivery and postpartum complications. *Int. J. Gynaecol. Obstet.* 2007;98(3):232-6.

[36] Anorlu RI, Maholwana B, Hofmeyr GJ. Methods of delivering the placenta at caesarean section. *Cochrane Database Syst. Rev.* 2008(3):CD004737.

[37] Soper DE. Postpartum endometritis. Pathophysiology and prevention. *J. Reprod. Med.* 1988;33(1 Suppl):97-100.

[38] Ahmed B, Abu Nahia F, Abushama M. Routine cervical dilatation during elective cesarean section and its influence on maternal morbidity: a randomized controlled study. *J. Perinat Med.* 2005;33(6):510-3.

[39] Koifman A, Harlev A, Sheiner E, Press F, Wiznitzer A. Routine cervical dilatation during elective cesarean delivery - Is it really necessary? *J. Matern Fetal. Neonatal. Med.* 2009;22(7):608-11.

[40] Jacobs-Jokhan D, Hofmeyr G. Extra-abdominal versus intra-abdominal repair of the uterine incision at caesarean section. *Cochrane Database Syst. Rev.* 2004(4):CD000085.

[41] Walsh CA, Walsh SR. Extraabdominal vs intraabdominal uterine repair at cesarean delivery: a metaanalysis. *Am. J. Obstet. Gynecol.* 2009;200(6):625 e1-8.

[42] Ohel G, Younis JS, Lang N, Levit A. Double-layer closure of uterine incision with visceral and parietal peritoneal closure: are they obligatory steps of routine cesarean sections? *J. Matern Fetal. Med.* 1996;5(6):366-9.

[43] Zareian Z, Zareian P. Non-closure versus closure of peritoneum during cesarean section: a randomized study. *Eur. J. Obstet. Gynecol. Reprod Biol* 2006;128(1-2):267-9.

[44] Cheong YC, Premkumar G, Metwally M, Peacock JL, Li TC. To close or not to close? A systematic review and a meta-analysis of peritoneal non-closure and adhesion formation after caesarean section. *Eur. J. Obstet. Gynecol. Reprod. Biol.* 2009;147(1):3-8.

[45] Komoto Y, Shimoya K, Shimizu T, et al. Prospective study of non-closure or closure of the peritoneum at cesarean delivery in 124 women: Impact of prior peritoneal closure at primary cesarean on the interval time between first cesarean section and the next pregnancy and significant adhesion at second cesarean. *J. Obstet. Gynaecol. Res.* 2006;32(4):396-402.

[46] Kapustian V, Anteby EY, Gdalevich M, Shenhav S, Lavie O, Gemer O. Effect of closure versus nonclosure of peritoneum at cesarean section on adhesions: a prospective randomized study. *Am. J. Obstet. Gynecol.* 2011.

[47] Malvasi A, Tinelli A, Farine D, et al. Effects of visceral peritoneal closure on scar formation at cesarean delivery. *Int. J. Gynaecol. Obstet.* 2009;105(2):131-5.

[48] Shahin AY, Hameed DA. Does visceral peritoneal closure affect post-cesarean urinary symptoms? A randomized clinical trial. *Int. Urogynecol. J.* 2010;21(1):33-41.

[49] Shahin AY, Osman AM. Parietal peritoneal closure and persistent postcesarean pain. *Int. J. Gynaecol. Obstet.* 2009;104(2):135-9.

[50] Shahin AY, Osman AM. Intraperitoneal lidocaine instillation and postcesarean pain after parietal peritoneal closure: a randomized double blind placebo-controlled trial. *Clin. J. Pain* 2010;26(2):121-7.

[51] Anderson ER, Gates S. Techniques and materials for closure of the abdominal wall in caesarean section. *Cochrane Database Syst. Rev.* 2004(4):CD004663.

[52] Chelmow D, Rodriguez EJ, Sabatini MM. Suture closure of subcutaneous fat and wound disruption after cesarean delivery: a meta-analysis. *Obstet. Gynecol.* 2004;103(5 Pt 1):974-80.

[53] Croce P, Frigoli A, Perotti D, Di Mario M. [Cesarean section, techniques and skin suture materials]. *Minerva Ginecol.* 2007;59(6):595-9.

[54] Frishman GN, Schwartz T, Hogan JW. Closure of Pfannenstiel skin incisions. Staples vs. subcuticular suture. *J. Reprod. Med.* 1997;42(10):627-30.

[55] Rousseau JA, Girard K, Turcot-Lemay L, Thomas N. A randomized study comparing skin closure in cesarean sections: staples vs subcuticular sutures. *Am. J. Obstet. Gynecol.* 2009;200(3):265 e1-4.

[56] Tuuli MG, Rampersad RM, Carbone JF, Stamilio D, Macones GA, Odibo AO. Staples compared with subcuticular suture for skin closure after cesarean delivery: a systematic review and meta-analysis. *Obstet. Gynecol.* 2011;117(3):682-90.

In: Cesarean Section: Procedures, Complications and Recovery ISBN: 978-1-62081-214-3
Editor: Eyal Sheiner

Chapter VII

STARK OR MISGAV LADACH CESAREAN SECTION

***Antonio Malvasi*[1], *Andrea Tinelli*[2] *and Michael Stark*[3]**

[1]Department of Obstetrics and Gynecology
Santa Maria Hospital, Lecce, Italy
[2]Department of Obstetrics and Gynecology
Vito Fazzi Hospital, Lecce, Italy
NESA Member and Diplomat
[3]New European Surgical Academy (NESA), Berlin
Scientific director, the European Commission –
SOFAR Tele-Surgical Project, Germany

ABSTRACT

Most abdominal operations today have an endoscopic alternative, except the Cesarean Section (CS), at a time when its use is increasing. It is therefore important to re-analyze, optimize and simplify this procedure and introduce evidence-based rather than tradition-based steps.

In a process of evaluation and comparison of alternative surgical steps at the Misgav Ladach hospital in Jerusalem, a modified method has been evolved.

In the early 1970s, Joel-Cohen (JC) described a transverse incision alternative to the traditional Pfannenstiel incision based on time and motion studies. The JC incision with some modifications is now used by obstetricians in more than 100 countries. With this method the longitudinal abdominal structures, muscles and blood vessels which have a lateral sway are stretched laterally and will return to their original positions at the end of the operation.

The peritoneum is opened by repeat bi-digital stretching. No abdominal towels are used, and after the delivery the uterus is sutured with one continuous layer. Both peritoneal layers are left un-sutured as a new peritoneum will be formed within short time.

Moreover, the suture of the visceral peritoneum causes a closed pocket between the bladder and the lower uterine segment, leading to bladder flap collection containing blood, edema, exudate, and fibrin, resulting in fibrosis, adhesions and possible urinary symptoms. The abdomen is closed in 2 layers only, fascia and skin. The worldwide distribution of this method is due to the beneficial outcome, quicker mobility, early hydration, lower febrile morbidity and lower costs, as only 10 instruments and usually only 3 suture materials are needed.

Introduction

The 20th century was accompanied by many innovative developments in gynecological and obstetrical surgery. Most of the used and known laparotomies were developed at the very end of the 19th century after the development of general and local anesthesia. As in many disciplines traditions started to prevail and routines became fixed. With admiration we observe the development of new surgical procedures in most of the surgical disciplines concerning the use of endoscopy.

The open laparotomies are still in use, and mostly without modifications. In obstetrics and gynecology most procedures have been replaced by these methods. This tendency will most probably continue. Possibly, in the future the cesarean section will be one of the very few laparotomies in use.

This is a good reason to ensure that the methods we are using are the most reasonable, optimal, efficient and cost-effective. For these reasons a re-evaluation of every single step in any gynecological operation as well as in cesarean section was made, in order to use steps based on evidence.

Each operation is composed of hundreds of movements. Each one has its origin and its way of performance, which influences the outcome. Each one of these steps should have its logic and rational.

The above mentioned traditions, even if producing a sense of security, might not be justified and even cause damage. Therefore, we should analyze each individual step in the cesarean section, and compare it to others in randomized prospective studies. This is the only way that only the irreplaceable steps with their right way of performance will remain, and unnecessary traditional steps will be omitted.

In this chapter each step in the cesarean section will be compared to its alternatives, and the logic behind the decision to perform it in the way it is described will be discussed.

Positioning of the Surgeon

Each small detail does have an influence on the outcome. The positioning of the surgeon is important. A right-handed surgeon should stand on the right side of the patient for the following reasons: It is optimal to deliver the head of the baby with the right hand because of the higher sensitivity in this hand.

This sensitivity will prevent extension of the uterine incision, and as a result fewer traumas and bleeding will occur. While suturing the uterus the needle points away from the bladder, preventing damage (Figure 1).

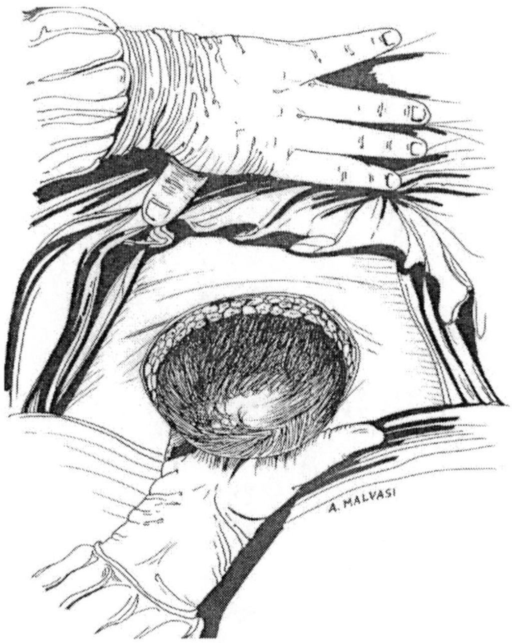

Figure 1. Positioning of the surgeon at the right side of the patient. It is optimal to delivery the head of the baby with the right hand.

Position of Parturient

Each decision in obstetrics must take into account the calculated risk involved. One of these examples is the positioning of the parturient. The positioning with her feet higher than her head (Trendelenburg position) makes the access to the lower segment easy. As will be mentioned later, in the Misgav Ladach (Stark) CS abdominal swabs are not used. The Trendelenburg position prevents the intestines to enter into the operative field. This position facilitates the distribution of the pharmacological agents used for anesthesia [1], but at the same time we have to take into account the rare risk of air-embolism. Should it happen, the patient should immediately be placed in an anti- Trendelenburg position and the operative area should be filled with normal saline [2]. The legs of the patient should lie parallel and not abducted. Parallel legs ensure that the closure of the Fascia will be done without tension.

Abdominal Swabs

There are good reasons why not to use abdominal swabs during cesarean section.

Usage of swabs might increase the rate of adhesions [3]. Experimental studies have shown that the use of surgical sponges in the peritoneal cavity in rats produced mesothelial trauma, therefore inflammatory response and adhesions may result [4]. In a series of 211 consecutive patients which were re-laparotomized 91% of the mothers had adhesions. In 66% of these textile particles were found [5] (Figure 2). Additional reason is that the amniotic fluid has a protective bacteriostatic action, mainly with elevated temperature [6,7] (Figure 3). As abdominal packs absorb fluids, this protective activity is lost. Additionally, when abdominal packs are not used, there is no risk of leaving them inside.

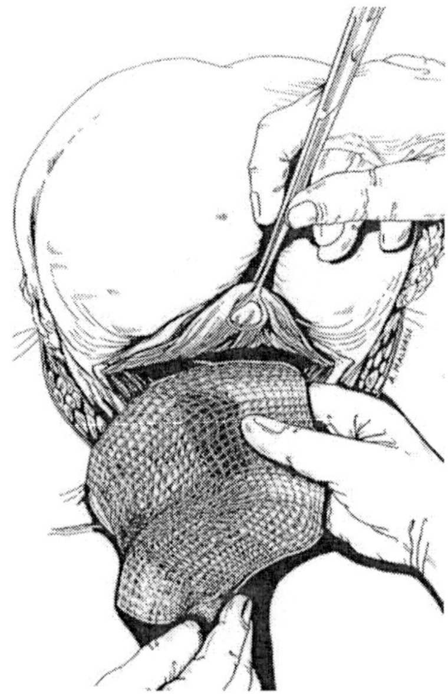

Figure 2. Swabs are not placed in the abdomen because they are abrasive to the tissue and might increase the risk of adhesions.

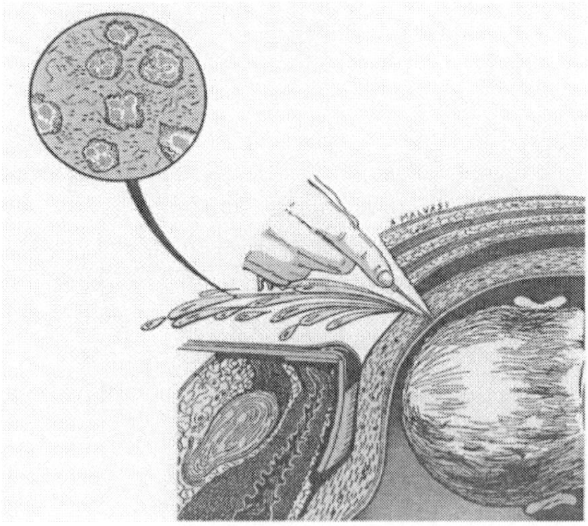

Figure 3. Swabs decrease the beneficial antibacterial proprieties of amniotic fluid.

Abdominal Incision

Throughout the 19th century, abdominal incisions for cesarean sections were longitudinal. Pfannenstiel described a transverse incision as an alternative in 1897 [8]. For many years both methods were used parallely without any controlled studies. The first known study was done

75 years after Pfannenstiel's description by Mowat and Bonnar [9] who found benefits in the transverse incision. This study was followed later by others [10-12]. In 1972, Joel-Cohen (JC) described an alternative transverse incision in hysterectomy [13]. The main difference was the location of the opening of the fascia which was above the Plica Arcuata, where the fascia moves freely over the muscles. At this level, the traumatic separation of the fascia from the muscles, which is the case in the Pfannenstiel incision, is not necessary. In 1994 we compared a modified Joel-Cohen incision with the Pfannenstiel incision. A significant lower febrile morbidity and the need for analgesics were shown [14]. For many years, obstetricians used to perform caesarean sections with longitudinal uterine incisions. In 1924 John Martin Munro-Kerr demonstrated the advantages of a transverse incision in the lower segment of the uterus over a longitudinal incision. Nowadays this approach is routine. Halperin et al., who used classical uterine incisions in preterm deliveries reported a frequency of 6% scar dehiscence in following pregnancies compared to none after transverse incisions [15]. The combination of the modified Joel-Cohen abdominal incision and the Munro-Kerr uterine incision provides optimal access to the lower segment. A superficial incision is done along a physiological skin fold transversely about 1 inch (3 cm) below the line between both anterior superior spinae iliacae (Figure 4).

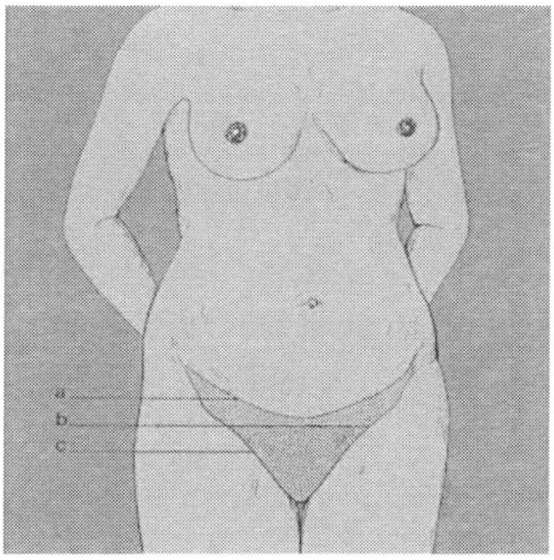

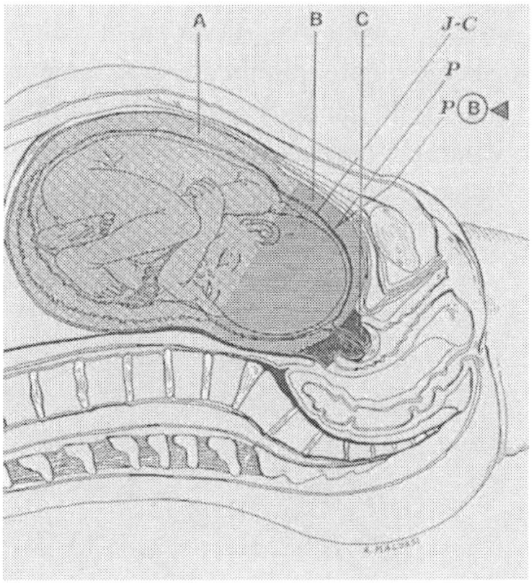

Figure 4. The Joel-Cohen laparotomy is performed by a straight superficial transverse incision in the skin, about 3 cm. below the spinae iliache anterior superior line, cutting only through the cutis. On the left the Malgaigne triangle used for cesareans is visualized with the inguinal femoural lines (on b and c). On the right the sagittal plane of pregnant uterus at term is visualized: a) uterine body; b) lower uterine segment; c) cervix; on the lower uterine segment: J-C) Joel-Cohen; P) Pfannestiel; PB) lower Pfannestiel.

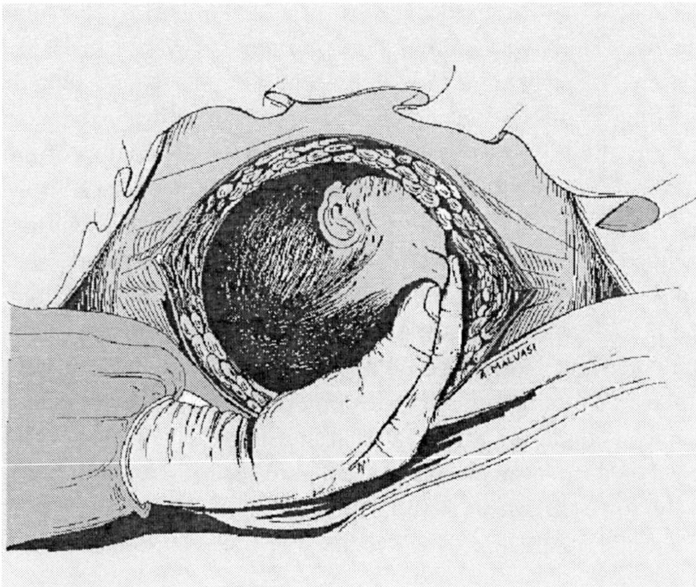

Figure 5. In breech presentation the cut should be more generous in order to avoid trapping fetal head.

This incision is done very superficial, cutting only through the cutis, as there are no major blood vessels at this level. The length of the cut should take into account the size of the baby. In breech deliveries it should be more generous in order to avoid trapping of the head (Figure 5).

In order to avoid distortions and facilitate the esthetical aspects of the scar, the line of incision should be programmed and marked within the physiological skin lines. This marking enables the (right-handed) surgeon to stretch the skin toward the left side in order to cut precisely into the optimal line. The pre-marking ensures that even by the stretching the result will be a precise and symmetrical cut.

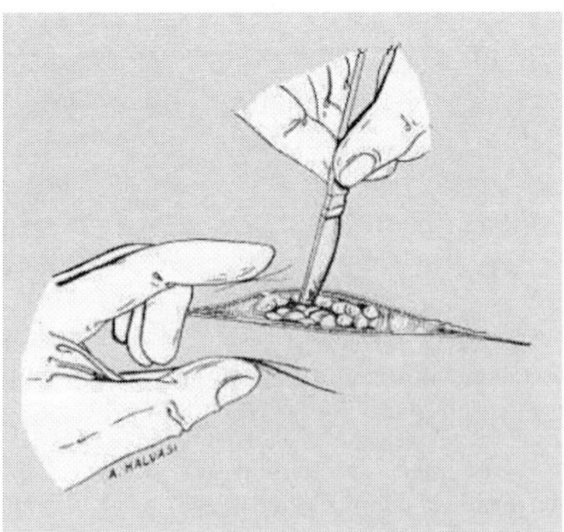

Figure 6. At the center, where there are no major blood vessels, the cut is deepened to the fascia.

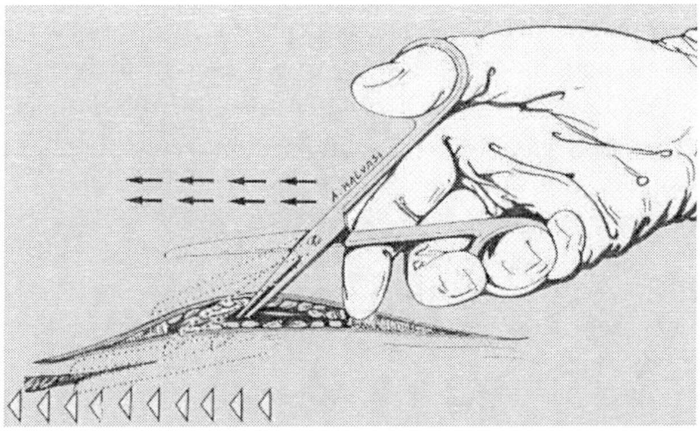

Figure 7. The slightly opened tips of a straight scissors are pushed transversely underneath the fat tissue in both directions.

In the middle part of the cut, where there are no major blood vessels, the opening is deepened with the scalpel until a cut of 2-3 mm in the fascia is done, through which the muscle can be seen (Figure 6). A pair of straight scissors with round edges are now been introduced into the opening in such a way, that one blade is placed below the fascia and one above. The opening between the blades should not be more than 3 mm. The scissors are now pushed towards the assistant, pointing up a little in order to prevent damage to the muscles, but respecting the curvature of the abdominal wall, as far as the opening of the fascia is needed, and then the same towards himself. The opening of the tip of the scissors should stay constant throughout these movements in order to prevent damage to the muscles and blood vessels (Figure 7).

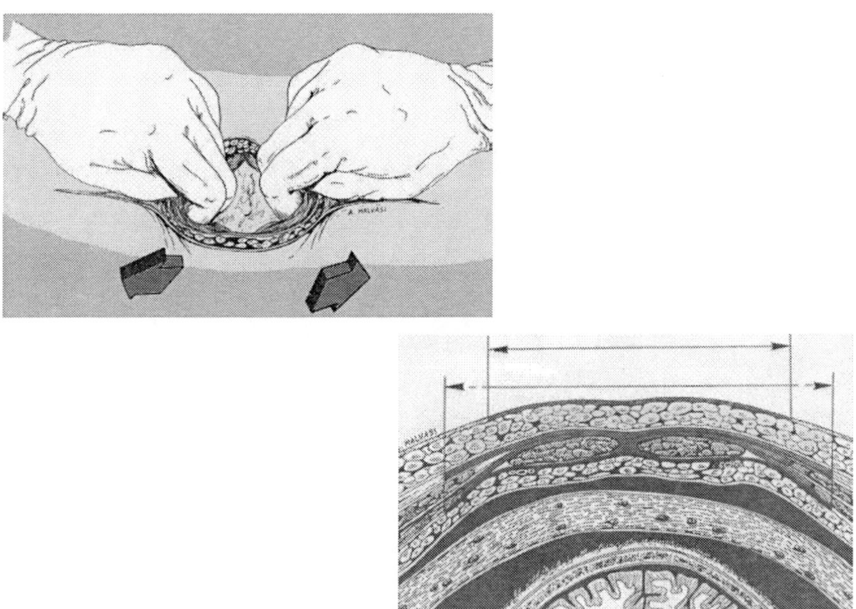

Figure 8. The surgeon and the assistant insert their index and middle fingers under the muscles and stretch the muscles with the overlying fat tissue by bilateral traction.

The surgeon now places his both index fingers pulling the fascia layers up and down. This enables the assistant, and later the surgeon, to put each of their index and middle fingers below the Mm. Recti and together, slowly, in order to enable the tissues to respond, to stretch the muscles to their sides until the desired opening is achieved (Figures 8).

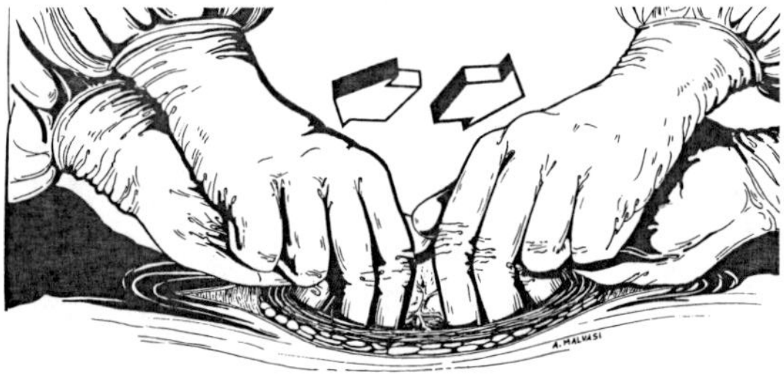

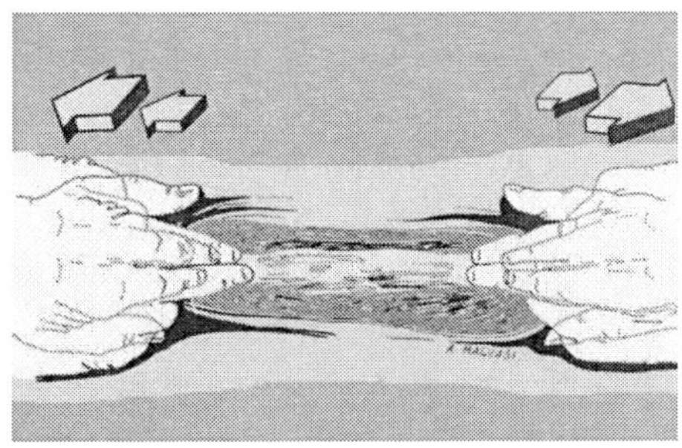

Figure 9. If more force is needed, for example in the case of obese women or in repeated cesarean section, the index and middle fingers of the other hand may be used and placed over the fingers of the first hand.

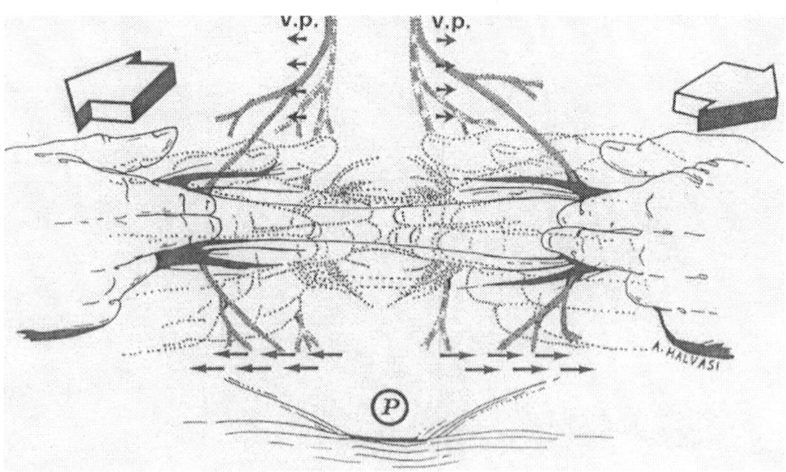

Figure 10. Anatomical structures such as muscles, nerves, and blood vessels have elasticity, and can be moved aside, falling back in place at the end of the procedure.

Sometimes, when the parturient is obese or when a repeat operation is being done, the power of the two fingers is not enough and a second hand should be used. The index and middle fingers of the left hand should be placed over those of the right hand, and the same traction should be done. The fingers of both hands should never be placed next to each other

(Figures 9), since blood vessels have a lateral sway but not a longitudinal one. Traction with both hands brings the tendency to separate the fingers from each other, which might cause tearing of blood vessels. The blood vessels and muscles, which have a lateral sway, now move laterally like strings in a music instrument. At the end of the operation they will return to their place (Figure 10). This method enables performing several operations without necessity of hemostasis.

Opening the Peritoneum

The peritoneum does not have its own blood vessels. Since it surrounds all the intra-abdominal structures, opening it with a sharp instrument might cause damage to the intestines, urine bladder or uterus. In order to prevent it one should open the peritoneum by stretching, high above the bladder in order to prevent damage, and with repeatedly stretching movements which results in a small hole. Stretching this hole up and down will cause a transverse opening of the peritoneum [16] (Figure 11).

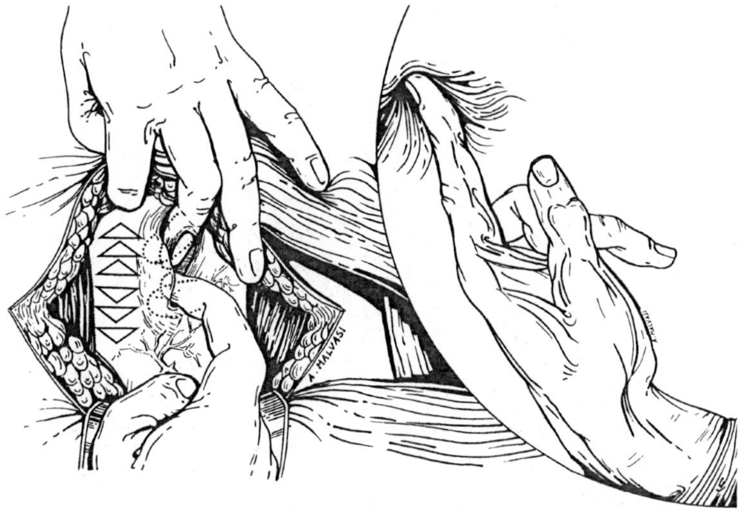

Figure 11. The parietal peritoneum is opened using both index fingers and stretching the peritoneum until a small hole is formed, and then- stretching it in a caudal-cranial direction.

Opening the Uterus

In 1924 Munro-Kerr (1868-1960) introduced the transverse incision of the lower segment of the uterus describing its advantages, less bleeding and lower incidence of scar dehiscence compared to the longitudinal uterine incision. [17]. This approach is more physiological because the fibers of the lower segment (developing toward the delivery) are positioned transversally, so the opening in this level will be along transverse fibers.

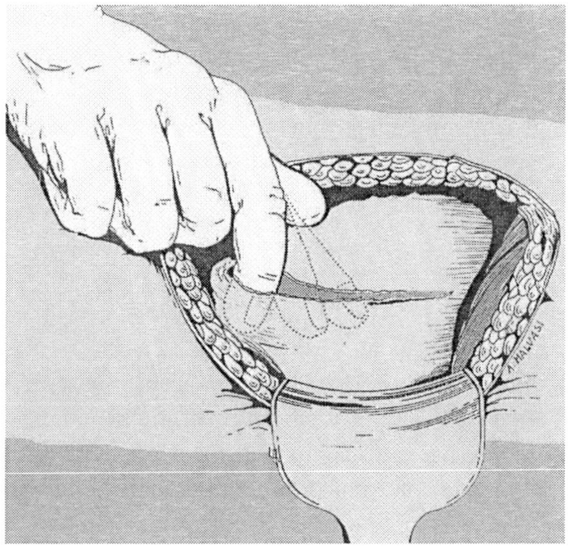

Figure 12. Opening the lower uterine segment (with and without pushing down the peritoneal plica).

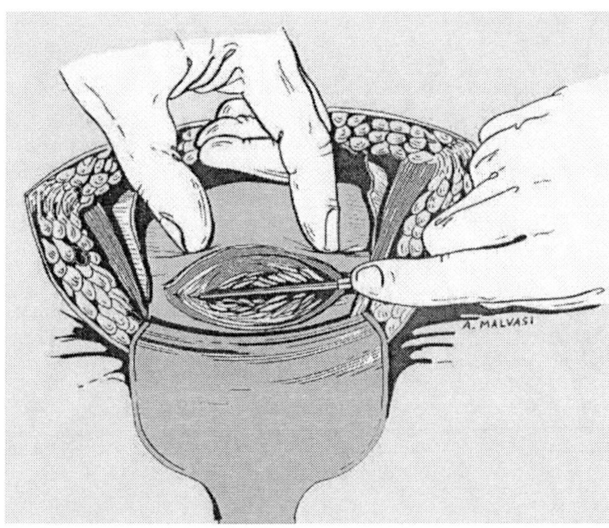

Figure 13. A transverse incision is performed using a scalpel. Penetration into the uterus is performed with the index finger.

Today the longitudinal incision has been abandoned because of the risks of ruptures in subsequent pregnancies [15,18]. There are, however, situations, where longitudinal incisions are still used [19]. The question if the plica should be pushed down or if the incision should be done above the plica is still open, despite some advantages concerning short outcomes when the uterus is opened above the bladder [20]. More prospective studies are needed. It is probably better to open the uterus as low as possible, knowing that the lower you are, the less muscle tissue and more fibrous tissue are present (Figure 12).

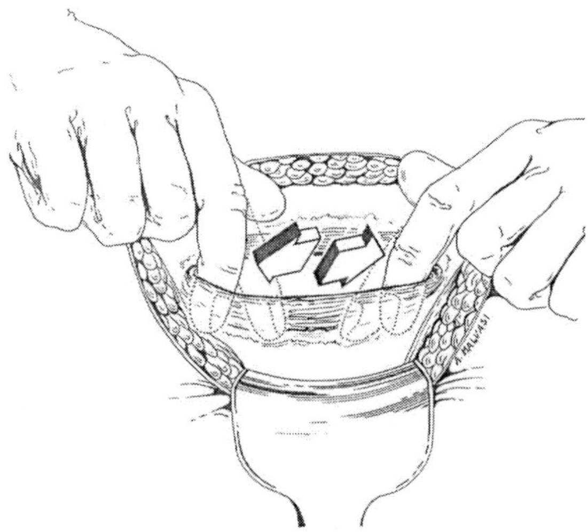

Figure 14. Placing the thumb of the right hand and the index finger of the left hand into the opening in order to open the uterus laterally by stretching.

In the midline a transverse incision is done with a scalpel. It is recommended not to cut the whole thickness of the wall of the uterus, but rather to penetrate it with the index finger (Figure 13), and then, to place the thumb of the right hand and the index finger of the left hand into the opening and to open the uterus laterally by stretching. This causes less bleeding than cutting the lower segment with scissors (Figure 14).

Removal of the Placenta

After the delivery the placenta can be removed either by traction of the umbilical cord while pushing the fundus from above, or by manual extraction. This step is not solved and there are different opinions [21] (Figure 15). According to the reviewers of the Cochrane Database, a manual extraction will cause more bleedings and will be followed by higher rate of endometritis [22] specifically when premature rupture of membranes occurred.

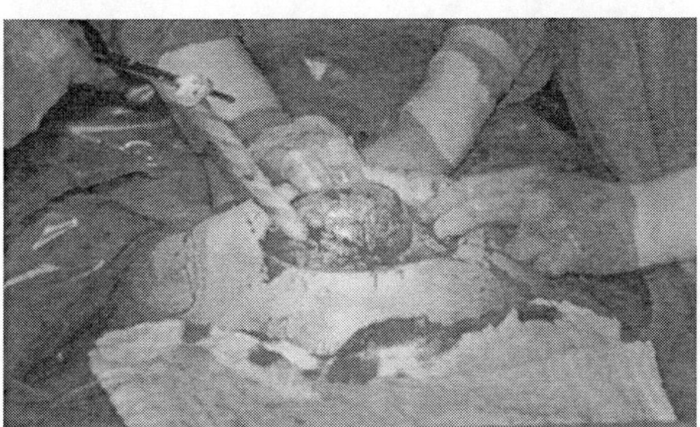

Figure 15. Removal of the placenta with umbilical cord traction and Credè maneuvers.

Suturing the Uterus

The uterus can be sutured while being exteriorized or while left in the abdomen. Both methods have their supporters and opponents. The exteriorization enables contracting the uterus manually and reducing bleeding, feeling more secure by preventing injuries of the intestines, and inspecting the ovaries (which should be done in every caesarean section). Exteriorization of the uterus was proved indeed to make operations faster, and to cause less bleeding when compared to suturing while the uterus is left inside the peritoneal cavity [23-25] (Figure 16).

Mostly, the cut edges of the uterus do not bleed heavily if the opening was done by stretching. If they do, hemostatic clamps should be placed on the bleeding points. If not, one uterine clamp in the middle on the lower cut edge is enough.

Many ways were described to suture the uterus, like two layers, the first continuous, and the second with single stitches, two continuous layers, or single stitches on the lateral edges and then two layers, etc. Over 30 years ago, the one-layer technique was introduced by Csucs, who showed better anatomical results with this method with less sacculations [26]. Other promoters of the single-layer method were Jelsema [27] and Hauth [28]. There are claims, that one-layer stitching will cause more ruptures in the following deliveries [29], but there are other evidence that one-layer suturing does not have disadvantages over two-layer suturing [30,31] (Figure 17).

Due to the physiology of the puerperium, where the uterus diminishes in size immediately after the delivery, any sutures placed will lie free over the edges of the cut, as they cannot shrink together with the uterus. Their function is only hemostatic in the first hours. This observation was also made by Allam using the B-Lynch method for the treatment of postpartum hemorrhage. He stressed the fact that after placing the B-Lynch suture, the uterus will undergo involution, and after 24 – 48 hours the sutures will loose tension without renewed bleeding [32].

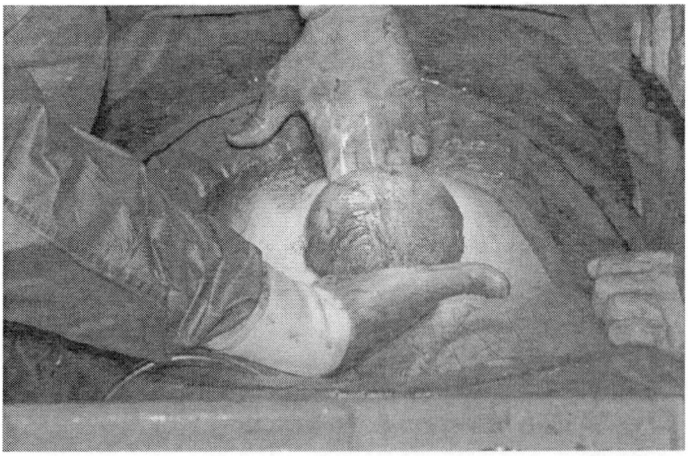

Figure 16. Uterine exteriorization after placental removal.

The more stitching material used, the more local inflammatory reaction will occur, which might weaken the scar and cause more pain. In the Stark cesarean section a big needle is used

(80 mm), which enables to suture the uterus with as few steps and a little foreign material as possible. Single stitches, even if less suturing material is used, are not advisable, as the knots may cause foreign body reaction.

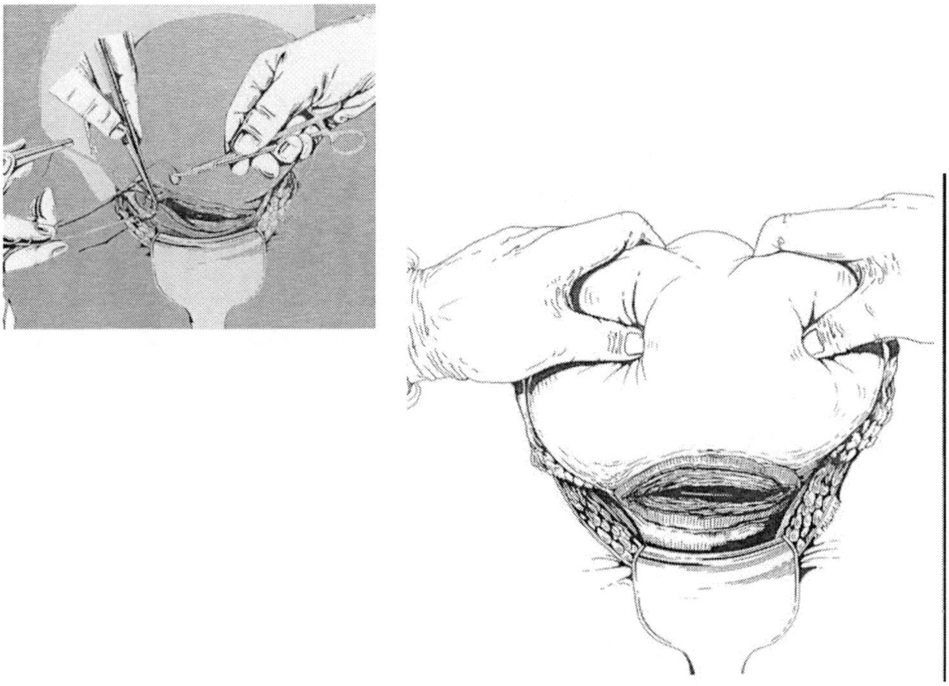

Figure 17. Suturing the uterus with a single continuous layer.

The suturing of the uterus as well as closing the fascia is done from the side of the surgeon towards the side of the assistant. Doing so, the hands never cross, and while holding the suturing material in the left hand, the surgeon can control the tension of the suturing material.

Free blood and amniotic fluid are now present in the abdominal cavity. Blood clots can be removed manually, as no packs should be introduced into the abdomen. Fluid blood will be absorbed by the peritoneum and lymph channels within a couple of hours. As mentioned before, amniotic fluid does have bacteriostatic reaction and therefore may be left in the peritoneal cavity. The abdomen should be washed with physiological water only in presence of amnionitis.

The Peritoneum

For many years surgeons believed that all anatomical layers should be returned to their situation as it was before the operation. Accordingly, they used to suture the peritoneum at the end of any abdominal operation (Figure 18).

Peritoneum should not be sutured, since its closure might lead to the creation of vascular bridges which later may become a focal of adhesions.

The coelum cells which are been present under the muscles, were shown by Harold Ellis to create a new peritoneum in a very short time [33] (Figure 19). In 1983 Stark started to leave the parietal peritoneum open, and in 1984 the visceral peritoneum as well. Leaving the peritoneum open resulted in fewer adhesions than when it was sutured [34].

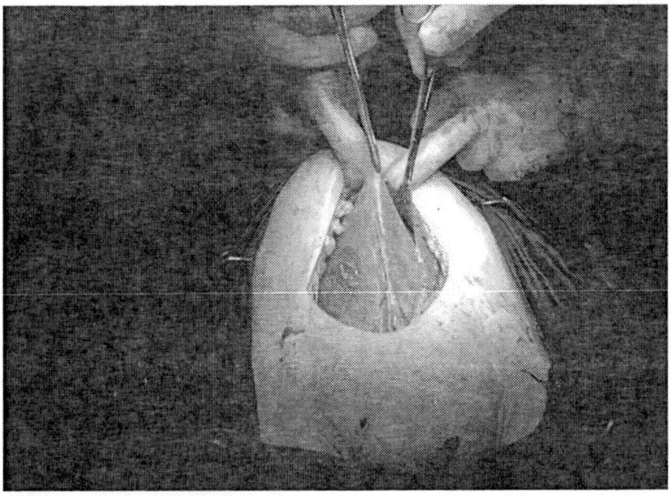

Figure 18. The parietal and visceral peritoneum.

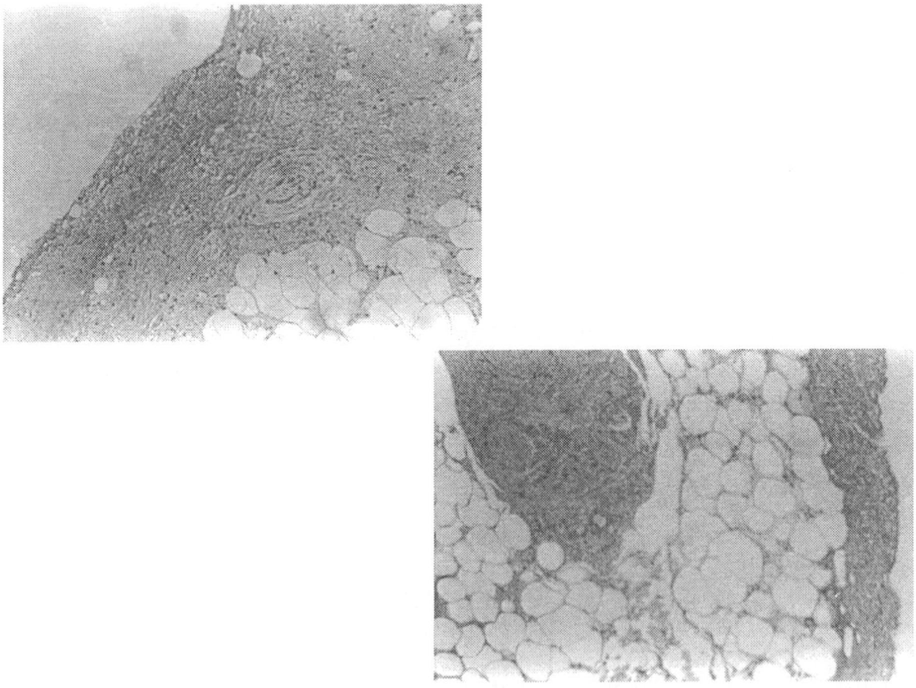

Figure 19. The visceral peritoneum four years after cesarean section. Histological differences were not observed. Left show the visceral peritoneum with closure and right show visceral peritoneum without closure in previous cesarean section.

Closing the peritoneum prolongs the operation time, causes more foreign body reaction and therefore more pain and adhesions.

This is valid for both, the visceral and parietal peritoneum. Leaving parietal and visceral peritoneum open was also recommended in 2002 by the Royal College of Obstetrics and Gynaecology [35].

Blood Pressure

The fascia should never be closed before the surgeon has been informed about the condition of the parturient and her blood pressure. Due to the influence of the pharmacological agents used and / or due to intra-operative bleeding, the operation field might look dry when the blood pressure is low. Possibly, after the operation, when the blood pressure rises, the cut edges will start to bleed again. For this reason, no abdomen should be closed when the blood pressure is low. The parturient should be treated and only after meticulous observations when the blood pressure returned to normal, the operation should continue.

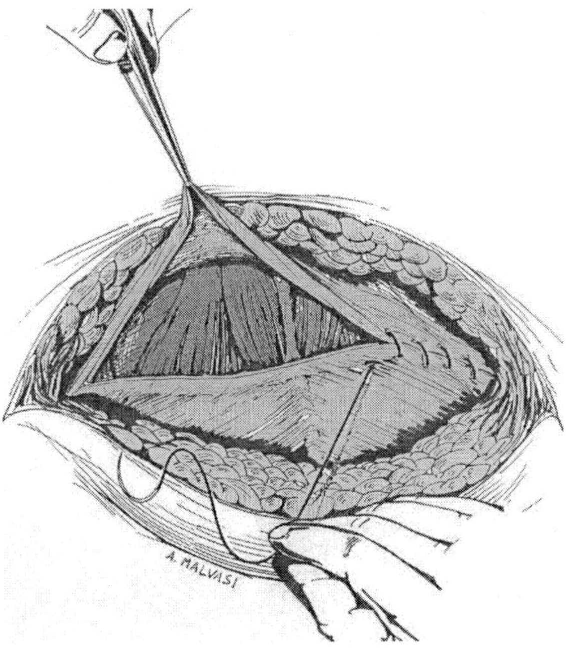

Figure 20. The surgical control of perforating blood vessels, before suturing the fascia.

Closure of the Fascia

As the Joel-Cohen incision is above the Plica Arcuata, one will find laterally two fascial layers. Four Pean forceps should be used. Two of them on both lateral sides, holding the two layers together, and the other two on the third quarter of the way toward the assistant, one holding the lower aspect, and the other the upper aspect of the fascia. The first knot should be done under the fascia in order to prevent a knot under the skin, which serves as a focus of foreign body reaction and pain.

To do so, the surgeon who stands on the right side of the parturient, starts the stitching of both layers of the fascia on the right side, from inside on the upper part of the fascia and then toward outside and then from outside towards inside on the lower aspect of the fascia. After placing the knot, the needle is guided out from inside outside on the upper aspect, and then continuously toward the assistant. The assistant holds both lateral instruments in his hands, close enough to prevent tension on the fascia, and open enough to enable the surgeon to look inside and make sure that no damage is been done to any intra-peritoneal structure. When the suturing arrives to the assistant, he removes both instruments lifting the lateral one close to him which will be removed only after making sure that both layers on the left side were included in the last step (Figure 20).

Closure of the Skin

When closing the skin using the Pfannenstiel incision, the intra-cutaneous suture proved to bring the best cosmetic results [36]. There are no studies comparing different suturing methods in the modified Joel-Cohen incision. It seems that the less sutures used, the better results are been expected due to better drainage (which prevents seromas and hematomas). Optionally, only three stitches might be used with a big cutting needle, two lateral stitches deep nearly until the fascia and one in the midline (Figure 21). Between them Allis clamps should be placed, holding the skin edges for a couple of minutes in order to achieve a good application. If this is not achieved, more superficial stitches can be placed. After the operation the cut edges do swell. The un-elastic sutures may therefore cause pain and longitudinal scars. To prevent this, both lateral (and the extra stitches) can be removed after 48 hours. It will be followed by immediate relief of pressure and pain. The middle stitch should be removed after five days.

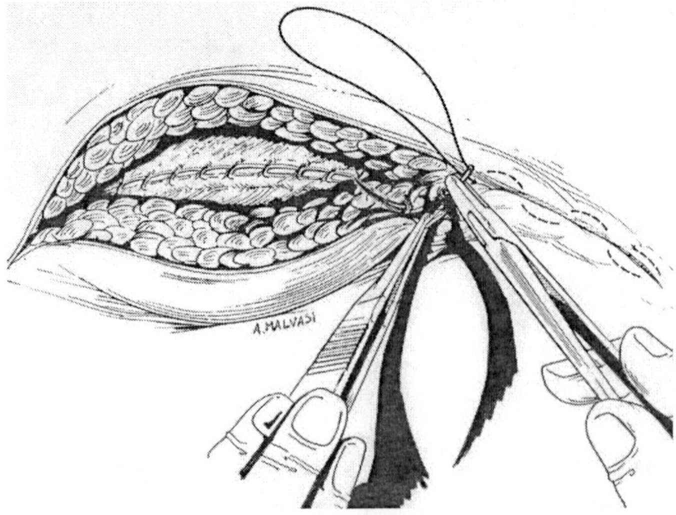

Figure 21. Closure of the skin with intra-cutan suture.

Outcome

After the first presentation and publication of this method [37, 38], it became wildly spread. It was shown that the mobilization of the patient is quicker than with the traditional methods, even when there are postoperative complications [39]. According to recent studies, this operation is short [40, 41], the parturients stay less time at the hospital [42], and need fewer analgesics [43]. A short acting anesthesia can be used (like 2% hyperbaric Mepivacaine) [43, 44]. Comparisons of results when using this method are not optimal as long as surgeons do not use exactly the same steps [45,46], however recent publications on this method [47-54] speak for themselves. It seems that the described method, as long as no other method proves more optimal, should become a standard procedure all over, to the benefit of the mothers and children.

References

[1] Setayesh AR, Kholdebarin AR, Moghadam MS, Setayesh HR. The Trendelenburg position increases the spread and accelerates the onset of epidural anesthesia for Cesarean section. *Can. J. Anaesth.* 2001;48(9):890-3.

[2] Lowenwirt IP, Chi DS, Handwerker SM. Nonfatal venous air embolism during cesarean section: a case report and review of the literature. *Obstet. Gynecol. Surv.* 1994;49(1):72-6.

[3] Down RH, Whitehead R, Watts JM. Do surgical packs cause peritoneal adhesions? *Aust. NZ J. Surg.* 1979;49(3):379-82.

[4] Down RH, Whitehead R, Watts JM. Why do surgical packs cause peritoneal adhesions? *Aust. NZ J. Surg.* 1980;50(1):83-5.

[5] Duron J, Olivier JJ. Foreign bodies and intra-peritoneal postoperative adhesions. *J. Long Term Eff. Med. Implants* 1997;7(3-4):235-42.

[6] Larsen B, Davis B. Enhancement of the antibacterial property of amniotic fluid by hyperthermia. *Obstet. Gynecol.* 1984;63(3):425-9.

[7] Larsen B, Galask RP. Host resistance to intra-amniotic infection. *Obstet. Gynecol. Surv.* 1975;30(10):675-91.

[8] Pfannestiel J. Über die Vorteile des suprasymphysären Faszienquerschnitt für die gynäkologischen Koliotomien, zugleich ein Beitrag zu der Indikationsstellung der Operationswege. *Samml Klein Vortr. Gynäkol.* 1897;68-98 (Klin Vortr NF Gynäk 1900;97:268).

[9] Mowat J, Bonnar J. Abdominal wound dehiscence after caesarean section. *Br. Med. J.* 1971;2(756):256-7.

[10] Ellis H, Coleridge-Smith PD, Joyce AD. Abdominal incisions – vertical or transverse ? *Postgrad Med. J.* 1984;60(704):407-10.

[11] Haeri AD. Comparison of transverse and vertical skin incisions for caesarean section. S. *Afr. Med. J.* 1976; 50(2):33-4.

[12] Hetzel H, Bichler A, Geir W, Dapunt O. Caesarean section: low transverse or middle incision? *Z. Geburtshilfe Perinatol.* 1979;183 (2):128-35.

[13] Joel-Cohen SJ. Abdominal and vaginal hysterectomy. New techniques based on time and motion studies. William Heinemann Medical Books, London, UK, 1992; pp. 170.
[14] Stark M Finkel AR. Comparison between the Joel-Cohen and Pfannestiel incision in caesarean sections. *Eur. J. Obstet. Gynaecol. Reprod. Biol.* 1994;53;121-122.
[15] Halperin ME, Moore DC, Hannah WJ. Classical versus low-segment transverse incision for preterm caesarean section: maternal complications and outcome of subsequent pregnancies. *Br. J. Obstet. Gynaecol.* 1988;95(10):990-6.
[16] Stark M. In the era of 'non-closure of the peritoneum', how to open it? (Not every simple method is optimal, but every optimal method is simple). *Acta Obstet. Gynecol. Scand.* 2009;88(1):119.
[17] Hewitt J. J.M. Munro Kerr. *J. Obstet. Gynaecol. Br. Emp.*1961;68:510-4.
[18] Borso A. Dehiscence of hysterotomy wounds after cesarean section performed with longitudinal incision of the lower segment. *Minerva Ginecol.* 1957;15;9(17):742-7.
[19] Neeser E, Niehues U, Hirsch HA- Maternal morbidity following cesarean section. Comparison of isthmo-corpus longitudinal section and isthmian transverse section in premature labor. *Geburtshilfe Frauenheilkd.* 1988;48(1):8-12.
[20] Hohlagschwandtner M, Ruecklinger E, Husslein P, Joura EA. Is the formation of a bladder flap at caesarean necessary ? A randomized trial. *Obstet. Gynecol.* 2001;98(6):1089-92.
[21] Lasley DS, Eblen A, Yancey MK, Duff P. The effect of placental removal method on the incidence of post-cesarean infections. *Am. J. Obstet. Gynecol.* 1997;176(6):1250-4.
[22] Wilkinson C, Enkin MW. Manual removal of placenta at caesarean section. *Cochrane Database Syst. Rev.*.2000;(2):CD000130.
[23] Darj E, Nordström ML. The Misgav Ladach method for cesarean section compared to the Pfannenstiel method. *Acta Obst. Gyn. Scand* 1999;78:37-41.
[24] Hershey DW, Quilligan EJ. Extraabdominal uterine exteriorization at cesarean section. *Obstet. Gynecol.* 1978;52(2):189-92.
[25] Wahab MA, Karantzis P, Eccersley PS, Russell IF, Thompson JW. A randomised, controlled study of uterine exteriorisation and repair at caesarean section. *Br. J. Obstet. Gynaecol.*1999;106(9):913-6.
[26] Csucs L, Kott I, Solt I. Mono-layer sutures of uterine incision in cesarean section based on clinical experience and animal experiments. *Zentralbl. Gynäkol* 1972;26; 94(34):1121-6.
[27] Jelsema RD, Wittingen JA, Vander Kolk KJ. Continuous, nonlocking, single-layer repair of the low transverse uterine incision. *J. Reprod. Med.* 1993;38(5):393-6.
[28] Hauth JC, Owen J, Davis RO. Transverse uterine incision closure: one versus two layers *Am. J. Obstet. Gynecol.* 1992;167(4 Pt 1):1108-11.
[29] Bujold E, Bujold C, Hamilton EF, Harel F, Gauthier RJ. The impact of a single-layer or double-layer closure on uterine rupture. *Am. J. Obstet. Gynecol* 2002;186(6):1326-30.
[30] Chapman SJ, Owen J, Hauth JC. One- versus two-layer closure of a low transverse cesarean: the next pregnancy. *Obstet. Gynecol.* 1997;89(1):16-8.
[31] Tucker JM, Hauth JC, Hodgkins P, Owen J, Winkler CL. Trial of labor after a one- or two-layer closure of a low transverse uterine incision. *Am. J. Obstet. Gynecol.* 1993;168(2):545-6.
[32] Allam MS, B-Lynch C. The B-Lynch and other uterine compression suture techniques. *Int. J. Gyn. Obstet.* 2005;89:236-241.

[33] Ellis H. Internal overhealing: the problem of intraperitoneal adhesions. *World. J. Surg.* 1980;4:303–306.

[34] Stark M. Clinical evidence that suturing the peritoneum after laparotomy is unnecessary for healing *World J. Surg.* 1993;17(3):419.

[35] Royal College of Obstetrics and Gynaecology. Peritoneal Closure. *RCOC Guideline* 2002;No. 15, July, 2002.

[36] Lindholt JS, Moller-Christensen T, Steele RE. The cosmetic outcome of the scar formation after cesarean section: percutaneous or intracutaneous suture? *Acta Obstet. Gynecol. Scand.* 1994;73(10):832-5.

[37] Stark M. Technique of caesarean section: Misgav Ladach method. In: Women`s Health Today, Perspectives on current research and clinical practice. Popkin DR, Peddle LJ, Eds. Proceedings of the XIV World Congress of Gynaecology and Obstetrics, Montreal. Parthenon Publishing group, New York, USA, 1994;pp: 81-5.

[38] Stark M, Chavkin Y, Kupfersztain C, Guedj P, Finkel AR. Evaluation of combinations of procedures in cesarean section. *Int. J. Gynaecol. Obstet.* 1995;48(3):273-6.

[39] Björklund K, Kimaro M, Urassa E, Lindmark G. Introduction of the Misgav Ladach caesarean section at an African tertiary centre: a randomised controlled trial. *Br. J. Obstet. Gynecol* 2000;107(2):209-216.

[40] Federici D, Lacelli B, Muggiasca L, Agarossi A, Cipolla L, Conti M. Cesarean section using the Misgav Ladach method *Int. J. Gynaecol. Obstet.* 1997;57(3):273-9.

[41] Li, M, Zou L, Zhu J. Study on modification of the Misgav Ladach method for cesarean section. *J. Tongji Med. Univ.* 2001;21(1):75-7.

[42] Ansaloni L, Brundisini R, Morino G, Kiura A. Prospective, randomized, comparative study of Misgav Ladach versus traditional cesarean section at Nazareth Hospital, Kenya. *World J. Surg.* 2001;25 (9):1164–1172.

[43] Meininger D, Byhahn C, Kessler P, Nordmeyer J, Alparslan Y, Hall BA, Bremerich DH. Intrathecal fentanyl, sufentanil, or placebo combined with hyperbaric mepivacaine 2% for parturients undergoing elective cesarean delivery. *Anesth Analg.* 2003;96(3):852-8.

[44] Moreira P, Moreau JC, Faye ME, Ka S, Kane Gueye SM, Faye EO, Dieng T, Diadjiou F. Comparison of two cesarean techniques: classic versus Misgav Ladach cesarean. *J. Gynecol. Obstet. Reprod.* 2002;31(6):572–576.

[45] Stark M. Optimised meta-analysis should be based on standardised methods. *BJOG* 2011 May;118(6):765-6.

[46] Stark M, Gerli S, Di Renzo GC. The importance of analyzing and standardizing surgical methods. *J. Minim. Invasive Gynecol.* 2009; 16(2):122-5.

[47] Walsh CA. Evidence-based cesarean technique. *Curr. Opin. Obstet. Gynecol.;* 2010 Apr;22(2):110-5.

[48] Malvasi A, Tinelli A, Pacella E. Mass closure of visceral peritoneum at cesarean section. A proposal method. *J. Matern Fetal. Neonatal. Med.;* 2010;23(4):345-6.

[49] Malvasi A, Tinelli A, Guido M, Zizza A, Farine D, Stark M. Should the visceral peritoneum at the bladder flap closed at cesarean sections? A post-partum sonographic and clinical assessment. *J. Matern Fetal. Neonatal. Med.*; 2010;23(7):662-9.

[50] Malvasi A, Tinelli A, Serio G, Tinelli R, Casciaro S, Cavallotti C. Comparison between the use of the Joel-Cohen incision and its modification during Stark's cesarean section. *J. Matern Fetal. Neonatal. Med.;* 2007;20(10):757-61.

[51] Malvasi A, Tinelli A, Tinelli R, Cavallotti C, Farine D. The diagnosis and management of post-cesarean section hemorrhagic shock. *J. Matern Fetal. Neonatal. Med.*; 2008;21(7):487-91.

[52] Malvasi A, Tinelli A, Tinelli R, Rahimi S, Resta L, Tinelli FG. The post-cesarean section symptomatic bladder flap hematoma: a modern reappraisal. *J. Matern Fetal. Neonatal. Med.*; 2007;20(10):709-14.

[53] Tinelli A, Malvasi A, Vittori G. Laparoscopic treatment of post-cesarean section bladder flap hematoma: A feasible and safe approach. *Minim. Invasive Ther. Allied Technol.*; 2009;18(6):356-60.

[54] Hofmeyr GJ, Mathai M, Shah A, Novikova N. Techniques for caesarean section. *Cochrane Database Syst. Rev.*; 2008;(1):CD004662.

In: Cesarean Section: Procedures, Complications and Recovery ISBN: 978-1-62081-214-3
Editor: Eyal Sheiner

Chapter VIII

TUBAL LIGATION DURING CESAREAN SECTION

Daniel Abehsera, Ignacio Zapardiel*
and Javier De Santiago
Obstetrics and Gynecology Department,
La Paz University Hospital, Madrid, Spain

INTRODUCTION

Tubal ligation during the course of a Caesarean section (CS) is technically simple and safe from the medical point of view, and does not adversely affect breastfeeding [1].Demand for tubal ligation by the patients is higher when offered in the context of CS instead of, when offered as a single act [2]. However, failure (i.e. pregnancy following the procedure) although extremely rare, is higher in puerperal tubal sterilization than in the interval tubal ligation, especially when using techniques of mechanical tubal occlusion [1].

Electrocoagulation by laparoscopy is associated with high efficacy, but with a potentially greater risk of complications and difficulties in the reversal of the tubal ligation. Tubal ligation has a number of advantages over other contraceptive methods, which require strict adherence to their use. Candidates for postpartum tubal sterilization should be carefully selected and assessed, since the technique is generally irreversible.

HISTORY

James Blundell was the first to propose salpingectomy during caesarean section to avoid future interventions (London, 1823). [3] Zweifel and Thomas were probably the first who tried it, but most authors agree that Lungren Samuel Smith made the first simple tubal ligation in 1880 in Ohio. Since then more than one hundred surgical techniques were described to achieve the interruption of tubal continuity of women, although their availability

* Correspondence: Ignacio Zapardiel MD, PhD, Obstetrics and Gynecology Department. La Paz University Hospital, Paseo de la Castellana 267, 28047 Madrid. SPAIN. Email: ignaciozapardiel@hotmail.com.

and acceptability were limited until the 1960's. In fact, tubal ligation for non-medical reasons was not available in all states of the United States until 1972, when federal courts legal abolished all restriction [4].

Epidemiology

Tubal ligation is one of the most frequently performed operations in the United States, after cesarean delivery (1.3 million / year), abortion (1.2 million / year), cholecystectomy (917,000 / year); coronary angioplasty (661,000 / year), and is more common than hysterectomy (569,000 / year) and episiotomy (454,000 / year). The number of tubal ligations performed annually in the United States has declined from 687,000 performed in 1995 to 643,000 in 2006, although the number of women between 15 and 44 years old has increased in 4%. This decline has also been reflected in Western Europe, Australia and Japan, probably due to an increase in the supply of contraceptive methods.

However, the number of postpartum tubal ligation performed has remained stable and performed in 8% - 9% of live birth deliveries in the United States [5].

Moreno et al. [6] found an increased rate of tubal ligations during cesarean section from the 80's, and specifically between the years 1978 and 1997 (Granada, Spain).

Surgical Technique

Performing tubal ligation during cesarean section is a great benefit to the patient who has fulfilled family planning, eliminating the morbidity of a future surgery. The increase in operation time has been estimated at 7 minutes by Wilson et al. [7], who perform a prospective observational study on a total of 331 cesarean sections.

Napolitano et al. [8] reported similar rates of ectopic pregnancy following tubal ligation performed either during CS or mini-laparotomy or laparoscopy.

1. Pomeroy's Method

The fallopian tube is identified and pulled up at the isthmic portion using a non traumatic forceps. Ligation is performed by using horn handle absorbable catgut suture of 0 or 2-0, and then resecting the handle. The resected portion of the tube should measure 1 to 2 cm. The ends should be tied inspected to ensure proper hemostasis, and confirm the presence of light tubes. The same procedure is completed in the contralateral side. When the suture is absorbed, the two ends of the tube are retracted and remain at a distance of 1 to 2 cm.

The use of suture material takes longer to resorb and the use of non-absorbable material reduces the likelihood of fistula formation and failure of the technique. The slip of the bands with retraction of the tubal stump is the most common complication of the Pomeroy technique. This risk is minimized by placing two stitches and exerts traction only in the distal suture.

Oligbo et al. [9] found a pregnancy rate of 0% after performing such tubal ligation during cesarean section after the performance of 203 tubal ligations between the years 1994 and 2007.

2. Parkland's Method (Modified Pomeroy)

Ligation is performed at two points instead of one. Ligation is performed in the proximal and distal portions of the tube with catgut absorbable suture of 0 or 2-0. The middle segment of the tube is removed.

Gálvez [10] found a success rate of 100% in 315 cases following this procedure; however follow- up of patients was only 36 months.

3. Labhardt-Uchida Method

The fallopian tube is identified and pulled up at the junction between isthmic and ampullary portion, by a non traumatic forceps. Injection of about 2 ml of saline in the antimesenteric border of the serosa along 2 cm is done and dissection of the tube is carried out. The purpose of the saline injection is to separate the serosal layer of the tube. Both ends of the tube portion are binded. The portion of the conduit between the two ligatures (1-2 cm) is resected. Then the serosa is closed between the two ends of the tube with a continuous suture of 4-0, leaving the proximal end of the buried conduit between the two layers of peritoneum mesosalpinx and the distal end of the suture outside, avoiding recanalization between the two extremes. To prevent retraction of the distal stump of the tube, which must remain outside the suture of the serosa, the stump can be sutured to the serosa, before carrying out the suture of the serosa of the tube.

By performing this procedure, Uchida [11] reported that there were no failures after completing more than 20,000 interventions.

4. Irving Method

The tubal ligation is performed in the isthmic portion which is partially resected. The resulting proximal stump is buried beneath the rear wall of the uterus and the distal stump is buried in mesosalpinx, similar to the technique of Labhardt-Uchida.

This technique has a high success rate, and Hall et al. [12] found no pregnancies following the completion of 634 procedures between 1969 and 1983.

5. Cook Method

The tubal ligation is performed in the isthmic portion which is partially resected. The resulting proximal stump is buried beneath the round ligament and the distal stump is left intraperitoneal, similar to the technique of Labhardt-Uchida.

6. Cornual Resection

The interstitial portion is resected and 1 cm of the isthmic portion is subsequently closed with sutures. The resulting distal stump of the tube is buried between layers of the broad ligament. Obviously, it is an irreversible method. It has a high risk of arterial bleeding from the uterine horn resection.

7. Kroener Method (Fimbriectomy)

Two ligatures are placed around the distal portion of the tube near the fimbriae, which are than resected. It is an irreversible method, but has failures due to the formation of fistulas. De la Garza [13] found a failure rate of 2.1%.

8. Madlener method

A loop with non-absorbable suture material at the ampullary portion of the tube is performed. It is done without removal of a segment of the tube. The failure rate of this technique is probably higher than other methods due to fistula formation under the suture material [14].

9. Oxford Method

Dissection of the tube is performed at the junction between the isthmic and ampullary portions. Subsequently, both ends are fixed to the round ligament.

10. Electrocoagulation

This is the preferred method today for laparoscopic tubal ligation.

11. Methods of Mechanical Occlusion

Typically these methods are not recommended for postpartum sterilization because the large size of the tubes can lead to technical failures and / or tubal damage. Oligbo et al. [9] found that the Pomeroy technique during cesarean showed less risk of failure than the application of Filshie clips. However, Kohaut et al. [15] compared the two methods and concluded that the use of clips requires less surgical time and is preferred by surgeons, but did not provide data on failures of the technique. The latest review of the Cochrane Database of 201116 on techniques for the interruption of tubal patency for female sterilization concluded that electrocoagulation was associated with less morbidity including post-operative pain when compared with the modified Pomeroy and tubal ring methods, despite the risk of burns to the small bowel. Nevertheless, they pointed out that data are basically based on studies with small sample size and lati with a relative short period of follow-up thus limiting the power to show clinical or statistical differences for failure rates.

Complications

1. Failure of the Technique

The main complication of tubal ligation is failure of the technique, which results in a pregnancy, either ectopic or intra-uterine. In a multicenter prospective cohort study, Peterson et al. [17] reported that postpartum salpingectomy had a failure rate of 2 (ectopic pregnancies) out of 1637 patients evaluated. Brenner et al. [18] suggested in their analysis of 100 ectopic pregnancies that the incidence of this complication is independent of the technique used for tubal ligation. Napolitano et al. [19] found an incidence of 36-67% of ectopic pregnancies after tubal ligation and suggested that there are no differences in the incidence of failure according to the technique used (minilaparotomy, cesarean section-associated sterilization, and laparoscopy).

2. Reversal of Sterilization

Regrets after sterilization occur in approximately 3% - 25% of patients. However, only about 1% - 2% seeks reversal of the technique [20-24]. The most commonly associated factor with the regrets is a change in marital status of the patient [25, 26]. It has also been linked with a conflict in the marriage at the time of performing the technique [27]. Other commonly associated factors are young maternal age and low parity while performing tubal ligation [28].

In order to identify patients at risk for regrets after performing the technique the Beck Depression Inventory was proposed [29]. Similarly, Demir et al. [30] proposed the use of Tubal Ligation Score for identifying such patients.

Those patients who wish to restore their fertility will have 2 options to get it: in vitro fertilization techniques, and sterilization reversal using microsurgery on the tubes. The advantages of microsurgical reconstruction on in vitro fertilization include the permanent restoration of the ability of women to conceive naturally (repeated pregnancies are possible without any additional therapy), as well as preventing the incidence of multiple births. Therefore, it is important to inform the patient about the possibility of reconstructive surgery of the tubes [31].

Microsurgical reversal of sterilization has a cumulative pregnancy rate of 40% to 84%, and monthly fertilization rate of 8% to 10%. Intrauterine pregnancy rates in women over age 40 range from 15% to 64%. In general, the risk of ectopic pregnancy is less than 10%. Prognostic factors include the type of sterilization procedure performed, the site of the anastomosis, and the length of the tubes after sterilization. Factors associated with higher likelihood of success include tubal occlusion with clips or rings, isthmic-isthmic anastomosis and tubal length greater than 5 cm [32].

The conventional technique of reversing tubal anastomosis is the microsurgery over the tube by laparotomy [33]. However, several authors have published series of patients using laparoscopic surgery [34, 35] and robot surgery [36], with good results.

3. Psychological Disorders and Sexual Dysfunctions

A study conducted in China [37] of 1000 patients (500 with and 500 without tubal ligation sterilization) between 35 and 39 years of age showed a statistically significant higher incidence of anxiety and depression in the group that underwent sterilization. However, it is possible that the incidence of these disorders is influenced by social factors in this specific target population.

With respect to sexual function, there are no data that this is diminished or altered. Smith et al. [38] conducted a prospective study of more than 4,500 patients who underwent tubal ligation, in which 82% of patients reported no changes in sexual function, and on the contrary, 18% reported an increase in their desire and sexual pleasure. However, the group of patients recruited underwent interval tubal ligation not during the course of a cesarean delivery.

4. Post-Tubal Ligation Syndrome

Several symptoms were described in patients following tubal ligation, including painful menstruation, menstrual dysfunction, and / or severe premenstrual syndrome. It has been hypothesized that menstrual bleeding disorders are the result of an alteration of ovarian blood flow with consecutive changes in hormone production [39, 40]. However this has not been demonstrated in a prospective study of five years duration that compared 9514 patients who underwent tubal ligation and 573 patients whose partners underwent vasectomy. Patients who underwent sterilization were more likely to have a reduction in days of menstruation, the amount of bleeding and menstrual pain. In addition, the incidence of breakthrough bleeding and menstrual cycle length was similar in both groups. However, patients who were sterilized had more irregularities in the cycle [41]. In a study of 976 patients Harlow et al. [42] showed no changes in hormone levels in women undergoing tubal ligation. Interestingly a significant and unclear association was noted between an increased incidence of hysterectomy in patients post tubal sterilization before the age of 30 [43, 44]. Post-ablation tubal sterilization syndrome refers to the development of an intensive, cyclical, unilateral or bilateral, pelvic pain, which usually occurs between five and ten months after endometrial ablation performed in women with previous tubal sterilization. This entity might be explained by the appearance of a cornual hematometra leading to hematosalpinx [45].

The Benefits of Tubal Ligation

Benefits of tubal ligation include an easy and reliable contraceptive method with low failure rate. Moreover, a lower risk of ovarian cancer was reported in women following tubal ligation [46]. There is also a reduction in serious pelvic inflammatory disease, although the procedure does not protect against sexually transmitted diseases [47]. Possibly, the mechanical obstruction of the tubes following ligation prevents the passage of germs and carcinogens into the peritoneal cavity.

REFERENCES

[1] Chi IC, Petta CA, McPheeters M. A review of safety, efficacy, pros and cons, and issues of puerperal tubal sterilization--an update. *Adv. Contracept.* 1995 Sep;11(3):187-206.

[2] Adesiyun AG. Female sterilization by tubal ligation: a re-appraisal of factors influencing decision making in a tropical setting. *Arch. Gynecol. Obstet.* 2007 Apr;275(4):241-4. Epub 2006 Sep 26.

[3] Speroff L, Marc AF. Planificación familiar, esterilización y aborto en endocrinología ginecológica, clínica y esterilidad pág 827-859. Ed. Lippincott Willians and Wilkins. Philadelphia 2006.

[4] Peterson HB. Sterilization. *Obstet. Gynecol.* 2008 Jan;111(1):189-203.

[5] Chan LM, Westhoff CL. Tubal sterilization trends in the United States. *Fertil Steril.* 2010 Jun;94(1):1-6.

[6] Moreno JM, Bartual E, Carmona M, Araico F, Miranda JA, Herruzo AJ. Changes in the rate of tubal ligation done after cesarean section. *Eur. J. Obstet. Gynecol. Reprod. Biol.* 2001 Aug;97(2):147-51.

[7] Wilson SH, Fecho K, Marshall J, Spielman F. Factors influencing cesarean delivery operative times: a prospective observational cohort study. *Int. J. Obstet. Anesth.* 2010 Oct;19(4):417-21.

[8] Napolitano PG, Vu K, Rosa C. Pregnancy after failed tubal sterilization. *J. Reprod. Med.* 1996 Aug;41(8):609-13.

[9] Oligbo N, Revicky V, Udeh R. Pomeroy technique or Filshie clips for postpartum sterilisation? Retrospective study on comparison between Pomeroy procedure and Filshie clips for a tubal occlusion at the time of Caesarean section. *Arch. Gynecol. Obstet.* 2010 Jun;281(6):1073-5.

[10] Gálvez Asún J. Postpartum tubal sterilization with the Parkland technique. *Rev. Chil. Obstet. Ginecol.* 1994;59(1):27-31.

[11] Uchida H. Uchida tubal sterilization. *Am. J. Obstet. Gynecol* 1975 Jan 15; 121(2):153-8.

[12] Hall JA, Hall BR, Hall KA. Irving tubal sterilization: report of 634 procedures. *Indiana Med.* 1988 Jun;81(6):520-4.

[13] De la Garza Quintanilla C. Tubal sterilization by postpartum minilaparotomy. *Ginecol. Obstet. Mex.* 1990 Nov;58:315-9.

[14] Bojović S. Spontaneous recanalization of tubes after surgical sterilization. *Jugosl Ginekol. Opstet.* 1980 May-Aug;20(3-4):153-6.

[15] Kohaut BA, Musselman BL, Sanchez-Ramos L, Kaunitz AM. Randomized trial to compare perioperative outcomes of Filshie clip vs. Pomeroy technique for postpartum

and intraoperative cesarean tubal sterilization: a pilot study. *Contraception.* 2004 Apr;69(4):267-70.

[16] Lawrie TA, Nardin JM, Kulier R, Boulvain M. Techniques for the interruption of tubal patency for female sterilisation. *Cochrane Database Syst. Rev.* 2011 Feb 16;(2):CD003034.

[17] Peterson HB, Xia Z, Hughes JM,Wilcox LS, Tylor LR, Trussell J. The risk of ectopic pregnancy after tubal sterilization. U.S. Collaborative Review of Sterilisation Working Group. *N. Engl. J. Med.* 1997;336(March (11)):796–7.

[18] Brenner PF, Benedetti T, Mishell Jr DR. Ectopic pregnancy following tubal sterilization surgery. *Obstet. Gynecol.* 1977;49(3):323–4.

[19] Napolitano PG, Vu K, Rosa C. Pregnancy after failed tubal sterilization. *J. Reprod. Med.* 1996 Aug;41(8):609-13.

[20] Grubb GS, Peterson HB, Layde PM, Rubin GL. Regret after decision to have a tubal sterilization. *Fertil Steril* 1985; 44(2):248-53.

[21] Henshaw SK, Singh S. Sterilization regret among U.S. couples. *Fam Plann Perspect* 1986 Sept-Oct; 18(5):238-40.

[22] Phillips JM, Hulka JF, Hulka B, Corson SL. 1979 AAGL membership survey. *J. Reprod. Med.* 1981Oct; 26(10):529-33.

[23] Allyn DP, Leton DA, Westcott NA, Hale RW. Presterilization counseling and women's regret about having been sterilized. *J. Reprod. Med.* 1986 Nov; 31(11):1027-32.

[24] Trussell, J, Guilbert, E, Hedley, A. Sterilization failure, sterilization reversal, and pregnancy after sterilization reversal in Quebec. *Obstet. Gynecol.* 2003 Apr; 101(4); 677-84.

[25] Divers WA Jr. Characteristics of women requesting reversal of sterilization. *Fertil Steril* 1984 Feb; 41(2):233-6.

[26] Winston RM. Why 103 women asked for reversal of sterilisation. *Br. Med. J.* 1977 Jul 30; 2(6082):305-7.

[27] Jamieson DJ, Kaufman SC, Costello C, Hillis SD, Marchbanks PA, Peterson HB; US Collaborative Review of Sterilization Working Group. A comparison of women's regret after vasectomy versus tubal sterilization. *Obstet. Gynecol.* 2002 Jun; 99(6):1073-9.

[28] Wilcox LS, Chu SY, Eaker ED, Zeger SL, Peterson HB. Risk factors for regret after tubal sterilization: 5 years of follow-up in a prospective study. *Fertil Steril* 1991 May; 55(55):927-33.

[29] Kelekçi S, Erdemoglu E, Kutluk S, Yilmaz B, Savan K. Risk factors for tubal ligation: regret and psychological effects impact of Beck Depression Inventory. *Contraception.* 2005 Jun;71(6):417-20.

[30] Demir SC, Cetin MT, Kadayifçi O. The effect of tubal ligation scoring and sterilization counseling on the request for tubal reanastomosis. *Eur. J. Contracept Reprod. Health Care.* 2006 Sep;11(3):215-9.

[31] Schippert C, Hille U, Bassler C, Soergel P, Hollwitz B, Garcia-Rocha GJ. Organ-preserving and reconstructive microsurgery of the fallopian tubes in tubal infertility: still an alternative to in vitro fertilization (IVF). *J. Reconstr. Microsurg.* 2010 Jul;26(5):317-23.

[32] Schippert C, Garcia-Rocha GJ. Is there still a role for reconstructive microsurgery in tubal infertility? *Curr. Opin. Obstet. Gynecol.* 2011 Jun;23(3):200-5.

[33] Zarei A, Al-Ghafri W, Tulandi T. Tubal surgery. *Clin. Obstet. Gynecol.* 2009 Sep;52(3):344-50.

[34] Hawkins J, Dube D, Kaplow M, Tulandi T. Cost analysis of tubal anastamosis by laparoscopy and by laparotomy. *J. Am. Assoc. Gynecol. Laparosc.* 2002;9:120–124.

[35] Cha SH, Lee MH, Kim JH, Lee CN, Yoon TK, Cha KY. Fertility outcome after tubal anastomosis by laparoscopy and laparotomy. *J. Am. Assoc Gynecol. Laparos.* 2001;8:348–352.

[36] Goldberg JM, Falcone T. Laparoscopic microsurgical tubal anastomosis with and without robotic assistance. *Hum. Reprod.* 2003;18:145–147.

[37] Luo L, Wu SZ, Zhu C, Fan Q, Liu K, Sun G. Psychological long-term effects of sterilization on anxiety and depression. *Contraception.* 1996 Dec;54(6):345-57.

[38] Smith A, Lyons A, Ferris J, Richters J, Pitts M, Shelley J. Are sexual problems more common in women who have had a tubal ligation? A population-based study of Australian women. *BJOG* 2010 Mar; 117(4):463-8.

[39] Revel A, Abramov Y, Yagel S, Nadjari M. Utero-ovarian morphology and blood flow after tubal ligation by the Pomeroy technique. *Contraception.* 2004 Feb;69(2):151-6.

[40] Kutlar I, Ozkur A, Balat O, Ugur MG, Genco Y, Aksoy F. Effects of three different sterilization methods on utero-ovarian Doppler blood flow and serum levels of ovarian hormones. *Eur. J. Obstet. Gynecol. Reprod. Biol.* 2005 Sep 1;122(1):112-7.

[41] Peterson HB, Jeng G, Folger SG, Hillis SA, Marchbanks PA, Wilcox LS; U.S. Collaborative Review of Sterilization Working Group. The risk of menstrual abnormalities after tubal sterilization. U.S. Collaborative Review of Sterilization Working Group. *N. Engl. J. Med.* 2000 Dec 7; 343(23):1681-7.

[42] Harlow BL, Missmer SA, Cramer DW, Barbieri RL. Does tubal sterilization influence the subsequent risk of menorrhagia or dysmenorrhea? *Fertil Steril.* 2002 Apr;77(4):754-60.

[43] Hillis SD, Marchbanks PA, Tylor LR, Peterson HB. Higher hysterectomy risk for sterilized than nonsterilized women: findings from the U.S. Collaborative Review of Sterilization. The U.S. Collaborative Review of Sterilization Working Group. *Obstet. Gynecol.* 1998 Feb; 91(2):241-6.

[44] Taffe J, Green A, Dudley E, Dennerstein L. Tubal ligation, hysterectomy and DandC: evidence from the Melbourne Women's Midlife Health Project. *Gynecol Obstet Invest* 2000; 50(2):117-22.

[45] McCausland AM, McCausland VM. Frequency of symptomatic cornual hematometra and postablation tubal sterilization syndrome after total rollerball endometrial ablation: a 10-year follow-up. *Am. J. Obstet. Gynecol.* 2002 Jun;186(6):1274-80; discussion 1280-3.

[46] Narod SA, Sun P, Ghadirian P, Lynch H, Isaacs C, Garber J, Weber B, Karlan B, Fishman D, Rosen B, Tung N, Neuhausen SL. Tubal ligation and risk of ovarian cancer in carriers of BRCA1 or BRCA2 mutations: a case-control study. *Lancet* 2001 May 12; 357(9267):1467-70.

[47] Abbuhl SB, Muskin EB, Shofer FS. Pelvic inflammatory disease in patients with bilateral tubal ligation. *Am. J. Emerg. Med.* 1997 May; 15(3):271-4.

In: Cesarean Section: Procedures, Complications and Recovery ISBN: 978-1-62081-214-3
Editor: Eyal Sheiner

Chapter IX

ANESTHESIA FOR CESAREAN SECTION

Alexander Zlotnik, Akiva Leibowitz and Yoram Shapira
Department of Anesthesiology and Critical Care,
Soroka University Medical Center, Beer Sheva, Israel

INTRODUCTION

Cesarean section possesses particular challenges to the anesthesiologist, derived from the unique physiological stare of pregnancy and its associated pathologies, the nature of the procedure, and, ultimately the need to care for two patients simultaneously – the mother and the fetus. Cesarean section may become a source for serious difficulties and complications, leading to increased maternal and fetal morbidity and mortality. Anesthesia, general or regional, induces a physiological imbalance, representing a significant deviation from the normal physiological state, requiring a deep understanding and knowledge of the induced changes, and specific effects of different interventions and treatment. In the present chapter we discuss the anesthetic implications of the physiological and pathophysiological changes throughout pregnancy and during delivery, their impact on the outcome, morbidity and mortality, the unique characteristics of the cesarean section candidate, particular anesthetic challenges, associated complications, and practical recommendations for anesthetic management of the cesarean section candidate.

ANATOMICAL AND PHYSIOLOGICAL CHANGES OF PREGNANCY, OF INTEREST TO THE ANESTHESIOLOGIST

Respiratory System

The respiratory system, is affected by pregnancy along its entire course, and includes anatomical changes of the oro-pharynx, edema of the respiratory tract mucosa, and a significant modulation of respiratory mechanics. Cesarean section, despite being a lower abdominal surgery, potentially leads to reduced lung volumes and capacities. While general anesthesia is known to induce further changes in respiratory mechanics, regional anesthesia, spinal or epidural might influence the respiratory system significantly as well.

The pregnant patient is at greater risk for airway management problems and difficult intubation compared to the nonpregnant patient. Anatomical and physiologic factors that place the pregnant patient at increased risk for airway management complications and difficult intubation include pregnancy-induced weight gain, increase in breast size, respiratory tract mucosal edema, and decreased functional residual capacity. Elevated body mass index (BMI) has been associated with an increased risk of airway management problems including difficult intubation. [1-4] Thus, cesarean section, often requiring general anesthesia poses the parturient at greater risks.

Both weight gain and uterine enlargement, lead to an increase in abdominal circumference and cephalad displacement of the diaphragm. By midterm, this leads to a decrease in the expiratory reserve volume and residual volume, causing a decrease in functional residual capacity (FRC). The decreased FRC, combined with the increased oxygen consumption associated with pregnancy accounts for the tendency to rapidly develop hypoxemia during short periods of hypoventilation or apnea. [5-8] While anatomical changes account for an approximate 20% decrease in FRC, posture may contribute to another 25% reduction in FRC, particularly when moving from the sitting position to supine. The supine position induces further alterations in abdominal and chest anatomy, mechanical properties of breathing, and flow-volume patterns. Pain and fatigue of labor, which may be present in parturients presenting for cesarean section due to non-progressive labor, may exacerbate the decrease in FRC as well. Assuming the Trendelenburg position, often required for good surgical exposure, further aggravates normal physiology. While these alterations may or may not be significant in the awake patient, the induction of general anesthesia has overt clinical sequel on the respiratory system. A FRC decrease below closing capacity leads to airway collapse and shunting of deoxygenated blood across the lungs, contributing to further hypoxemia. [6] The impaired hypoxic pulmonary vasoconstriction caused by volatile anesthetics, may have further impact. Hormonal changes induced by pregnancy increase the subcostal angle of the ribs. The antero-posterior and transverse diameters of the thoracic cage increase resulting in only a small net decrease in total lung capacity. The work of breathing is increased in obese parturients due to increased chest wall weight and decreased chest wall compliance, leading to higher ventilatory requirements and increased oxygen demand, which may exceed 50%. [9,10] Lung compliance and total airway resistance, remain unchanged. Excess body weight increases oxygen consumption and CO_2 production in a linear fashion. Increased maternal metabolic and respiratory requirements combined with fetal metabolic needs result in increased maternal oxygen consumption and significantly shorten the safe time until maternal and fetal hypoxia develops [3,4,7].

Reduced chest wall compliance leads to difficulties with positive pressure ventilation, necessitating higher pressures to overcome reduced compliance. Vigorous mask ventilation may increase risk of stomach distention, and subsequent aspiration.

Airway

Controlling patient's airway remains a major responsibility of the anesthesiologist, while loss of control may have serious implications on morbidity and mortality of mother and fetus.

The parturient presenting for emergent cesarean section may arrive with little reserve, due to hemorrhage thus leaving little lax for dealing with loss of airway. Any additional hypoxia, may be deleterious to the fetus who is already compromised.

Pregnancy results in significant increase in breast size. In the supine position, the enlarged breasts tend to fall back against the neck, thus interfering with insertion of the laryngoscope and intubation. Therefore, use of a short-handled laryngoscope has been widely recommended in obstetric patients [4,7].

Vascular engorgement of the respiratory tract during pregnancy leads to edema of the nasal and oral pharynx, larynx, and trachea, resulting in bleeding at the time of airway manipulation or nasogastric tube placement, consequently usage of nasal airway is relatively contraindicated in pregnant patients.[6] Laryngeal edema may inhibit the passage of a standard size endotracheal tube, despite adequate vocal cord visualization upon laryngoscopy, requiring a smaller tube size. [4] Pregnant patients have elevated gastric acid content, with decreased pH, and reduced function of the gastroesophageal sphincter secondary to the mechanical and hormonal effects (predominantly progesterone) of pregnancy. [11] Gastric emptying is traditionally believed to be delayed in pregnant obese women, but this belief has been challenged, and recent studies demonstrate normal emptying times for fluids even in pregnant obese term parturients. [11] Studies performed on obese and non-obese pregnant women in labor not discriminating fluids from solids, showed that gastric volume in obese parturients was five times greater than in controls. [12-15] Acidic gastric content (whether elevated or not) predisposes patients to the development of severe pneumonitis in case of aspiration. Pain and stress, lead to activation of the sympathetic nervous system slowing gastric motility, and should therefore be avoided whenever possible. Despite all precautions, parturients with expected difficult airways should be given neuroaxial anesthesia when possible. When necessary, airway should be secured, adhering to the ASA difficult airway algorithm. [10] Current recommendations and guidelines advocate approaching parturients undergoing cesarean section as having full stomachs, requiring the known anesthetic precautions (rapid sequence induction, RSA). [3,4,7,11] Anesthesia should always be induced with application of cricoid pressure to decrease the risk of regurgitation of gastric contents in the pharynx. Denitrogenation with the administration of 100% oxygen is mandatory before rapid-sequence induction of general anesthesia [2].

Cardiovascular System

Late pregnancy is associated with unique adaptive changes in cardiovascular system. Those changes significantly affect course of perioperative period and shall be taken into consideration by anesthesiologist. Cardiac output increases as much as by 50 percent compared to non-pregnant condition. Twenty five percent to this elevation is contributed by elevation of stroke volume, while another 25% is a sequence of elevated heart rate. Elevated oxygen consumption and reduced myocardial perfusion time may exacerbate cardiovascular problems in compromised patients suffering from cardiovascular disease. Elevated circulating blood volume and anemia of pregnancy additionally contribute to this problem. Despite significantly increased cardiac output, arterial blood pressure remains unchanged or even decreases as a result of considerable decrease in systemic vascular resistance. Co-existing pregnancy-induced hypertension might further decrease cardiovascular reserve and precipitate heart failure.

Unlike the respiratory system, where pregnancy may offer some favorable effects in obese patients, the cardiovascular system is compromised and further stressed, in the event of these two coexisting states [12].

Pregnancy is associated with a significant reduction in systemic afterload. When pregnancy is associated with obesity, however, afterload reduction is significantly impaired due to increased peripheral resistance. [9] Volume load initially brings about left ventricular hypertrophy followed by subsequent myocardium dilation due to the increased pressure overload [12,16,17].

Increase in heart rate is a component of the elevated cardiac output, thereby decreasing the diastolic interval, thus shortening the myocardial perfusion time. Impaired myocardial diastolic relaxation leads to diastolic dysfunction. If fat deposition occurs in myocardial tissue, conduction and contractility may be seriously affected. Hence, it is not uncommon to encounter systolic, diastolic or combined systolic and diastolic dysfunction of the left ventricle. Right ventricular failure may be found be present in patients with pulmonary hypertension and OSA. [17,18] Congestive heart failure becomes clinically visible in the presence of any additional stress [19].

Subclinical right ventricular dysfunction in the overweight and obese population is present even in those without cardiac or sleep apnea problems. These subclinical changes add to the spectrum of overt clinical disorders of hypertension, ischemic heart disease, cardiomyopathy and heart failure. Hence careful assessment of the cardiovascular and respiratory systems is warranted [20].

Aorto-Caval compression, the well-known effect of an enlarged uterus compressing abdominal major vessels and causing supine hypotension syndrome, is common in the parturient presenting for cesarean-section. Assuming the supine position, a non-physiological position for the parturient, and the Trendelenburg position required for good surgical exposure contribute greatly to this syndrome.

Thrombo-embolic episodes remain one of the leading causes of direct maternal deaths. Surgical stress, bleeding, administration of blood products and clotting factors, immobilization may increase the risk significantly. Although data regarding the benefits of routine DVT prophylaxis for parturients undergoing cesarean section under general anesthesia is not firm, deep vein thrombosis prophylaxis, including both pharmacological (Heparin or Low molecular weight heparin) and mechanical (self-inflating device, IPC) strategies are advocated by some. [12,21] Parturients with elevated risks for thromboembolic events should be treated according to guidelines, taking into account their particular state and background. Regional anesthesia for cesarean-section in patients receiving DVT prophylaxis should be administered according to current guidelines [22-24].

Anesthesia Related Peripartum Mortality

A 2003 analysis of the ASA Closed Claims database revealed that 635 of the 5300 cases (12%) were associated with obstetric anesthesia care; 71% of these 635 cases were associated with cesarean section. The most common claim was maternal death (22%), which was more frequently associated with general anesthesia than regional anesthesia. Critical events involving the respiratory system were the most common precipitants of injury in these cases. [25] Respiratory system problems included difficult intubation, aspiration, esophageal intubation, inadequate ventilation/oxygenation, bronchospasm, airway obstruction, inadequate fractional inspired oxygen (FiO2), seizures, and problems with equipment. [10] Therefore, it is important to focus attention on the prevention and treatment of difficult airway in obstetric practice.

Maternal mortality rate is frequently regarded as a direct indicator of the health-care level of a nation. Estimated global maternal mortality is more than 500,000 per year. Nearly 99% of maternal mortality occurs in developing countries and 1% in developed ones [10].

Although infant mortality has declined steadily due to increased survival of preterm infants and prevention of sudden infant death syndrome, maternal mortality in the United Kingdom has remained approximately 7.5 maternal deaths per 100,000 live births over the last 15 years. The reason for the lack of improvement is unclear. Over half of maternal deaths are preventable - hemorrhage, pregnancy-induced hypertension, infection, and ectopic pregnancy (account for 59%). Anesthetic causes are numbered 6 on the list of causes for maternal mortality in the United States and UK and contribute to 3% of overall maternal mortality [26,27].

General anesthesia related death rates remained stable until 1990, [28,29] while the number of deaths associated with regional anesthesia declined markedly. [27,29] This occurred despite the fact that regional anesthesia was being used more often for cesarean delivery in virtually every hospital. [26,30,31] The decline in regional anesthetic related deaths occurred in the mid-80s, coinciding with the withdrawal of 0.75% bupivacaine and the increasing awareness of local anesthetic toxicity, and implementation of test dosing [30].

General anesthesia for obstetric patients carries greater risks for mother and fetus than does regional anesthesia. Team members involved in treatment should be made aware that the current low incidence of obstetric anesthesia complications is due predominantly to the increasing use of neuraxial anesthesia (including spinal and epidural ones), which is associated with 17-fold reduction in complication rates compared to general anesthesia. [32] Several factors affect the relative safety of regional vs. general anesthesia:

1. Decreased risk of aspiration due to maintenance if intact protective airway reflexes. The chances of developing severe, often lethal ARDS is greatly reduced compared to general anesthesia.
2. Since airway problems are the most common cause of anesthesia-related deaths, avoiding the need to manipulate the airway decreases these risks.
3. General anesthesia in obstetrics is often performed in emergencies, when preparation and examination of the patient are not optimal.
4. General anesthesia is used in patients who have failed regional anesthesia (e.g., obesity) or have contraindications to its use due to medical conditions (e.g., hemorrhage, HELLP syndrome).
5. Residency training programs may not provide residents with adequate exposure to general anesthesia on their obstetric rotations because anesthesiologists, patients, and obstetricians prefer regional anesthesia.
6. Selection bias: general anesthesia is often reserved for women with poor compliance or communication difficulties. Typically these patients suffer poor health conditions,

limited access to medical services, and lack proper medical observation during the pregnancy.

It would appear that maternal mortality will decrease further only by continuing to encourage the use of regional anesthesia and providing organized airway management programs for residents and practitioners so they are prepared for obstetric airway emergencies. [33] Further emphasis on airway management is justified, due to the fact that even some of the deaths during regional anesthesia are attributable to airway management complications. Several reports of death during regional anesthesia entail a "high" neuroaxial block, impairing adequate ventilation, followed by failed attempts to secure the airway, leading to hypoxia and/or aspiration.

While regional anesthesia is the mainstream approach, several circumstances warrant the preference of general anesthesia over regional anesthesia, such as hemorrhage accompanied by hemodynamic instability or umbilical cord prolapse. Recent data suggest a mortality rate was of only 2.8-17 per *million* general anesthetics. [34] This number is expected to decrease as additional tools for managing difficult airways (laryngeal mask airway, fiber optic devices, camera assisted laryngoscopes, etc.) become more widely available, and the American Society of Anesthesiologists (ASA) Difficult Airway Algorithm becomes familiar to all practitioners [31].

Minimizing the Risk for Anesthetic Caused Maternal Mortality

Difficult Airway

The incidence of failed intubation in obstetric patients is 1:280 while the incidence of failed intubation in the general population undergoing elective surgery is 1:2,230. [31] All anesthesia providers should be familiar with the ASA Difficult Airway Algorithm [35-38].

Placement of "prophylactic regional anesthesia" is recommended when a difficult airway is anticipated. [39] Timely preparation requires that all patients be screened for a predictive difficult airway, and a continuous epidural or spinal catheter should be inserted as soon as the parturient has committed to delivery. In the event of fetal distress or other reason mandating emergent proceeding to the operating room, regional anesthesia can be provided expediently. Since in most institutions, obstetricians and midwives interact with the parturient earlier in the birthing process, they should be aware and warn an anesthesiologist when they recognize or suspect a parturient with a difficult airway or, when a woman has documented history of difficult airway in the past. Obstetric staff should be familiar with signs of predictable difficult airway, be knowledgeable about the risks of airway complications and should involve an anesthesiologist as early as possible when such a suspicion exists, providing extra time to provide a regional anesthetic or to secure the airway. [40] Aspiration prophylaxis should be administered to any patient with a potentially difficult airway as soon as operative delivery is anticipated. Medications for aspiration prophylaxis are discussed later at this chapter. It shall be noted that it may take an hour for maximum effectiveness if intubation is necessary. General anesthesia should not be attempted alone, and experienced "extra hands" should be available at induction of general anesthesia.

The ACOG's committee opinion states that obstetricians should obtain an early consultation with an anesthesiologist in high-risk patients, particularly those with a potentially difficult airway, so that the anesthesiologist can properly prepare the patient for anesthesia. [41] ACOG's committee opinion entitled "Anesthesia for Emergency Deliveries" recommends that strategies be developed to minimize the need for emergency induction of general anesthesia in women for whom it would be hazardous. Patients at risk for whom cesarean delivery is anticipated, planned placement of an epidural catheter should be considered in early labor, with confirmation that the catheter is functional.

Mutual attempts of anesthesiologists, obstetricians and midwives to recognize difficult airways in advance, may decrease the risks involved with unprepared dealing with an unrecognized difficult airway, and are more likely to be successful when conducted in advance, without urgency [32].

Gastric Content Aspiration

This complication remains one of the leading causes of death in obstetric anesthesia, frequently associated with difficult or failed intubation. Risk for aspiration is increased significantly during pregnancy as a result of the combined effect of progesterone on gastric empting, decreased tonus of the lower esophageal sphincter and direct pressure of the gravid uterus [11].

This life-threatening complication may be prevented in several ways. Risk of aspiration is obviously lower when regional anesthetic techniques are applied, compared with general anesthesia. Rarely, aspiration can occur during a high spinal, high epidural block or development of local anesthetic toxicity. Decreasing the volume and acidity of gastric contents pharmacologically has been advocated, but there are no outcome studies to prove that this is beneficial. In parturients with no contraindications, minimizing the risk of aspiration per-se by applying neuraxial anesthesia is preferable. Both the ASA *Practice Guidelines for Obstetrical* Anesthesia [39] and several American College of Obstetricians and Gynecologists statements support modest amounts of clear liquids in labor but oppose any intake of solid foods. [42-46] The ASA Guidelines go on to say, "patients with additional risk factors of aspiration (e.g., morbid obesity, diabetes, difficult airway) or patients at increased risk for operative delivery (e.g., non-reassuring fetal heart rate pattern) may have further restrictions of oral intake, determined on a case-by-case basis." Parturients who are planned for elective cesarean-section, should adhere to the accepted pre-operative guidelines, even when neuraxial anesthesia is planned.

Local Anesthetic Toxicity

Local anesthetic toxicity is the leading cause of death during regional anesthesia; [31] however, its occurrence has decreased markedly in the last decade. Newer local anesthetics such as ropivacaine and levobupivacaine may have a better safety profile than bupivacaine, but their place in obstetric anesthesia remains unclear. Lidocaine remains the amide local anesthetic drug bearing the best safety profile, although of limited use in single shot spinal anesthesia. Prevention of local anesthetic toxicity is based on incremental dosing and injecting a "test dose." The "test dose" is usually comprised of small amount of local anesthetic (3 ml of 2% lidocaine or 0.5% bupivacaine) with or without addition of epinephrine.

High spinal or epidural block: A misplaced or displaced catheter may cause inadvertent injection of an epidural intended volume into the subarachnoid space. Probably the best indicator of a subarachnoid injection is the speed onset and block depth. If the laboring patient is comfortable within one contraction, the catheter is in the CSF until proven otherwise. The Trendelenburg position required for surgical exposure, may impact the spread of local anesthetic, both in subdural and epidural spaces. [47] Posture, as well as baricity of local anesthetic was found to impact spread and level of block, with hypobaric bupivacaine in the sitting position producing the highest rate of hypotension and cervical blocks. [48] Thus, when changing patients' position intraoperatively, one should consider whether local anesthetic is isobaric, hypobaric or hyperbaric. As noted earlier, airway management equipment, vasopressors and resuscitation fluids must be readily available.

A "complete" spinal poses two major problems: i) Hemodynamic instability: a drastic decrease in preload and an empty heart causing hypotension and decreased cardiac output. ii) Respiratory dysfunction: paralysis of the respiratory muscles leading to hypoxia and aspiration.

The mainstay of treatment is supportive i.e. airway management, mechanical ventilation support, fluids, vasopressors, left uterine displacement, and elevation of the legs to promote venous return and improve cardiac output.

Oxytocin

The principal clinical uses of oxytocin are to induce labor at term and to counter uterine hypotonicity and decrease hemorrhage in the postpartum or postabortion period. Nevertheless use of this drug in patients with blunted cardiovascular reflexes, such as under regional or general anesthesia, may elicit serious side effects. High doses of oxytocin produce a direct relaxant effect on vascular smooth muscles that manifests as a decrease in systolic and diastolic blood pressure and the appearance of flushing. Reflex tachycardia and increased cardiac output accompany the transient decrease in systemic blood pressure. A marked decrease in blood pressure, however, may occur if oxytocin is administered to patients with blunted compensatory reflex responses, as may be produced by anesthesia. Likewise, hypovolemic patients may be particularly susceptible to oxytocin-induced hypotension [49].

Following the 1997–1999 "Confidential Enquiry Report" majority of anesthesiologists have changed their practice, from using a single intravenous bolus injection of 10 units of oxytocin to using the recommended dose of 5 units [50].

Many anesthesiologists promote use of oxytocin only in a continuous drip rather than small bolus doses. This may be perceived as a conflict of interest arising between obstetricians and anesthesiologists, the former preoccupied with maintenance of uterus and decreasing post-partum bleeding, and the latter concerned about maintaining cardiovascular stability. These two approaches are not incompatible, and both concerns are in many instances important factors in maintaining cardiovascular stability and maternal well-being. In otherwise stable patients, uterine tone should initially be stimulated by slow administration of intravenous 5 IU oxytocin, maintaining cardiovascular stability and thereafter maintained by continuous infusion of oxytocin, intramuscular administration of ergometrine and intramuscular carboprost as necessary [34].

Obesity

The health risks of obese women dramatically increase during the antepartum and peripartum periods. In Why Mothers Die 2000–2002, 35% of all the women who died were obese, 50% more than in the general population [20,34,51]. Analysis of maternal mortality in the UK in 2003-2005 revealed that of 150 cases of maternal death, six women died from direct anesthetic causes, and in 31 additional cases, poor perioperative anesthetic management may have contributed to the outcome. Obesity was a factor in four of these women who died. Two of these six deaths were in women in early pregnancy, who received general anesthesia for gynecological surgery by inexperienced anesthesiologists who failed to manage the airway and provide adequate ventilation. When trainee anesthesiologists are relatively inexperienced their consultants must be aware of the limits of their competence, and provide close supervision and help. In the 31 deaths in which anesthetic management contributed to the outcome, obesity was again a relevant factor. [34,51] Based on the collected data, authors of the report concluded that in obese parturients the next steps may contribute to decrease in the risk of mortality:

- All obstetric units should develop protocols for the management of morbidly obese women. These should include pre-assessment procedures, special community, ward and operating theatre equipment such as large sphygmomanometer cuffs, hoists, beds and operating tables and long regional block needles.
- Morbidly obese women should be referred for anesthetic assessment and advice as part of their antenatal care. [1,52]
- Management by consultant anesthetists is essential.
- Difficulties with airway management and intubation should be anticipated. [53] No manipulation on airway in case of expected difficult airway shall be undertaken by trainee without supervision and help of attending anesthesiologist experienced in management of difficult airway [54].
- Positioning the patient requires skill and sufficient manpower in the event of a need for induction of general anesthesia.
- Direct arterial pressure measurement may be useful in the morbidly obese women where sphygmomanometry is often inaccurate.
- All morbidly obese women in childbirth should be given prophylactic low molecular weight heparin and the duration of therapy needs to be determined in view of likely immobility. Thromboembolic stockings of appropriate size need to be available [34].

In another retrospective analysis of outcome in morbidly obese patients authors found that although successful epidural anesthesia was equally likely for both obese and non-obese parturients, morbidly obese patients required more repeat placements of epidural catheters to achieve success. [55] The first placement attempt epidural catheters failed in 42% of morbidly obese parturients, but in only 6% of control patients. Three accidental dural punctures occurred in the morbidly obese group, and none occurred in the control group.

The rate of difficult intubation was significantly higher in the obese as compared to the control group. [55] Authors concluded that performing successful epidural or spinal anesthesia in morbidly obese parturients was difficult. Misidentification of appropriate landmarks and anatomic distortion contributed to high initial failure rate.

However careful insertion and replacement of questionable epidural catheters produced improved regional anesthesia success rate for morbidly obese patients [55].

Analysis of maternal mortality in Michigan in 1985-2003 revealed that of 855 pregnancy-associated deaths, eight cases were anesthesia related deaths and seven cases were anesthesia-contributed deaths. [56] There were no deaths during induction of general anesthesia. Five resulted from hypoventilation or airway obstruction during emergence, extubation, or recovery. Lapses in either postoperative monitoring or anesthesiology supervision seemed to contribute to 5 of the 8 anesthesia-related deaths. Other characteristics common to these cases included obesity (n = 6) and African-American race (n = 6). Four of eight cases were related to airway problems on emergency from general anesthesia, four other cases were related to high spinal anesthesia, leading to respiratory and cardiac arrest as a result of spinal or epidural anesthesia. Again, obesity figured in six of eight of anesthesia related deaths, indicating that obesity is an important contributing factor for anesthesia related maternal mortality.

Obese women continue to face unacceptably high risk for anesthesia related mortality. [56] Results of the study lead the authors to conclude that the following actions might further reduce mortality: (1) recognize the relatively high potential for anesthetic disaster during emergence and recovery from general anesthesia; (2) ensure appropriate monitoring throughout the perioperative period, particularly for postoperative hypoventilation and airway obstruction; (3) use strategies to maximize safety for obese and morbidly obese women; and (4) advocate for workforce policies that ensure appropriate involvement of anesthesiologists in developing clinical protocols and in delivering patient care [56].

Approach to the Airway in the Obstetric Population

Airway Assessment in the Obstetric Population

Nearly two thirds of the cesarean-sections present as an emergent cesarean section. [57] General anesthesia for cesarean section, often in the setting of fetal distress, is the most common indication for endotracheal intubation in the obstetric patient. [58] However, a failed regional technique, high spinal or high epidural block, local anesthetic toxicity, cardiac arrest, and respiratory and neurological emergencies may each result in the need for endotracheal intubation. Therefore, airway evaluation is paramount in the preoperative evaluation. Airway assessment must be performed irrespective of kind of anesthesia has been chosen. [59] Some advocate, that all patients on the labor floor should undergo an airway assessment examination upon admission. The American College of Obstetricians and Gynecologists recommends that the obstetric care team should "be alert" for the general anesthesia risk factors, and if present, specialist consultation should be obtained, and consideration be given for the placement of an epidural catheter in early labor [60,61]. In assessing the obstetric airway it is important to take into account maternal congenital abnormalities; for example, Noonan syndrome, Pierre Robin syndrome, hereditary telangiectasia, and neurofibromatosis. Important acquired maternal conditions include preeclampsia, morbid obesity, and obstructive sleep apnea.

Both congenital and acquired conditions may contribute to the difficult obstetric airway.

Anatomical features associated with difficult intubation include: facial edema, swollen tongue, obesity and short neck, limited flexion and/or extension in cervical spine, short thyromental distance (less than 6.5 cm), limited mouth opening, dentition- protruding maxillary incisors, missing teeth, receding mandible, short neck, limited oropharyngeal view (Mallampaty class 3-4). [3,10,62] It is of interest to note that neck circumference (more than 40 cm), and not BMI, is more predictive of a difficult intubation in morbidly obese patients [57].

Mallampati grading is performed with the patient in upright position. The patient is asked to open her mouth and protrude the tongue maximally without phonation. The oropharyngeal structures are visualized and classified as follows: class I-soft palate, fauces, uvula, and tonsillar pillars; class II- soft palate and fauces seen, tip of uvula obscured; class III- soft palate and only base of tongue seen; and class IV- soft palate not visible. [62] Although widely utilized, Mallampati grading has been shown to have low sensitivity, moderate specificity, and very low positive predictive value [62].

However, among obstetric patients, the combination of Mallampati score and thyromental distance has been shown to have a sensitivity of 100% and positive predictive value of 61.5% for prediction of difficult laryngoscopy [9].

Certain anatomical features may also render mask ventilation difficult or impossible. They include very large breasts and heavy chest wall, obesity, obstructive sleep apnea, large tongue, no teeth and sunken cheeks, limited head or neck flexion, massive jaw, upper airway mass [3].

Management of Recognized Difficult Airway

The principal decision algorithm in case of recognized difficult airway is offered in figure 1 [10].

If there is any doubt regarding the ability to maintain airway patency during general anesthesia, alternative methods of anesthesia should be considered. Options include the use of regional anesthesia, local infiltration anesthesia, or, if there is adequate time, an awake intubation followed by induction of general anesthesia.

Regional anesthesia: The ongoing debate of general versus regional neuraxial anesthesia, regarding major maternal and neonatal outcomes in the general population has not been decided upon, and recent data suggests both approaches are safe. [63-66] Nevertheless, data suggest that regional anesthesia is the best choice for cesarean section in most cases of anticipated difficulty with endotracheal intubation. [67,68] All regional techniques including spinal, epidural or combined spinal-epidural anesthesia are acceptable providing there is no contraindication. All the techniques allow the mother to be awake and minimize the potential for hypoxia and gastric acid aspiration. [69] However, the anesthesiologist should understand that regional anesthesia itself does not solve the problem of a difficult airway, anticipate potential complications (*e.g.,* failed anesthesia, total spinal anesthesia), and be fully prepared (both mentally and technically) to administer general anesthesia, and therefore to perform tracheal intubation in suboptimal emergent conditions and urgently deal with difficult airway. [4,7] All necessary equipment and drugs must be immediately available, including the recommended equipment for difficult intubation.

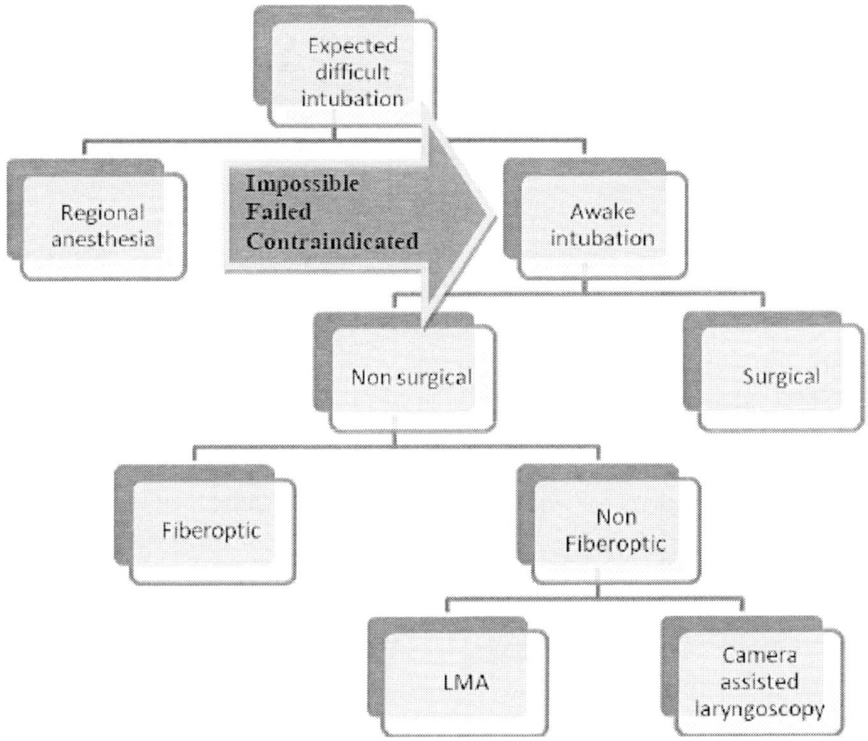

Figure 1. Expected difficult intubation algorithm. Adapted from Vasdev, G. M., B. A. Harrison, et al. (2008). "Management of the difficult and failed airway in obstetric anesthesia." J Anesth 22(1): 38-48. According to American Society of Anesthesiology guidelines.

Hawksworth and Purdie described a patient with a failed combined spinal epidural technique who failed an endotracheal intubation, and was then woken up and underwent an awake fiberoptic intubation. [70] This is one of many case reports illustrating the potential difficulties of regional anesthesia. When deciding upon the regional technique, it is important to select the technique that minimizes the potential for airway, cardiac, and respiratory emergencies for the individual parturient. When anesthesia is administered by an anesthesiologist inexperienced in the management of obstetric regional anesthesia and difficult airway, consultation with an obstetric anesthesiologist is strongly recommended [10].

Nausea and vomiting are common complications during administration of regional anesthesia for cesarean section. In addition, in the event of a failed block, general anesthesia may be required. Therefore, all patients should receive pharmacologic prophylaxis against gastric acid aspiration. [69] All patients should also receive supplemental oxygen during administration of spinal or epidural anesthesia for cesarean section. The increased maternal fractional inspired oxygen concentration increases fetal oxygenation. [3,71] Additionally, good oxygenation during the case may prolong safe time in case a complication develops leading to loss of airway and hypoxia.

Some anesthesiologists prefer awake fiberoptic intubation over regional anesthesia in the predicted difficult airway parturient. They argue that the use of regional anesthesia in a patient with an expected difficult airway does not solve the airway problem, and regional anesthesia related problems may lead to an emergency difficult airway situation [10].

Local anesthesia. Local anesthetic infiltration is warranted as the primary anesthetic technique, when patients with a predicted difficult airway which have a contraindication to the use of spinal or epidural anesthesia, require urgent cesarean section. However, local anesthetic infiltration is a technique rarely used today for cesarean section in developed countries. This technique requires skillful surgery, patient compliance and time. It is more often used in undeveloped countries with an inadequate number of experienced anesthesia providers and/or limited anesthesia equipment and supplies [3].

Awake Intubation Followed by General Anesthesia

Awake intubation is considered a safe approach for management of anticipated difficult airways. In this approach, the airway is secured by insertion of an ETT while the patient remains awake. [3,7] Although awake intubation can be somewhat time-consuming, there are several compelling reasons to perform the procedure in a patient with a recognized difficult airway: 1) the natural airway is better maintained in an awake patient; 2) the presence of normal muscle tone helps maintain the natural separation of the upper airway structures, which facilitates the identification of anatomical landmarks; and 3) induction of general anesthesia and muscle paralysis results in anterior movement of the larynx, which impedes visualization of the larynx during direct laryngoscopy.

Successful awake endotracheal intubation requires proper preparation of the patient. Ideal preparation results in a quiet and cooperative patient and a larynx that is non-reactive to physical stimuli. The first step is psychological preparation. The patient who knows what is going to happen is usually more receptive and cooperative. Minimal monitoring should include the use of an automated blood pressure cuff, pulse oximetry, and electrocardiogram. Supplemental oxygen should be administered at all times during the procedure.

Administration of an anticholinergic drying agent (*e.g.*, glycopyrrolate) allows better application of local anesthetic spray to the airway mucosa, improves visualization, and inhibits vagal reflexes. Glycopyrrolate is poorly transferred across the placenta, and its maternal administration does not result in a detectable fetal hemodynamic response. Judicious use of intravenous (IV) sedation helps relieve anxiety and increases the pain threshold in an awake patient. This situation facilitates patient tolerance of the application of the topical anesthetic as well as the performance of nerve blocks and endotracheal intubation. It is essential to titrate analgesic and sedative drugs carefully so as to maintain continual verbal communication between the anesthesiologist and the patient. Midazolam is the benzodiazepine recommended for these purposes. To date, no adverse fetal effects have been reported [3,7].

Topical anesthesia is the primary anesthetic for awake intubation. In some patients, topical anesthesia is the only anesthetic needed, provided sufficient time is allowed to anesthetize all portions of the airway adequately. Blockade of the internal branch of the superior laryngeal nerve represents a second upper airway nerve block that is a helpful supplement to the use of topical anesthesia and block of the lingual branch of the glossopharyngeal nerve. This block consists of application of local anesthetic superficial or deep to the thyrohyoid membrane between the superior lateral cornu of the thyroid cartilage and the inferior lateral margin of the cornu of the hyoid bone. In obese parturients it may be difficult to perform this block, because the landmarks might be often obscured. [7] Transtracheal administration of local anesthetic (administered through the cricothyroid membrane) may also be performed easily. Cough effectively spreads local anesthetic in the trachea and subglotic area.

There is some controversy as to the appropriate use and extent of local anesthesia for awake intubation in a patient with a presumed full stomach. Block of the superior larynx may theoretically allow food and water to enter the trachea during deglutition. Some researchers have recommended that airway anesthesia be limited to the transtracheal injection of local anesthetic in patients with a full stomach. However, many studies showed that appliance of superior laryngeal nerve block in the patients with full stomach had not led to any case of aspiration during awake intubation [10].

The key to evade aspiration is to avoid oversedation; *i.e.,* there is a low-risk of aspiration of gastric contents in an awake, alert, and rational patient, regardless of the extent of topical anesthesia. Attempts to ventilate the patients with positive pressure lead to inflation of stomach, and in turn, significantly increase the risk of regurgitation and aspiration. The risk of aspiration in an awake locally anesthetized patient can be further minimized by IV administration of an H2-receptor antagonist, metoclopramide and oral administration of a nonparticulate antacid before beginning the procedure. [69] H2-receptor antagonists block histamine receptors on the oxyntic cells, thus decreasing gastric acid production. When given IV, H2-receptor antagonists are effective within 30 minutes, but 30 to 60 minutes are required for maximal effect. Metoclopramide is a procainamide derivative that is a cholinergic agonist peripherally and a dopamine receptor antagonist centrally. A 10-mg IV dose of metoclopramide increases lower esophageal sphincter tone and reduces gastric volume by increasing gastric peristalsis. Metoclopramide can have a significant effect on gastric volume in as little as 15 minutes. Metoclopramide crosses the placenta, but researchers have reported no significant effects on the fetus. Oral administration of sodium citrate at dose of 30 ml of 0.3M solution may be used for neutralization of acidity, but is known to increase volume of gastric content. H2 antagonists cimetidine and ranitidine effectively decrease secretion of acid and therefore increasing pH of gastric content, but it takes much time to achieve desired effect.

The major impediments to success are significant amounts of blood or secretions and lack of patient preparation and cooperation. The fiberoptic bronchoscope/laryngoscope can aspirate only small amounts of secretions. It may be recommended to insufflate oxygen through the suction port. The insufflation blows secretions away from the tip of the bronchoscope, which facilitates optimal visualization of the anatomical structures of the airway. Insufflation of oxygen through the suction port also serves as a defogging mechanism, and it provides supplemental oxygen, which results in a higher FIO2 for the patient. Immersion of the tip of the bronchoscope into warm saline (or antifog solution) before insertion into the patient also decreases fogging. Extension of the cervical spine provides the optimal position for performance of fiberoptic laryngoscopy. Extension tilts the larynx anteriorly and lifts the epiglottis off the posterior pharyngeal wall. Bit protector shall be always used to prevent injury to fiberoptic scope.

An appropriately sized, well-lubricated ETT is placed over the bronchoscope before its insertion. Once the fiberoptic bronchoscope is passed into the trachea, the ETT is threaded off the fiberoptic bronchoscope, the bronchoscope is withdrawn, the ETT adaptor is reattached, and the ETT is connected to the breathing circuit. Even with the fiberoptic bronchoscope in the correct position, the ETT may not always follow easily into the trachea because the right arytenoid or right vocal cord may obstruct the ETT as it is passed off the fiberoptic bronchoscope. This problem is corrected by withdrawing the tube slightly and then rotating it 90 degrees counterclockwise so that the bevel tip is at 12 o'clock. After the ETT has been passed over the fiberoptic bronchoscope into the trachea, the distance between the carina and the tip of the ETT should be noted to ensure proper positioning of the tube.[3] The gold standard for verification of proper position of ETT is direct visualization of carina with bronchoscope ensuring that the tip of the ETT is located 3-4 cm above carina.

Management of Unrecognized Difficult Airway

In the event of an unsuccessful intubation, the anesthesiologist should have a well-formulated plan in mind, and the appropriate equipment and supplies should be immediately available to implement that plan. Practice Guidelines for Obstetrical Anesthesia developed by the ASA state that the availability of equipment for the management of airway emergencies is associated with reduced incidence of maternal complications. Practice Guidelines recommend that labor and delivery units have equipment and personnel readily available to manage airway emergencies. Basic airway management equipment should be immediately available during the provision of regional anesthesia. In addition, portable equipment for difficult airway management should be readily available in the operative area of labor and delivery units.

The principal decision algorithm in case of unrecognized difficult airway is offered in figure 2 [10].

When intubation is difficult, as demonstrated by the laryngeal view, or when there is failure to intubate, mask ventilation must be attempted to ensure oxygenation and ventilation. One should be aware that serious complications develop as a result of hypoxia rather a result of inability to intubate the patient. [72] Because of the increased weight in pregnancy, and oro-pharygeal edema, mask ventilation can be difficult. Oral airways are introduced to improve the efficiency of mask ventilation. Nasal airways can also be utilized, but the increased vascularity of the nasal mucosa increases the potential for bleeding. Manipulation of the airway with the aim of improving the seal of the mask is important. Many algorithms and authors suggest that two people may be necessary, one to maintain a seal of the mask and airway while the other (less experienced provider) ventilates the patient. [10] It is advocated that cricoid pressure be maintained while this is occurring. If mask ventilation is inadequate with cricoid pressure, the cricoid pressure should be relieved to see if ventilation improves.

The first step in the difficult or failed obstetric airway is to maintain oxygenation and ventilation through bag mask ventilation. [72] Once this first essential step has been performed, further assessment of the maternal and fetal status is undertaken. The obstetric team should guide the anesthesiologist regarding the necessity for immediate or nonurgent delivery of the baby. [10] If there is no fetal distress, the patient is hemodynamically stable, there is adequate gas exchange *via* mask, and only one anesthesiologist has attempted

Percutaneous insertion of a large-gauge IV catheter through the cricothyroid membrane is simple, quick, and relatively safe in most patients. This technique represents an effective method to facilitate TTJV in the desperate situation in which the patient cannot be intubated or ventilated by mask. Compared with emergency surgical cricothyrotomy or tracheostomy, establishment of percutaneous TTJV is quicker, simpler, and more efficacious. This technique permits continuous, uninterrupted oxygenation while allowing unhurried access to secure the patient's airway. First, the cricothyroid membrane is palpated with the neck of the patient extended. Then a 14-gauge IV catheter is used to puncture the cricothyroid membrane with the needle pointed 30 degrees caudal from the perpendicular. A 20 mL syringe is then attached to the catheter, and aspiration of air confirms its transtracheal location. The needle stylet is then removed, and the catheter is advanced into the trachea until the hub of the catheter is at the skin line. The TTJV catheter should be reaspirated to reconfirm intratracheal lumen location. The hub of the IV catheter is then connected to a TTJV system. A designated individual should be responsible for holding the hub of the TTJV catheter secure to the skin. During TTJV, it is important to maintain the natural airway by using bilateral jaw thrust and oropharyngeal and nasopharyngeal airways to allow for exhalation of inspired gas and to prevent air trapping and lung hyperinflation. If TTJV system is not available, insufflation of 100% oxygen via the catheter at high flow makes possible to maintain certain level of oxygenation until the patient will start breathing spontaneously.

Open cricothyrotomy should be considered the last resort maneuver, in case of failed-airway. Surgical assistance should always be summoned or available if these procedures are performed by non-surgeons. The call for surgical assistance must occur early in the management of the difficult airway so that assistance will be available at the appropriate time [3,4,7].

Anesthesia and Analgesia for Cesarean Section and Postoperative Pain

Regional Anesthesia for Cesarean Delivery

Cesarean section is an independent risk factor for both maternal and neonatal morbidity and mortality. [73] Surgical access may be difficult, while the semi-recumbent rather than supine position may need to be maintained in order to ensure adequate ventilation. Cesarean delivery, particularly when associated with placenta previa, vasa previa and placenta accreta which may involve significant bleeding, can cause severe cardiovascular compromise. Regional anesthesia and the associated vasoplegia and sympathetic block may induce cardiovascular instability disproportional to blood loss. Close liaison between obstetric and anesthetic teams is required.

Regional anesthetic techniques remain the most commonly used and preferred techniques for caesarean delivery. They include single shot spinal, epidural and combined spinal-epidural anesthesia [74].

Single shot spinal anesthesia offers the advantage of dense reliable block with rapid onset. Consequent paralysis of intercostal muscles, along with assumption of the supine position and cephaled retraction of viscera, may compound cardiovascular compromise and provoke respiratory failure [12]. Other relevant issues include technical difficulties, potential for high blockade, and the inability to prolong the blockade. Spinal anesthesia causes a BMI-dependent decrease in lung function of both pregnant and nonpregnant obese females. An attempt to adjust the intrathecal dose according to height and weight resulted in less maternal hypotension but a lengthy onset time for adequate sensory blockade. This delay may be critical in emergency scenarios.

A dense regional block to the level of the fourth thoracic dermatome is required for caesarean section and may aggravate cardiovascular compromise.

Technical difficulties are the same as those for locating the epidural space. However, it is often easier to identify the epidural space with a large gauge stiff epidural needle than with a smaller gauge flexible spinal needle. Many anesthesiologists use an epidural needle as an introducer for a spinal needle in difficult cases.

It is widely accepted that local anesthetic requirements (as well as general anesthetics requirements) are decreased in pregnant patients. [75] Proposed mechanisms for the enhanced neural blockade in pregnancy include hormone-related changes in the action of spinal cord neurotransmitters, potentiation of the analgesic effect of endogenous analgesic systems, increased permeability of the neural sheath or other pharmacokinetic / dynamic differences. Both pregnancy and obesity increase intra-abdominal pressure and cause compression of the inferior vena cava, which leads to engorgement of the epidural venous plexus and increased epidural space pressure. This in turn reduces the volume of cerebrospinal fluid in the subarachnoid space. Compared with spinal anesthesia, epidural anesthesia offers several advantages, including an easily titratable local anesthetic dose and level of anesthesia, ability to extend the block for prolonged surgery, slower hemodynamic changes which are better controlled, decreased risk for excess motor blockade, and utilization of the catheter for postoperative analgesia. [76,77] However, clear cut evidence regarding the superiority of one over the other remains undecided. [78-81] The height of blockade for a given volume of local anesthetic agent is proportional to BMI and weight but not height. [82] The decreased volume of the epidural space, for reasons discussed above, may contribute to excessive spread of local anesthetic agents in obese parturients [83].

Extending existing labor epidural analgesia for caesarean section requires the addition of a local anesthetic agent at higher concentrations. Both 2% lidocaine and 0.5% bupivacaine may be useful for this purpose. The optimum dose for this remains undetermined, but data suggest that speed of onset calls for use of lidocaine and quality of block advocates the use of bupivacaine [84].

Prevention of local anesthetic toxicity is centered on incremental dosing and the introduction of a "test dose." The "test dose", comprising of a small volume of local anesthetic (3 ml of 2% lidocaine or 0.5% bupivacaine) is usually used with or without addition of epinephrine.

Epinephrine may detect inadvertent injection of the solution into a blood vessel by the appearance of maternal tachycardia. Concerns have been expressed that it may be difficult to differentiate epinephrine induced tachycardia from pain and contraction tachycardia. The effect of epinephrine on maternal-placental circulation has not been clearly elucidated. [31] Early signs of sympathetic (decrease of blood pressure) or motor block (weakness in lower extremities) after injection of the test-dose of local anesthetic may be a positive sign of inadvertent injection into subarachnoid space. A gentle careful aspiration should be attempted before injection of local anesthetic into epidural space. Appearance of CSF or blood in epidural catheter necessitates repositioning of the catheter. Injection of local anesthetic into epidural space should be performed gradually in incremental doses of about five to seven ml.

Single-shot spinal anesthesia is the most popular anesthetic technique practiced worldwide for cesarean section. Combined spinal-epidural technique is a reasonable alternative, combining the advantages of rapid onset and dense block with the ability to prolong the block when the surgery is technically difficult and use postoperatively. Furthermore, use of smaller doses of local anesthetic agent intrathecally, may circumvent the problems of sudden onset of hypotension. [9] However, the technical challenge of correctly placing an epidural catheter remains [12].

General Anesthesia for Cesarean Section

As mentioned previously, regional anesthesia is the preferred anesthetic approach for cesarean section in the obese patient, albeit current data does not unequivocally demonstrate this advantage in the general population. [62-66,74] Several situations preclude use of neuraxial blockade such as patient refusal or definite or relative contraindications to neuraxial blocks, and mandate the induction of general anesthesia.

In an otherwise normal airway, administration of general anesthesia begins with effective denitrogenation of the lungs, as since the combination of decreased FRC and increased oxygen consumption lead to rapid desaturation when patient is apneic. Denitrogenation can be performed by either 3 min of tidal breathing with 100% oxygen or by four maximal breaths with 100% oxygen. There is little evidence to support one technique over the other. [12] Hence, it is reasonable that urgency of cesarean section dictates the technique of denitrogenation.

The choice of intravenous induction agent is relatively unimportant if there are no co-existing medical problems. In the event of repeated dosing, special attention should be given, due to prolonged elimination. An induction dose of 4-5 mg/kg providing good intubation conditions is recommended for cesarean section. The pharmacokinetics of propofol remain relatively unchanged in obese patients, and initial dosing should be calculated according to lean body weight [9].

Succinylcholine remains the muscle relaxant of choice for intubation. It is recommended that anesthesiologists administer succinylcholine according to total rather than lean body weight in adult patients. The dose of succinylcholine 1.5-2 mg/kg up to a maximum of 200 mg is reasonable and this dose is higher than recommended to nonpregnant patient due to increased volume of distribution. [12] Both depolarizing and non depolarizing muscle relaxants (NDMR) are ionized and do not readily cross the placenta. Administration of NMDR facilitates mechanical ventilation and provides adequate surgical relaxation.

Tracheal intubation should be confirmed by the repetitive and characteristic capnographic waveform in addition to auscultation. One lung intubation should be promptly recognized and corrected to avoid intra- and postoperative pulmonary complications. In the event of failure to intubate the trachea after rapid sequence induction, it is imperative to institute a failed intubation drill without delay. Repeated attempts and a second dose of succinylcholine are seldom beneficial and often detrimental. The primary objective in the management of failed intubation is to ensure adequate maternal oxygenation despite the concerns of fetal well-being or risk of regurgitation. The detailed discussion of appropriate treatment of difficult airway and failed intubation and ventilation is discussed earlier in this chapter.

Various techniques such as greater tidal volumes, high inspired oxygen concentration and PEEP have been used to maintain adequate oxygenation. In high-risk cases, emptying of the stomach and administration of sodium citrate via an orogastric tube before extubation may be helpful. In order to prevent aspiration of gastric content, extubation should be attempted only when the patient is awake and alert, with adequate reversal of neuromuscular blockade. All protective airway reflexes must be restored. A 30 degrees head-up tilt is a more favorable position for extubation than supine in the obese population.

Most commonly, use of intraoperative opiates is delayed until extraction the fetus, to minimize the effects of systemic opiates, which readily cross the placenta, on the newborn. More recently, there has been interest regarding the use of remifentanil in obstetric anesthesia and analgesia, due to its unique pharmacologic attributes. [85,86], although data regarding routine use of this agent is still scarce [87,88].

Postoperative Care

Analysis of maternal mortality in Michigan in 1985-2003 revealed that five of eight of deaths directly related to anesthesia resulted from hypoventilation or airway obstruction during emergence, extubation, or recovery and were a direct sequence of lapses in either postoperative monitoring or anesthetic supervision. [56] The majority of these patients were obese. Therefore, the importance of proper monitoring and adequate observation in postoperative period in obese patients cannot be overemphasized.

Parturients are at increased risk of postoperative complications such as hypoxemia, atelectasis and pneumonia, deep vein thrombosis and pulmonary embolism, pulmonary edema, and postpartum cardiomyopathy. Early mobilization, DVT prophylaxis, aggressive chest physiotherapy and adequate pain control are the key to the success of effective postoperative care. Early mobilization has been shown to improve the respiratory volumes in the immediate postoperative phase.

Computerized tomography has demonstrated that obesity predisposes to the formation of pulmonary atelectasis per se and even more so under general anesthesia, persisting into the postoperative period. Moreover, following spinal anesthesia, there is a BMI dependent decrease in respiratory function [89].

When the patient suffers from OSA and uses a continuous positive airway pressure device during her night sleep, use of same equipment in postoperative period in order to improve respiratory function is advocated [90].

Thrombo-embolic episodes remain one of the leading causes of direct maternal deaths. Both pharmacological and mechanical strategies are used for DVT prophylaxis and an adequate dose of an anticoagulant for an appropriate duration is recommended.

Postoperative Analgesia

Pain control should be adequate in the postoperative period. Aside from increasing patient comfort, good analgesia facilitates mobilization and chest physiotherapy, which are determinants of postoperative maternal morbidity. A wide variety of analgesic approaches have been used and recommended. [91,92] Narcotics and sedatives should be used judiciously, especially in the patient with obstructive sleep apnea. Narcotics can be titrated to respiratory rate. Patient controlled intravenous opioids have also been successfully used for postoperative pain relief. Multimodal pain therapy such as the use of NSAIDs and local anesthesia infiltration at the surgical incision site can be helpful in reducing the use of postoperative opioids. [57] Transversus abdominis plane blocks have been shown to provide adequate analgesia, lasting 24-48 hours post-operatively, while enabling early mobilization and increasing patient satisfaction. [93-95] Epidural analgesia and intrathecal opioids have been shown to provide good postoperative analgesia, and is a popular choice in instances where and epidural catheter was placed for neuraxial anesthesia. Neuraxial analgesia has been shown to improve postoperative respiratory function in patients undergoing abdominal surgery. Epidural infusion of local anesthetic with opioids improves the quality of dynamic postoperative pain relief [12].

Local infiltration of surgical wound, prior to closure has been shown to be effective and reduces systemic opioid consumption [96-98].

Conclusion

In current obstetric practice, cesarean section is becoming more common due to a multitude of reasons such as patient population, early detection of fetal distress, and medic-legal concerns. Within such a framework, administration of anesthesia for cesarean section is growing rapidly, frequently called upon for emergent and urgent sections, in suboptimal conditions. [99] Under such circumstances, the anesthesiologist should be well prepared with knowledge and equipment to provide the safest anesthesia in a timely manner, reducing risks for the patient. Several approaches including general, regional and local anesthesia exist and should be tailored to suite maternal and fetal considerations, as well as surgical approach. Being well prepared to attend the difficult airway is of paramount importance, and having proper training and access to the different devices cannot be under estimated. Postoperative care, including adequate analgesia is an important factor in maternal well-being and outcomes.

References

[1] Mhyre JM, Greenfield ML, Polley LS: Survey of obstetric providers' views on the anesthetic risks of maternal obesity. *Int. J. Obstet. Anesth.* 2007; 16: 316-22.

[2] McClelland SH, Bogod DG, Hardman JG: Pre-oxygenation and apnoea in pregnancy: changes during labour and with obstetric morbidity in a computational simulation. *Anaesthesia* 2009; 64: 371-7.

[3] Kuczkowski KM: Practice guidelines and prevention of obstetric anesthesia-related maternal mortality. *Middle East J. Anesthesiol.* 2009; 20: 325-6.

[4] Kuczkowski KM: Labor analgesia for the morbidly obese parturient: an old problem--new solution. *Arch. Gynecol. Obstet.* 2005; 271: 302-3.

[5] Unterborn J: Pulmonary function testing in obesity, pregnancy, and extremes of body habitus. *Clin. Chest Med.* 2001; 22: 759-67.
[6] Eng M, Butler J, Bonica JJ: Respiratory function in pregnant obese women. *Am. J. Obstet. Gynecol.* 1975; 123: 241-5.
[7] Kuczkowski KM, Reisner LS, Benumof JL: Airway problems and new solutions for the obstetric patient. *J. Clin. Anesth.* 2003; 15: 552-63.
[8] Sroczynski T: [Evaluation of respiratory tract function in healthy women in the last month of uncomplicated pregnancy]. *Ann. Acad. Med. Stetin* 2002; 48: 331-50.
[9] Roofthooft E: Anesthesia for the morbidly obese parturient. *Curr. Opin. Anaesthesiol.* 2009; 22: 341-6.
[10] Vasdev GM, Harrison BA, Keegan MT, Burkle CM: Management of the difficult and failed airway in obstetric anesthesia. *J. Anesth.* 2008; 22: 38-48.
[11] Wong CA, McCarthy RJ, Fitzgerald PC, Raikoff K, Avram MJ: Gastric emptying of water in obese pregnant women at term. *Anesth. Analg.* 2007; 105: 751-5.
[12] Saravanakumar K, Rao SG, Cooper GM: Obesity and obstetric anaesthesia. *Anaesthesia* 2006; 61: 36-48.
[13] Roberts RB: Aspiration and its prevention in obstetrical patients. *Int. Anesthesiol. Clin.* 1977; 15: 49-70.
[14] Roberts RB, Shirley MA: The obstetrician's role in reducing the risk of aspiration pneumonitis. With particular reference to the use of oral antacids. *Am. J. Obstet. Gynecol.* 1976; 124: 611-7.
[15] Roberts RB, Shirley MA: Reducing the risk of acid aspiration during cesarean section. *Anesth. Analg.* 1974; 53: 859-68.
[16] Tomoda S, Tamura T, Sudo Y, Ogita S: Effects of obesity on pregnant women: maternal hemodynamic change. *Am. J. Perinatol.* 1996; 13: 73-8.
[17] Mabie WC, Ratts TE, Ramanathan KB, Sibai BM: Circulatory congestion in obese hypertensive women: a subset of pulmonary edema in pregnancy. *Obstet. Gynecol.* 1988; 72: 553-8.
[18] Hodgkinson R, Husain FJ, Hayashi RH: Systemic and pulmonary blood pressure during caesarean section in parturients with gestational hypertension. *Can. Anaesth Soc. J.* 1980; 27: 389-94.
[19] Veille JC, Hanson R: Obesity, pregnancy, and left ventricular functioning during the third trimester. *Am. J. Obstet. Gynecol.* 1994; 171: 980-3.
[20] Saravanakumar K, Rao SG, Cooper GM: The challenges of obesity and obstetric anaesthesia. *Curr. Opin. Obstet. Gynecol.* 2006; 18: 631-5.
[21] Duhl AJ, Paidas MJ, Ural SH, Branch W, Casele H, Cox-Gill J, Hamersley SL, Hyers TM, Katz V, Kuhlmann R, Nutescu EA, Thorp JA, Zehnder JL: Antithrombotic therapy and pregnancy: consensus report and recommendations for prevention and treatment of venous thromboembolism and adverse pregnancy outcomes. *Am. J. Obstet. Gynecol.* 2007; 197: 457 e1-21.
[22] Horlocker TT, Wedel DJ, Rowlingson JC, Enneking FK: Executive summary: regional anesthesia in the patient receiving antithrombotic or thrombolytic therapy: American Society of Regional Anesthesia and Pain Medicine Evidence-Based Guidelines (Third Edition). *Reg. Anesth. Pain Med.* 2010; 35: 102-5.
[23] Horlocker TT, Wedel DJ, Rowlingson JC, Enneking FK, Kopp SL, Benzon HT, Brown DL, Heit JA, Mulroy MF, Rosenquist RW, Tryba M, Yuan CS: Regional anesthesia in

the patient receiving antithrombotic or thrombolytic therapy: American Society of Regional Anesthesia and Pain Medicine Evidence-Based Guidelines (Third Edition). *Reg. Anesth. Pain Med.* 2010; 35: 64-101.

[24] Gogarten W, Vandermeulen E, Van Aken H, Kozek S, Llau JV, Samama CM: Regional anaesthesia and antithrombotic agents: recommendations of the European Society of Anaesthesiology. *European Journal of Anaesthesiology* (EJA) 2010; 27: 999-1015 10.1097/ EJA.0b013e32833f6f6f.

[25] Cheng HC, Chen KB, Liu YC, Wu RS: Birth asphyxia during general anesthesia for a morbidly obese parturient with gestational diabetes mellitus undergoing cesarean section--a case report. *Acta Anaesthesiol. Taiwan* 2007; 45: 53-7.

[26] Hawkins JL: Maternal mortality: anesthetic implications. *Int. Anesthesiol. Clin.* 2002; 40: 1-11.

[27] Marx GF, Berman JA: Anesthesia-related maternal mortality. *Bull N. Y. Acad. Med.* 1985; 61: 323-30.

[28] Endler GC, Mariona FG, Sokol RJ, Stevenson LB: Anesthesia-related maternal mortality in Michigan, 1972 to 1984. *Am. J. Obstet. Gynecol.* 1988; 159: 187-93.

[29] Gevirtz CM, Sanapati MR, Lebowitz P: Anesthesia-related deaths during obstetric delivery in the United States. 1979-1990. *Anesthesiology* 1997; 87: 1007-8.

[30] Dick W, Traub E, Baur H, Konietzke D: [Anesthesia-related maternal mortality during labor. Results of a survey in the Federal Republic of Germany 1971-1980]. *Anaesthesist* 1985; 34: 481-8.

[31] Hawkins JL: Anesthesia-related maternal mortality. *Clin. Obstet. Gynecol.* 2003; 46: 679-87.

[32] Bamgbade OA, Khalaf WM, Ajai O, Sharma R, Chidambaram V, Madhavan G: Obstetric anaesthesia outcome in obese and non-obese parturients undergoing caesarean delivery: an observational study. *Int. J. Obstet. Anesth.* 2009; 18: 221-5.

[33] Butwick AJ, Carvalho B: Can we improve maternal outcome for high-risk obstetric patients? *Int. J. Obstet. Anesth.* 2007; 16: 311-3.

[34] Cooper GM, McClure JH: Anaesthesia chapter from Saving mothers' lives; reviewing maternal deaths to make pregnancy safer. *Br. J. Anaesth.* 2008; 100: 17-22.

[35] Frova G, Sorbello M: Algorithms for difficult airway management: a review. *Minerva Anestesiol.* 2009; 75: 201-9.

[36] Langeron O, Amour J, Vivien B, Aubrun F: Clinical review: management of difficult airways. *Crit. Care 2006*; 10: 243.

[37] Munnur U, Suresh MS: Airway problems in pregnancy. *Crit. Care Clin.* 2004; 20: 617-42.

[38] Practice guidelines for management of the difficult airway: an updated report by the American Society of Anesthesiologists Task Force on Management of the Difficult Airway. *Anesthesiology* 2003; 98: 1269-77.

[39] Practice guidelines for obstetrical anesthesia: a report by the American Society of Anesthesiologists Task Force on Obstetrical Anesthesia. *Anesthesiology* 1999; 90: 600-11.

[40] D'Angelo R: Anesthesia-related maternal mortality: a pat on the back or a call to arms? *Anesthesiology* 2007; 106: 1082-4.

[41] Anesthesia for emergency deliveries. ACOG committee opinion: committee on obstetrics: maternal and fetal medicine. Number 104--March 1992. *Int. J. Gynaecol. Obstet.* 1992; 39: 148.

[42] Maharaj D: Eating and drinking in labor: should it be allowed? *Eur. J. Obstet. Gynecol. Reprod. Biol.* 2009; 146: 3-7.

[43] Breuer JP, Correns I, Spies C: [Preoperative fasting in labour]. *Anasthesiol Intensivmed Notfallmed Schmerzther* 2007; 42: 192-8.

[44] O'Sullivan G, Liu B, Shennan AH: Oral Intake During Labor. *International Anesthesiology Clinics* 2007; 45: 133-147 10.1097/AIA.0b013e31802b8dea.

[45] Soreide E, Eriksson LI, Hirlekar G, Eriksson H, Henneberg SW, Sandin R, Raeder J: Pre-operative fasting guidelines: an update. *Acta Anaesthesiol Scand.* 2005; 49: 1041-7.

[46] Soreide E, Ljungqvist O: Modern preoperative fasting guidelines: a summary of the present recommendations and remaining questions. *Best Pract. Res. Clin. Anaesthesiol.* 2006; 20: 483-91.

[47] Setayesh AR, Kholdebarin AR, Moghadam MS, Setayesh HR: The Trendelenburg position increases the spread and accelerates the onset of epidural anesthesia for Cesarean section. *Can. J. Anaesth.* 2001; 48: 890-3.

[48] Hallworth SP, Fernando R, Columb MO, Stocks GM: The effect of posture and baricity on the spread of intrathecal bupivacaine for elective cesarean delivery. *Anesth. Analg.* 2005; 100: 1159-65.

[49] Stoelting RK, Hillier S: Handbook of pharmacology and physiology in anesthetic practice, 2nd edition. Philadelphia, Lippincott Williams and Wilkins, 2006.

[50] Lewis G, Drife J: Why Mothers Die 1997-1999 - The fifth report of the Confidential Enquiries into Maternal Deaths in the United Kingdom, *Royal College of Obstetricians and Gynaecologists* 2001.

[51] Lewis G, CEMACH: Why Mothers Die 2000-2002 - The sisxth report of the Confidential Enquiries into Maternal Deaths in the United Kingdom, *Royal College of Obstetricians and Gynaecologists* 2004.

[52] Jones T: Morbid obesity: a risk factor for maternal mortality. *Int. J. Obstet. Anesth.* 2007; 16: 384-5.

[53] McCrae AF: Morbidly obese patients should not be anaesthetised by trainees without supervision. *Int. J. Obstet. Anesth.* 2009; 18: 373-6.

[54] Dresner M: Opposer to 'Morbidly obese patients should not be anaesthetised by trainees without supervision'. *Int. J. Obstet. Anesth.* 2009; 18: 376-8.

[55] Hood DD, Dewan DM: Anesthetic and obstetric outcome in morbidly obese parturients. *Anesthesiology* 1993; 79: 1210-8.

[56] Mhyre JM, Riesner MN, Polley LS, Naughton NN: A series of anesthesia-related maternal deaths in Michigan, 1985-2003. *Anesthesiology* 2007; 106: 1096-104.

[57] Vallejo MC: Anesthetic management of the morbidly obese parturient. *Curr. Opin. Anaesthesiol.* 2007; 20: 175-80.

[58] Hodgkinson R, Husain FJ: Caesarean section associated with gross obesity. *Br. J. Anaesth.* 1980; 52: 919-23.

[59] Edomwonyi NP, Osaigbovo PE: Incidence of obesity in parturients scheduled for caesarean section, intra-operative complications, management and outcome. *East Afr. Med. J.* 2006; 83: 112-9.

[60] ACOG Committee Opinion. Committee on Obstetric Practice. Optimal goals for anesthesia care in obstetrics. *Obstet. Gynecol.* 2001; 97: suppl 1-3.

[61] Herring SJ, Platek DN, Elliott P, Riley LE, Stuebe AM, Oken E: Addressing obesity in pregnancy: what do obstetric providers recommend? *J. Womens Health* (Larchmt) 2010; 19: 65-70.

[62] Rocke DA, Murray WB, Rout CC, Gouws E: Relative risk analysis of factors associated with difficult intubation in obstetric anesthesia. *Anesthesiology* 1992; 77: 67-73.

[63] Afolabi BB, Lesi FE, Merah NA: Regional versus general anaesthesia for caesarean section. *Cochrane Database Syst. Rev.* 2006: CD004350.

[64] Algert CS, Bowen JR, Giles WB, Knoblanche GE, Lain SJ, Roberts CL: Regional block versus general anaesthesia for caesarean section and neonatal outcomes: a population-based study. *BMC Med.* 2009; 7: 20.

[65] Gulur P, Nishimori M, Ballantyne JC: Regional anaesthesia versus general anaesthesia, morbidity and mortality. *Best Pract. Res. Clin. Anaesthesiol.* 2006; 20: 249-63.

[66] Mancuso A, De Vivo A, Giacobbe A, Priola V, Maggio Savasta L, Guzzo M, De Vivo D: General versus spinal anaesthesia for elective caesarean sections: effects on neonatal short-term outcome. A prospective randomised study. *J. Matern Fetal Neonatal Med.* 2010; 23: 1114-8.

[67] Jones TL: Morbid obesity, regional anaesthesia and mode of delivery. *Int. J. Obstet. Anesth.* 2008; 17: 188-9.

[68] Hawkins JL, Koonin LM, Palmer SK, Gibbs CP: Anesthesia-related deaths during obstetric delivery in the United States, 1979-1990. *Anesthesiology* 1997; 86: 277-84.

[69] Paranjothy S, Griffiths JD, Broughton HK, Gyte GM, Brown HC, Thomas J: Interventions at caesarean section for reducing the risk of aspiration pneumonitis. *Int. J. Obstet. Anesth.* 2011; 20: 142-8.

[70] Hawksworth CR, Purdie J: Failed combined spinal epidural then failed intubation at an elective caesarean section. *Hosp. Med.* 1998; 59: 173.

[71] Gunaydin B, Nas T, Biri A, Koc E, Koc A, McCusker K: Effects of maternal supplementary oxygen on the newborn for elective cesarean deliveries under spinal anesthesia. *J. Anesth.* 2011; 25: 363-8.

[72] Cormack RS, Rocke DA, Latto IP, Cooper GM: Failed intubation in obstetric anaesthesia. *Anaesthesia* 2006; 61: 192-3; author reply 193-4.

[73] Boutsikou T, Malamitsi-Puchner A: Caesarean section: impact on mother and child. *Acta Paediatr* 2011.

[74] Sia AT, Fun WL, Tan TU: The ongoing challenges of regional and general anaesthesia in obstetrics. *Best Pract Res. Clin. Obstet. Gynaecol.* 2010; 24: 303-12.

[75] Fassoulaki A, Gatzou V, Petropoulos G, Siafaka I: Spread of subarachnoid block, intraoperative local anaesthetic requirements and postoperative analgesic requirements in Caesarean section and total abdominal hysterectomy. *Br. J. Anaesth.* 2004; 93: 678-82.

[76] Hodgkinson R: Repeat caesarean section associated with gross obesity. *Br. J. Anaesth.* 1981; 53: 1108.

[77] Konishi R, Akazawa S, Mitsuhata H, Hiruta M, Suzuki H, Saitoh K, Igarashi T, Shimizu R: [Cesarean section in a morbidly obese parturient under epidural anesthesia]. *Masui* 1996; 45: 1503-6.

[78] Schewe JC, Komusin A, Zinserling J, Nadstawek J, Hoeft A, Hering R: Effects of spinal anaesthesia versus epidural anaesthesia for caesarean section on postoperative analgesic consumption and postoperative pain. *Eur. J. Anaesthesiol.* 2009; 26: 52-9.

[79] Chiu CL, Mansor M, Ng KP, Chan YK: Retrospective review of spinal versus epidural anaesthesia for caesarean section in preeclamptic patients. *Int. J. Obstet. Anesth.* 2003; 12: 23-7.

[80] Ng K, Parsons J, Cyna AM, Middleton P: Spinal versus epidural anaesthesia for caesarean section. *Cochrane Database Syst. Rev.* 2004: CD003765.

[81] Macfarlane AJ, Pryn A, Litchfield KN, Bryden F, Young S, Weir C, McGrady EM: Randomised controlled trial of combined spinal epidural vs. spinal anaesthesia for elective caesarean section: vasopressor requirements and cardiovascular changes. *Eur. J. Anaesthesiol.* 2009; 26: 47-51.

[82] Hodgkinson R, Husain FJ: Obesity and the cephalad spread of analgesia following epidural administration of bupivacaine for Cesarean section. *Anesth. Analg.* 1980; 59: 89-92.

[83] Panni MK, Columb MO: Obese parturients have lower epidural local anaesthetic requirements for analgesia in labour. *Br. J. Anaesth.* 2006; 96: 106-10.

[84] Hillyard SG, Bate TE, Corcoran TB, Paech MJ, O'Sullivan G: Extending epidural analgesia for emergency Caesarean section: a meta-analysis. *Br. J. Anaesth.* 2011; 107: 668-78.

[85] Hill D: Remifentanil in obstetrics. *Curr. Opin. Anaesthesiol.* 2008; 21: 270-4.

[86] Hill D: The use of remifentanil in obstetrics. *Anesthesiol. Clin.* 2008; 26: 169-82, viii.

[87] Park BY, Jeong CW, Jang EA, Kim SJ, Jeong ST, Shin MH, Lee J, Yoo KY: Dose-related attenuation of cardiovascular responses to tracheal intubation by intravenous remifentanil bolus in severe pre-eclamptic patients undergoing Caesarean delivery. *Br. J. Anaesth.* 2011; 106: 82-7.

[88] Amini S, Yaghmaei M: The use of remifentanil in general anesthesia for cesarean section in a parturient with severe mitral stenosis and pulmonary edema. *Middle East J. Anesthesiol.* 2010; 20: 585-8.

[89] von Ungern-Sternberg BS, Regli A, Bucher E, Reber A, Schneider MC: Impact of spinal anaesthesia and obesity on maternal respiratory function during elective Caesarean section. *Anaesthesia* 2004; 59: 743-9.

[90] Sinha AC: Some anesthetic aspects of morbid obesity. *Curr. Opin. Anaesthesiol* 2009; 22: 442-446.

[91] Gadsden J, Hart S, Santos AC: Post-cesarean delivery analgesia. *Anesth. Analg.* 2005; 101: S62-9.

[92] Kuczkowski KM: Postoperative pain control in the parturient: new challenges in the new millennium. *J. Matern Fetal Neonatal Med.* 2011; 24: 301-4.

[93] Baaj JM, Alsatli RA, Majaj HA, Babay ZA, Thallaj AK: Efficacy of ultrasound-guided transversus abdominis plane (TAP) block for postcesarean section delivery analgesia--a double-blind, placebo-controlled, randomized study. *Middle East J. Anesthesiol.* 2010; 20: 821-6.

[94] Belavy D, Cowlishaw PJ, Howes M, Phillips F: Ultrasound-guided transversus abdominis plane block for analgesia after Caesarean delivery. *Br. J. Anaesth.* 2009; 103: 726-30.

[95] Kanazi GE, Aouad MT, Abdallah FW, Khatib MI, Adham AM, Harfoush DW, Siddik-Sayyid SM: The analgesic efficacy of subarachnoid morphine in comparison with ultrasound-guided transversus abdominis plane block after cesarean delivery: a randomized controlled trial. *Anesth. Analg.* 2010; 111: 475-81.

[96] Nguyen NK, Landais A, Barbaryan A, M'Barek M A, Benbaghdad Y, McGee K, Lanba P: Analgesic Efficacy of Pfannenstiel Incision Infiltration with Ropivacaine 7.5 mg/mL for Caesarean Section. *Anesthesiol. Res. Pract.* 2010; 2010.

[97] Bamigboye AA, Hofmeyr GJ: Local anaesthetic wound infiltration and abdominal nerves block during caesarean section for postoperative pain relief. *Cochrane Database Syst. Rev.* 2009: CD006954.

[98] Bamigboye AA, Hofmeyr GJ: Caesarean section wound infiltration with local anaesthesia for postoperative pain relief - any benefit? *S. Afr. Med. J.* 2010; 100: 313-9.

In: Cesarean Section: Procedures, Complications and Recovery ISBN: 978-1-62081-214-3
Editor: Eyal Sheiner

Chapter X

MATERNAL COMPLICATIONS OF CESAREAN DELIVERY

Naomi Schneid-Kofman*
Outpatient Obstetrics and Gynecology,
Meuhedet Health Services, Israel

INTRODUCTION

Cesarean delivery (CD) currently accounts for the most common major surgical procedure for women in the United States. The percentage of deliveries by CD increased substantially in recent years, from 20.7% in 1996 to an all-time high of 31.1% in 2006. The rate of CD increases with maternal age, nearly half of all deliveries in women over 40 years of age are by CD. Whilst in recent years the rate of CD has increased for all gestational ages, the highest rate (46%) is found in premature deliveries prior to 34 weeks while merely one quarter of postdate deliveries (>40 weeks) are cesarean [1].

Cesarean section has provided a life-saving form of delivery since medieval history. In those times the fetal life saved was at the expense of the mother's life. With development of safe anesthesia and modern surgery, cesarean delivery has become a delivery method of choice [2]. CDs on maternal request are estimated to make up 4% to 18% of all CDs. These are defined as a CD for a singleton pregnancy at term in the absence of medical or obstetric indications, done upon maternal request. In 2006, the National Institute of Child Health and Human Development (NICHD), held a panel in the subject of CD upon maternal request. The panel acknowledged that a large gap exists between current knowledge and clinical practice and expressed concern that this surgery is being chosen without rigorously evaluating the evidence [3].

In this chapter we will review latest literature regarding cesarean delivery complications. A full view of maternal and fetal short and long term complications is crucial for achieving a

* Author: Naomi Schneid Kofman. Address: Sansana, D.N. Negev 3, 85334, Phone and Fax: 972-8-6519325, Email: shir2k@zahav.net.il.

patients' informed consent for CD when it is an indicated surgical procedure, and further while electing cesarean section as the preferred mode of delivery.

Complications may result from the surgical process as well as from the general or regional anesthesia preformed. Pre-delivery fetal or maternal conditions may influence the nature and rate of complications (as in the case of fetal anomaly or maternal obesity); the fetal- neonatal aspects will be discussed in a separate chapter.

Evidence concerning under-reporting of medical risk factors and complications of labor and delivery on birth certificates of both CD and vaginal deliveries has been published [4]. Whether the missing data is a result of loss of follow up after hospital discharge, loose communication between neonatal and maternal departments, liability issues or other reasons is not well established. It is possible that future comprehensive, reliable documentation may have an affect upon published research in the subject and hence alter the trend of increasing CD rates.

Traditionally, surgical complications are subdivided into short and long term complications. While most types of surgery involve a single patient CD affects the life and wellbeing of two. Different titles in this chapter will deal with each subset of complications for the sake of comprehensive review yet we must keep in mind that a single event or cause may account for several complications, and interconnections may exist.

Short Term Complications

Short term complications of general abdominal surgery consist of blood loss, infection, paralytic ileus, length of procedure, hospital stay, thromboembolic events and distinct procedure complications. Post cesarean specific short term complications include post partum hemorrhage.

a. Post Partum Hemorrhage

Obstetric hemorrhage is a leading cause of maternal morbidity and mortality worldwide, with more substantial impact in developing countries. An estimated 140,000 women worldwide die per year from postpartum hemorrhage, over 50% occur within the first 24 hours of delivery. Postpartum hemorrhage (PPH) remains among the top three causes of maternal deaths in the United Stated. Estimation of blood loss is frequently an inaccurate visual estimation by a medical staff member. Overestimation as well as underestimation delay diagnosis and treatment [5]. As a result there is no precise definition for postpartum hemorrhage. The lack of a standardized method of defining and measuring obstetric hemorrhage affects clinical practice and hinders research efforts into this condition.

The average blood loss after cesarean delivery has been shown to be 1000 mL. Traditionally, postpartum hemorrhage after cesarean delivery has been defined as any loss more than this amount. A decline in hematocrit level of 10% after delivery has been proposed as a definition of postpartum hemorrhage. Although potentially useful for quality assurance and research, this retrospective laboratory diagnosis is not valuable in the acute management of obstetric hemorrhage. Hemoconcentration resulting from intrapartum dehydration or preeclampsia also may lead to a significant fall in hematocrit in the postpartum period in the absence of significant blood loss. In addition, this degree of decline may not lead to symptoms in all patients. Severe hemorrhage can also be defined by the requirement of blood transfusion or excessive bleeding that results in symptoms (dizziness, syncope) or signs (hypotension, tachycardia, oliguria) of hypovolemia. Though a patient's overall health and preoperative status can alter these descriptions, in most cases, the degree of hemodynamic compromise or shock parallels the volume of blood lost. Most women experience mild symptoms with no signs of hypovolemia after blood loss of 1000 mL (15% of blood volume). Conversely, a loss of 3000 mL (45% of blood volume) leads to severe shock and cardiovascular collapse in most patients.

In the large prospective cohort study on cesarean delivery by the Maternal Fetal Medicine Units Network, 2.6% of approximately 57,000 women studied received a transfusion. More women received a blood transfusion after primary cesarean delivery (3.2%) than repeat cesarean delivery (2.2%), probably since additional risk factors for hemorrhage exist in primary CD, including labor. A history of PPH increases the risk of hemorrhage in a subsequent pregnancy approximately threefold [6].

Predisposing factors and causes for PPH may be grouped by the site of bleeding:

Uterus:

1) Uterine atony: This is a general description of a hypotonic myometrium. Predisposing factors include:
   - Problems in the perfusion of the uterine muscle
     - Hemorrhage resulting in hypotensive shock
     - Some anesthetics used in conduction analgesia
   - Over-distended uterus having trouble contracting after it is emptied
     - large fetus
     - multifetal pregnancy
     - hydramnios - excessive amniotic fluid.
     - high parity
   - Prolonged or precipitate labor
   - Chorioamnionitis

2) Retained placental fragments or pathological adherence like placenta accreta.
3) Uterine rupture

Genital tract:

- Lacerations of the cervix, vagina, or perineum
- Surgical tear of genital tract

Coagulation abnormalities which may be revealed for the first time in the woman's life during labor and could intensify all of the above [7].

In a study from a large labor and delivery department (over 12,000 deliveries per year), a rate of 0.33% of CDs and 0.55% of vaginal deliveries where complicated with PPH, respectively. The authors found an increased risk of PPH in repeated CD and speculated that rising rates of CDs and repeat CDs may contribute to the general rise in PPH over the years [7].

Elective CD is associated with a lower rate of PPH (2.1%) than emergency cesarean deliveries (3.3%). Among maternal factors examined placenta previa (adjusted odds ration (aOR) 19.7; 95% CI 5.4-72.2) and transverse lie (aOR 4.9; 95% CI 0.9-26.5) were the only risk factors for extensive blood loss in elective operations, whereas placenta previa (aOR 8.4; 95% CI 2.4-29.9), placental abruption (aOR 2.0; 95% CI 2.0-14.5), intervention at full cervical dilation (aOR 3.2; 95% CI 1.4-7.1) and high BMI (aOR 3.4; 95% CI 1.6-7.2) were risks in emergency operations. The authors concluded that different risk pattern for excessive bleeding in CDs should be recognized when planning for surgery [8].

Excessive blood loss associated with CD is from various origins. Among uterine causes are injury to blood vessels, retained placental parts and uterine atony. Atony of the uterus, contributing 80% of PPH may result from preoperative conditions as mentioned above and furthermore from the surgical manipulation. Uterine atony can also affect a focal area of the uterus. Control of bleeding after delivery occurs primarily through myometrial contraction, since the lower uterine segment and cervix have a paucity of myometrial fibers, spiral arteries in the lower segment cannot be compressed as effectively. In addition, as medical treatment of uterine atony is mainly targeted at enhancing myometrial contraction, the lower segment may not respond appropriately to this therapy [6].

Hemostasis during CD can typically be achieved through a combination of pressure, electrocoagulation, and suture ligation. Topical hemostatic agents often assist in achieving adequate hemostasis, particularly for patients with a coagulopathy or after hysterectomy. Both mechanical and active hemostatic agents are available for use. The mechanical agents are applied locally with pressure. Gelatin (Gelfoam) is a purified gelatin solution available as powder, spong and sheet it provides effective small-vessel hemostasis. Cellulose (Oxycel, Surgicel) oxidized regenerated cellulose is produced from plant fiber and is available in different vehicles. Collagen (Avitene) a bovine microfibrillar collagen product is available in different vehicles. Active agents include Thrombin (Thrombostat) which converts fibrinogen to fibrin, a key element in clot formation. Other products of this group include Bovine thrombin and Fibrin sealants (combine thrombin and fibrinogen-Tisseel, Evicel, Vitagel). Another combination agent is Gelatin and thrombin (FloSeal) a combination of bovine collagen and pooled human thrombin. And finally, Albumin and glutaraldehyde (BioGlue), a surgical adhesive used for repair of large vessels.

When medical therapy does not prove effective, a surgical approach is required.

Although hysterectomy ultimately should control postpartum hemorrhage, several other approaches attempt to manage hemorrhage while preserving fertility. Compression techniques are primarily employed to encourage the uterine myometrium to compress spiral arteries and venous sinuses that supply the placental bed. Uterine packing was the first technique used for this purpose, lately discarded for concerns of infection and concealed bleeding. Recent techniques are intrauterine balloon placement and various suture compressive techniques, with the B-Lynch suture most commonly used.

Uterine artery ligation was first described in the 1950s. A reduction of 90% of blood flow to the uterus enables control of PPH in the vast majority of cases. Complications are broad ligament hematoma, failure to separate the ureters from the blood vessels prior to ligation. Recanalization is expected after resorption of suture and hence permanent damage to uterus or ovaries is rarely described. High ligation affecting ovarian artery anastomoses may enhance the risk. Bilateral hypogastric artery ligation is a more advanced surgical technique performed to achieve a reduction in perfusion pressure and subsequent control of the PPH. There are several serious risks of this procedure, including ischemia of the gluteal muscles (from ligation of the posterior division), injury to the ureter, accidental ligation of the external iliac artery leading to ischemia of the lower limb, and laceration of the internal iliac vein. Fertility does not seem to be compromised.

Invasive radiology can be used to occlude bleeding vessels, this usually requires preoperative setup for high risk patients (as placentation defects diagnosed or suspected prior to delivery) [6].

Several studies have examined correlation between surgical technique and uterine atony their recommendation vary greatly. In-situ uterine repair (repair of uterine incision without extracting the uterus trough the abdominal wall incision) was preferred to extra-abdominal uterine repair resulting in less atony, a shorter operating time, a faster return of bowel function, a lesser need for postoperative analgesics, and lower rates of wound infection [9]. Yet a meta-analysis comparing extra-abdominal and intra-abdominal repair of uterine incision, found no difference in postoperative and intra-operative complications. Operative time, estimated blood loss, and hospital stay were all unaffected by repair technique [10]. In a study comparing the effect of closure and non-closure of the parietal peritoneum, an increased rate of PPH was found with open peritoneum. The authors advise closure of the parietal peritoneum and warn of a delay in detection of severe PPH since the open Rezius space may accumulate a significant volume of blood [11]. Administration of Tranexamic acid prior to CD or during surgery lowers blood loss [12]. This finding is in accordance with a beneficial effect of Tranexamic acid upon PPH after vaginal deliveries and reduction of intra-operative bleeding in trauma and orthopedic surgery.

When severe PPH occurs post CD, and when there is an unstable hemodynamic patient an indication for re-laparotomy exists. A low incidence of reopening the surgical site was reported at 0.12%. Risk factors for re-laparotomy were placental abruption and repeated CD ≥3 increasing risk by 15 fold. Common procedures during re-laparotomy include drainage of blood from peritoneum, resuturing of uterus and hemostasis control with stitches. Less frequent are bladder repair, herniation repair and hysterectomy. Further complications are admission into the intensive care unit and rarely maternal mortality [13].

Cesarean hysterectomy is a major complication of CD. In a review of 158 cesarean hysterectomies (incidence 0.78 per 1000 deliveries), most frequent risk factors were previous CD (76%) and placenta previa (35%). Abnormal placenta adherence was the indication for cesarean hysterectomy in 50.7%, followed by uterine atony in 34.7% and uterine rupture in 16.7% of the cases. Post operative complications were febrile morbidity (44.4%) and disseminated intravascular coagulopathy (22.9%) [14]. Another major complication is uterine inversion during CD. It is a rare occurrence that may follow vigorous traction of a normal placenta or an undiagnosed placenta accreta. Cardiac arrest might pursue, requiring cardiopulmonary resuscitation [15]. Treatment is restoration of anatomic build by use of muscle relaxants. A delay in treatment may result in a refractory uterine atony and uncontrollable PPH.

b. Wound Complications and Infectious Morbidity

Post cesarean infectious morbidity includes a variety of diseases; febrile morbidity, wound infection and wound disruption, endometritis, and peritonitis. In a rare, catastrophic event Burst abdomen occurs, in this situation beyond wound disruption, the inner fascia layer is interrupted exposing peritoneal organs to extracorporeal conditions. Failure to identify and urgently treat Burst abdomen may turn fatal.

Wound morbidities as seroma, hematoma, infection, and separation can lead to significant pain and discomfort, delay in a return to normal function, longer hospital stay, and possible readmission to hospital.

Endometritis complicates the postoperative course of a cesarean delivery 6-27% of the time. Post cesarean endometritis, up to 10 times more frequent than after vaginal delivery, can lead to serious complications such as bacteremia, peritonitis, intra-abdominal abscess, and sepsis.

Postpartum febrile morbidity is associated with length of ruptured membranes, length of labor, and number of vaginal examinations. The causal organisms in endometritis and infectious morbidity often arise from ascending inoculation of the upper genital tract by cervicovaginal flora [16].

Risk factors for early wound infection (diagnosed prior to discharge) following CD, were identified in a population-based study of 19,416 CDs, conducted by the author and colleagues, 3.7% (n=726) were complicated by wound infection. A multivariable logistic regression model identified these independent risk factors: Obesity (OR 2.2, CI 1.6-3.1), hypertensive disorders (OR 1.7, CI 1.4-2.1), premature rupture of membranes (PROM) (OR 1.5, CI 1.2-1.9), diabetes mellitus (OR 1.4, CI 1.1-1.7), emergent CD (OR 1.3, CI 1.1-1.5), and twin deliveries (OR 1.6, CI 1.3-2.0). Combining obesity and diabetes mellitus (gestational and pre-gestational) increased the risk for wound infection to 9.3-fold (95% CI 4.5-19.2; $P<0.001$). Information regarding higher risk of wound infection should be provided to obese patients undergoing CD, specifically when diabetes coexists [17]. In another study, a much higher rate of surgical site infection was documented, at 23.5%. Of these 95% (!) became apparent after discharge from hospital, mostly within the first 15 days following surgery [18]. The inclusion of wound infection diagnosed after discharge may explain the divergence between these studies. Much research was done to define risk factors for surgical site wound infection. In another study, post cesarean infectious morbidity within 30 days was diagnosed in 18.4% of women. Only 7.0% were diagnosed in-hospital. Once more, a higher risk of infection was among obese women. Diabetes further strengthens the association between obesity and infection [19]. Others have found different risk factors for surgical site infection. In a study with 5% risk of surgical site infection among low transverse CD, risk factors included the occurrence of a subcutaneous hematoma (aOR, 11.6 (95% CI, 4.1-33.2), operation performed by the university teaching service (aOR, 2.7 (95% CI, 1.4-5.2)), and a higher body mass index at admission (aOR, 1.1 (95% CI, 1.0-1.1)). A lower risk of surgical site infection was found following cephalosporin therapy before or after the operation (aOR, 0.2 (95% CI, 0.1-0.5)). Use of staples for skin closure was associated with a marginally increased risk [20]. In their study regarding massively obese women (BMI>50 kg/m2) Alanis et al reported a very high CD rate of 60%. Thirty percent were diagnosed with post CD infectious complications. Of these, 90% were wound disruption, 87% diagnosed after hospital discharge. Subcutaneous drains and smoking were associated with wound complications while, in this study, labor or ruptured membranes were not [21]. Following the high rates of infectious complications, many recent studies aimed to further identify the subpopulation at risk and correlated surgical technique. Three major risk factors were suggested; body mass index (BMI) over 31.1 at term, (OR of 2.28 (95% CI 1.18-4.39; $p = 0.013$)), wound length over 166 mm, (OR 4.3 (95% CI 2.2-8.6; $p < 0.001$)) and corticosteroid administration prior to delivery, (OR 3.4 (95% CI 1.5-7.9; $p = 0.004$)). Cautious administration of steroid drugs prior to cesarean was recommended [22].

A debate on the subject of the optimal cesarean technique to minimize surgical morbidity is ongoing. For a full view of the debate, a general explanation of the common surgical techniques for cesarean delivery will follow.

The Joel-Cohen technique includes straight transverse incision through skin only 3 cm below the level of the anterior superior ileac spines (higher than the Pfannenstiel incision). The subcutaneous tissues are opened only in the middle 3 cm. The fascia is incised transversely in the midline then extended laterally with blunt finger. Finger dissection is used to separate the rectus muscles vertically and laterally and open the peritoneum. All the layers of the abdominal wall are stretched manually to the extent of the skin incision. The bladder is reflected inferiorly. The myometrium is incised transversely in the midline but not to breach the amniotic sac, then opened and extended laterally with finger dissection. Interrupted sutures are used for the closure of the myometrium.

The Misgav-Ladach technique is a modification of the Joel-Cohen technique developed by Stark. The Joel-Cohen abdominal incision is used. The uterus is opened as for the Joel-Cohen method. The placenta is removed manually. The uterus is exteriorized. The myometrial incision is closed with a single-layer locking continuous suture. The peritoneal layers are not sutured. The fascia is sutured with a continuous suture. The skin is closed with 2 or 3 mattress sutures. Between these sutures, the skin edges are approximated with Allis forceps, which are left in place for about 5 minutes while the drapes are being removed.

The Pelosi-type CS includes a Pfannenstiel abdominal incision. Electrocautery is used to divide the subcutaneous tissues and the fascia transversely. The rectus muscles are separated by blunt dissection to provide space for both index fingers, which free the fascia vertically and transversely. The peritoneum is opened by blunt finger dissection and all the layers of the abdominal wall are stretched manually to the extent of the skin incision. The bladder is not reflected inferiorly. A small transverse lower segment incision is made through the myometrium, and extended laterally, curving upward, with blunt finger dissection or scissors. The baby is delivered with external fundal pressure, oxytocin is administered and the placenta removed after spontaneous separation. The uterus is massaged. The myometrial incision is closed with a single-layer chromic catgut 0 continuous locking suture. Neither peritoneal layer is sutured. The fascia is closed with a continuous synthetic absorbable suture. If the subcutaneous layer is thick, interrupted 3-0 absorbable sutures are used to obliterate the dead space. The skin is closed with staples.

Available evidence suggests that the Joel-Cohen–based techniques (Joel-Cohen, Misgav-Ladach, and modified Misgav-Ladach) have advantages over Pfannenstiel and traditional CS techniques in relation to short-term outcomes: less blood loss, shorter operating time, less fever, less use of antibiotics, lower duration of postoperative pain and less use of analgesia. Furthermore, shorter time from skin incision to birth of the baby (a reduction of approximately 3 minutes) was demonstrated though no difference in Apgar score or neonatal intensive care admission was noted. No overall difference in the occurrence of wound infections or postoperative hematocrit level and hemoglobin decrease >4 g/dL. Modified Misgav-Ladach showed a trend to increased wound hematoma. No significant difference in wound breakdown between the different techniques nor in time to recover basic functions of bowel function, mobilization and breast feeding. A Cochrane review gave the following recommendations:

1) No preoperative hair removal; or clipping or depilatory creams on the day of surgery or the preceding day (no shaving).
2) Antibiotic prophylaxis with ampicillin or a first-generation cephalosporin.
3) Chlorhexidine for skin preparation.
4) Double gloving is advised in areas with high rates of blood-borne infections to achieve fewer perforations in inner glove and prevent needle stick injuries.
5) Transverse lower abdominal wall opening and uterine opening using Joel-Cohen–based methods.
6) Placental removal with cord traction.
7) Uterine closure with interrupted or single-layer continuous locking suture has short-term benefits. However, the evidence from observational studies of an increased risk of scar rupture may favor the use of double-layer closure pending evidence on this outcome from randomized trials.
8) Non closure of both peritoneal layers.
9) Closure of the subcutaneous tissues.
10) No routine drainage of the subcutaneous tissues.
11) Skin closure with subcuticular or interrupted sutures, staples, or tissue adhesive.
12) No withholding of oral fluids after surgery [23,24]. An evidence-based checklist was suggested to reduce surgical site complications. Removal of hair at the site of surgical incision by electric clippers rather than a razor and washing the skin with a chlorhexidine solution were advised to reduce rates of wound infection. Administering broad-spectrum antibiotic prophylaxis before the start of surgery rather than after the neonate's umbilical cord has been clamped and removal of the placenta by traction on the umbilical cord rather than by manual extraction were proposed to reduce the frequency of endometritis. Closure of the deep subcutaneous layer was proposed in patients whose subcutaneous tissue is greater than 2 cm in thickness to reduce the risk of seroma, hematoma, and subsequent wound disruption. Institution of thromboprophilaxis in intermediate and high-risk patients was recommended to reduce the risk of subsequent thromboembolic events [25]. Different methods of skin closure were compared in several studies. In a randomized prospective trial, subcuticular Monocryl suture was considered versus stainless steel staples. Staple closure was associated with a 4-fold increased risk of wound separation in this study (aOR 4.66; 95% CI, 2.07–10.52; $P<.001$) [26]. In one metaanalysis primary outcomes were rates of wound dehiscence (separation) and a composite wound complication rate. Secondary outcomes were patient satisfaction, operating time, and postoperative pain. A total of 877 women from 5 trials were included. Both wound separation (pooled odds ratio, 4.01; $P < .0001$) and composite wound complication (pooled odds ratio, 2.11; $P = .003$) rates were higher with staples. The use of staples reduced operating time (weighted mean difference, -5.05 minutes; $P = .021$). Data on postoperative pain and patient satisfaction were

insufficient for the analysis. This metaanalysis suggests a possible benefit with subcuticular sutures compared to skin staples [27]. Accordingly, in another recent meta-analysis, staple closure of skin incision was associated with a twofold higher risk of wound infection or separation compared with subcuticular suture closure (13.4% versus 6.6%, pooled OR 2.06, 95% CI 1.43-2.98). The number needed to harm associated with staple closure was 16. Staple closure was associated with shorter duration of surgery, whereas the techniques were similar regarding pain, cosmetic result, and patient satisfaction [28].

Routine cervical dilatation before closure of uterine scar was studied. Postpartum febrile morbidity (5.1 and 3.1%, respectively; p = 0.071), hospitalization duration (4.1 +/- 1.4 and 4.1 +/- 2.0 days; p = 0.95), wound infection (0.9% and 1.25%, p = 0.451) or anemia rate (9.50 +/- 0.73 and 9.54 +/- 0.65, p = 0.91) were similar between women who underwent cervical dilatation and those who did not. Nevertheless, among patients following a previous vaginal delivery, cervical dilatation was significantly associated with post-operative fever (OR = 5.8; 95%CI 1.2-38.0; p = 0.021) [29].

In a few studies, vaginal cleansing with poviodine prior to CD reduced infectious complications yet not statistically significant [30,31]. Yet in a literature review, vaginal cleansing with povidone-iodine immediately prior to CD significantly reduces the incidence of post-cesarean endometritis (from 9.4% to 5.2% (risk ratio 0.57, 95% CI 0.38 to 0.87). The risk reduction was particularly strong for women with ruptured membranes (from 15.4% to1.4% in the vaginal cleansing group; risk ratio 0.13, 95% CI 0.02 to 0.66). No adverse effects were reported with the povidone-iodine vaginal cleansing [32].

In the issue of prophylactic antibiotic treatment, a Cochrane review of 86 studies, administration of antibiotics was found to significantly reduce wound infection, febrile morbidity and endometritis, however no impact was attributed to the time of administration [33,34]. Accordingly, the Committee on Obstetric Practice (2010) recommended antimicrobial prophylaxis for all cesarean deliveries, administered within 60 minutes of the start of the cesarean delivery [35].

Infrequent infectious complication sites have been published. For instance, a case report of a primiparous woman diagnosed with a Streptococcus group B subphrenic abscess consequent to an emergency CD. Prior to surgery chorioamnionitis during labor was documented [36].

Rare pathogens have been described in the literature responsible for various infectious complications post CD, although most pathogens arise from the genital tract flora. Recently reported pathogens include Mycoplasma Hominis as a rare primary causative organism in an abscess formed at a surgical site hematoma after surgical drainage. The abscess formation was attributed to the fact that M. hominis is resistant to several antimicrobial agents that are usually used to treat obstetric infections and to the length of time that is required for identifying the pathogen [37]. Mucormycosis is a rare cause of necrotizing fasciitis in immunocompromised patients. A report of rhizopus necrotizing fasciitis of a caesarean wound resulting in maternal mortality was published. Cause of death was non-responding sepsis and irreversible multi-organ failure. High index of suspicion can lead to early diagnosis by frozen section of histopathology and fungal culture technique. Aggressive surgical debridement and intravenous anti-fungal medication is the main stay of treatment. A delay in diagnosis and treatment may cause multi-organ failure leading to high mortality [38].

c. Bladder Injury

In a retrospective analysis, a rate of 0.44% of bladder injury during CD was found. Primary CD accounted for 41.2% of the injuries while 58.8% resulted of repeat CD. Overall incidence was 0.27% of primary surgery and 0.81% for repeated CD. Bladder injury occurs when normal anatomy is interrupted and subsequent surgical efforts are then required during opening of the peritoneal cavity and while developing the bladder flap over the lower uterine segment, mainly due to adhesions and scar tissue resulting from previous abdominal surgery. All the bladder injuries in this study were recognized intra-operatively and repaired with an overall satisfactory outcome [39]. Another study reported an overall incidence of 0.13%. Women with a bladder injury were more likely to have had a prior caesarean delivery, as compared with the control group (72.4% vs 34.2%; $p < 0.001$). Similarly, were also more likely to have had prior pelvic surgery. Bladder injury was correlated with higher rates of adhesions during the procedure. Other risk factors were labor, progressed station of the presenting fetal part (deeper than or equal to +1) and a large baby [40]. Bladder-flap hematoma (BFH) has been described. This is a puerperal complication that may develop within a week after CD. A blood collection in the vesicouterine space as a result from bleeding at the uterine suture. A proposed treatment comprises of laparoscopic drainage and washing and peritoneal suturing. No clear, defined and standardized protocols exist for the clinical and surgical management of post-caesarean section BFH. Hysterectomy should be reserved for severe uterine necrosis, myometritis or abscess formations [41]. Rare complications of the bladder have been published as fungus infection of the bladder following uterine artery embolization during CD, the authors speculated the embolization resulted in ischemia of the bladder wall which enabled a fungal infection to develop [42]. Diverticula of bladder, resulting from CD was reported, diagnosed due to urinary tract infection that resolved following diverticulotomy [43].

d. Paralytic Ileus and Bowel Injury

Postoperative ileus is one of the common problems after abdominal and pelvic surgeries to the extent that most patients will experience some degree of intestinal ileus. Exact mechanism is unknown yet it is attributed to the opening of the peritoneal cavity and further aggravated by manipulation of the intestines, treatment with narcotic drugs for analgesia and electrolyte imbalances. Symptoms and signs include abdominal distension, anorrhexia, nausea, vomiting and diminished bowel sounds. Radiographic findings are dilated loops of small and large intestines, as well as air-fluid levels while X-ray is taken in the upright position. It contributes to delayed recovery and prolongs hospital stay. Differential diagnosis should always include bowel obstruction and bowel injury. One should keep in mind that evidence of free air on abdominal x ray does not necessarily mean perforation of viscus and may result from the surgical process. Traditional therapy for paralytic ileus is placement of nasogastric tube, correction of fluid and electrolyte imbalance, and return to feeding gradually. Lately new approaches have been trialed, including early re-feeding [44]. Sham feeding, such as gum chewing, as well as other methods were suggested to accelerate return of bowel function and reduce morbidity and length of hospital stay [45]. Bowel injury should be suspected following complex surgery, after repeated CD, and when the patient fails to improve with conservative treatment.

e. Thromboembolic Complications

Venous thromboembolism (VTE) is one of the leading causes of maternal mortality in the United States. Cesarean delivery is a known risk factor for thromboembolism. The contributing factors are the thrombogenic pregnancy state and the immobilization after surgery. In one study, deep vein thrombosis rate after cesarean delivery was 0.5%. [46]. In a case control study, the incidence of venous thromboembolism was 1 per 1000 pregnancies. The ante- and postnatal incidences were similar. Antenatal risk factors were assisted reproduction, gestational diabetes, age older than 35 years, multiple pregnancies, and 1st pregnancy. Postnatal risk factors were CD, preeclampsia, assisted reproduction, abruption of placenta, and placenta previa [47]. A higher risk of 0.22% was found in a retrospective review of 33,311 deliveries. There were 40 incidents of deep vein thrombosis (DVT) (0.12%) and 37 of pulmonary embolism (PE) (0.11%). DVT involved the iliac veins (6), the femoral or popliteal veins (16), the infrapopliteal veins (17), and the axillary vein (1). Most (57.5%) of the DVTs involved the left lower extremity. 51.6% occurred in the postnatal period, mostly (87%) within 1 week of delivery. 68% of postnatal VTE were seen in patients who underwent a CD. Risk factors were age, a hypercoagulable disorder, prior history of VTE, oral contraceptive therapy or hormonal stimulation therapy before pregnancy were also more common among women who developed VTE. These findings are in accord with previously published rates of DVT: 0.04-0.14% and PE: 0.003-0.04% [48].

As activation of the coagulation pathway is a physiological response to injury, the development of disseminated intravascular coagulopathy (DIC) is a warning signal to the clinician that the primary pathological disease state is decompensating. In pregnancy, DIC can occur in several settings, which include emergencies such as placental abruption and amniotic fluid embolism as well as complications such as pre-eclampsia. The proportion of the coagulant and the opposing fibrinolytic response may vary and result in different conditions. Yet a common theme for pregnancy-associated DIC is the essential role played by the placenta. Removal of the placenta and appropriate blood product support are the keys to management [49]. Compared to the last decade, CDs performed more recently were less likely to be complicated by (DIC) [50]. Yet DIC it remains a life threatening complication that may appear in low risk patients as well as those with coagulation predisposing conditions.

Unfractionated subcutaneous heparin or low molecular weight heparin (LMWH) are drugs administered for prevention of thrombosis after cesarean [51]. A worrisome consideration is development of consequent hemorrhage soon after surgery. Since incidence of VTE after CD is 0.22%, and the hemorrhagic risk related to LMWH is 0.24% the treatment is safe but only marginally more effective in women with no risk factors. With the addition of other risk factors, reductions in VTE greatly outnumbered the increase in major hemorrhages. At this point of data available, assessment of the individual thrombotic risk should guide treatment decisions [52]. Laboratory prolongation of APTT is seen with unfractionated subcutaneous heparin in 7% of women to the level of 150% of preoperative APTT value, suggesting a sub group with an elevated risk for hemorrhagic complications following the anticoagulation treatment, yet in this sub group rarely do hemorrhagic complications occur. A proposal to check APTT one day after surgery may detect high risk cases [53].

Hemorrhagic stroke after cesarean delivery under combined spinal-epidural anesthesia was reported as a case report. A woman was treated with anticoagulants for protein C deficiency. The hemorrhagic stroke followed administration of vasopressor therapy for intraoperative hypotension [54]. Similarly, post cesarean cerebral venous thrombosis is reported, mainly in women with preexisting coagulation defects. Both postpartum period and immobilization after CD increase the risk for cerebral venous thrombosis, angiographic MRI (venous phase) is the preferred diagnostic tool and treatment is low molecular weight heparin. Since preventive thromboprophylaxis drugs are available, peripartum cerebral vein thrombosis is not a detrimental to future pregnancies [55].

Long Term Complications of Cesarean Delivery

The long term complications will be further addressed in the following chapter.

For the wholeness of the review they are mentioned as an integral part of CD complications.

Long term complications are defined differently in several reports. Some regard the postpartum period (following six weeks after delivery) as the early related period, and any complication beyond 6 weeks as a late complication while others rely upon general surgery definition of complications first diagnosed after 30 post operative days [56].

The incidence of late surgical interventions (after puerperium) following CD is 0.4%, the complications treated included skin lesions, urogenital fistula, gastrointestinal problems, Omentum masses and pelvic lesions [57]. Incision hernia may occur in 10-15% of abdominal wounds usually appearing within the first year but can be delayed by up to 15 years after surgery. Risk factors include obesity, distension and poor muscle tone, wound infection and multiple use of same incision site. The hernia presents as bulge in abdominal wall close to previous wound, usually asymptomatic but there may be pain, especially if strangulation of small bowel occurs. Hernias tend to enlarge over time and become a nuisance. Management includes surgical repair where there is pain, strangulation or nuisance. Type of repair should take into account if there is intent for future use of the same incision site (family planning) [56].

The most important and least regarded in the process of informed consent for CD, are late complications which influence future pregnancy and delivery.

Future Pregnancy and Labor

A cesarean delivery at first birth is followed in subsequent pregnancy by increased risks of preeclampsia 1.7 (CI 1.6-1.8), small for gestational age (OR 1.3 (CI 1.3-1.4), placenta previa (OR 1.4 (CI 1.2-1.7), placenta accreta (OR 1.9 (CI 1.3-2.8), placental abruption (OR 1.7 (CI 1.6-1.9), and uterine rupture (OR 37.2 (CI 24.7-55.9), compared with a vaginal delivery at first birth. ORs after repeat CD were similar to or lower than the ORs after one CD [58]. These findings suggest a profound effect of primary CD upon obstetric future, regardless of the indication for surgery. The impact of a scarred uterus upon succeeding second-trimester surgical abortion complications was established in the literature. In the study of Frick et al. two or more previous CDs increased the risk for a major complication during a 2nd trimester abortion (e.g. transfusion, disseminated intravascular coagulation, and re-operation) compared with previous vaginal delivery by sevenfold (OR 7.4, 95% CI 3.4-15.8). This was the strongest independent risk factor detected [59]. In a recent study, no increased risk was found with termination of late second-trimester pregnancy by Laminaria dilatation (the insertion of absorbent material through the cervix and evacuation after previous CD or multiple CDs, the authors advised larger studies are needed to empower these findings [60].

Uterine rupture at site of previous cesarean incision may occur during pregnancy, however, this is rare, frequently accompanying other risk factors are present (abnormal placentation, previous infection or mal-suturing). While most ruptures occur during a trial of labor. A case report of a 30-year-old gravida 2 para 1 was admitted to hospital 2 years after CD, at 20 weeks' gestation with acute onset of abdominal pain and hypovolemic shock. Emergency laparotomy revealed a uterine rupture located in the anterior uterine wall caused by a placenta percreta. Supracervical hysterectomy was performed. This uterine wall site of invasion of placenta and finally rupture was in projection of the previous lower-segment CD [61].

Uterine rupture is the most serious complication for women undergoing trial of labor after prior CD. The reported risk for this complication ranges between 0.5 and 4%. Previous vaginal delivery and prior successful vaginal birth after cesarean delivery (VBAC) confer the lowest risk of rupture on women attempting trial of labor. In contrast, multiple prior cesareans, short interval between pregnancies, single layer uterine closure, prior preterm cesarean, labor induction and augmentation have all been suggested in some studies as factors which may increase the rate of uterine rupture. While considering these risk factors is important in counseling women regarding childbirth following CD, the infrequency of uterine rupture coupled with relatively weak associations for most risk factors has prevented the development of an accurate prediction tool for uterine rupture. Preliminary studies suggest that sonographic evaluation of the uterine scar may hold some promise for identifying women at risk [62].

Up to the 1970s, deliveries by CD were considered as indication for repeat CD in the future pregnancies. In the 1980s, the dictum "once a cesarean, always a cesarean" (by Craigin 1916), was put to a test and a trial of labor was proposed in subsequent pregnancies in an attempt to reduce CD rates [63].

Vaginal birth after cesarean (VBAC) increased after the first National Institutes of Health Consensus Conference on Cesarean Childbirth in 1981. The rate of vaginal delivery after cesarean increased from 3% to a maximum rate of 28.3% in 1996. Despite studies reporting stable success rates of approximately 70% and low complication rates (<1%), concerns about patient safety and physician liability have led to more restrictive policies and a decrease in vaginal birth after cesarean use [64]. A reported increase in the incidence of uterine rupture shifted the pendulum back to repeated CD.

Conflicting evidence in several metaanalysis articles during the late 1980s have left the medical community at debate [63]. The current rate of VBACs is approximately 8.5%, and decreased rates have been noted for all ages and ethnic groups. A concern for patient safety as well as physician liability issues have resulted in decreased availability of VBAC [64]. In a metaanalysis late into the next decade vaginal delivery was found to be successful in 17,905 of 24,349 women (73%). Maternal mortality was similar in women attempting vaginal delivery or planned CD. Uterine rupture and dehiscence were 0.4 and 1.3%, respectively. Failed trial of labor resulted in higher rates of morbidity, uterine rupture, blood transfusions and hysterectomy. (17%, 4.4%, 3%; 0.5%) than after successful vaginal delivery (3.1%, 0.2%, 1.1%, 0.1%) or planned CD (4.3%, 0.4%, 1%, 0.3%). These findings show that a higher risk of uterine rupture in women planning trial of labor than planned CD is counterbalanced by reduction of morbidity, uterine rupture, blood transfusion and hysterectomy when vaginal delivery is successful. Therefore, identification of risk factors for failure of a trial of labor will minimize the incidence of maternal complications. Several studies demonstrated an association between clinical factors, maternal characteristics, and unsuccessful vaginal delivery, yet data to date does not support these factors as predictors [64].

High risk subpopulations were targeted in order to reduce rate of complications, hence vaginal birth after cesarean was examined in the multiparous population. Rates of trial of labor after cesarean have decreased largely in multiparous women in recent years because of maternal and neonatal complications. The clinical management of grand multiparous (GMP) women (>5 births) with a prior CD is even less clear. In a retrospective study of 1,102 women repeated CD was compared to a vaginal delivery after CD in GMP. A successful VBAC was achieved in 56% of trials. 14% failed a trail of labor and had repeated CD and 30% had an elective repeated CS. Women who had a successful VBAC required less blood transfusion, and had less puerperal fever diseases ($P < 0.001$). Induction or augmentation of labor was associated with failure of VBAC ($P < 0.001$). No significant differences in neonatal complications were observed between the groups. No significant difference in uterine dehiscence, uterine rupture, amnionitis, postpartum hemorrhage, hysterectomy, puerperal fever and thromboembolic diseases was observed between the groups. A successful VBAC in the GMP population was not associated with a higher risk of maternal complications in comparison with a repeated elective CS [65].

Avoiding uterine rupture as a complication in subsequent pregnancies is crucial, in particular in developing countries, where access to repeated CD may not be available at all times. Higher rates of uterine rupture were reported in Africa in comparison with North America. It has been suggested that double-layer closure of the uterine wall shows some advantage over single layer closure in lowering the rate of uterine scar rupture, though not established [23].

Uterine scar dehiscence is failure of the uterine scar to remain intact in a following pregnancy. Mostly dehiscence is diagnosed during subsequent labor or delivery, yet unclear definition results in inconsistent rates of dehiscence reported in the literature.

A uterine scar dehiscence rate of 1.03% among women with repeated CD was established in one study. Risk factors included unprogressive first stage of labor, increasing number of previous CDs, preterm delivery and low Apgar scores at 5 minutes. In contrast, parity was a protective factor [66]. In accordance, a nested case control study with a multivariable model could not accurately predict major maternal morbidity, although women attempting VBAC with a history of abdominal surgery or those who undergo augmentation or induction of labor are at an increased risk for major maternal morbidity, and women with a prior vaginal delivery have a decreased risk of major morbidity [67].

How many CDs establish a contraindication for trial of labor? Safety of vaginal delivery after three or more prior CDs was compared to trial of labor after fewer CDs. Of 25 005 women, 860 had three or more prior caesarean deliveries: 89 attempted VBAC and 771 elected for repeat caesarean. Of the 89 who attempted VBAC, there were no cases of composite maternal morbidity (uterine rupture, bladder or bowel injury, or uterine artery laceration). Successful vaginal delivery rate was similar to that of women with one prior caesarean (79.8% versus 75.5%, adjusted OR 1.4, 95% CI 0.81-2.41, P = 0.22). The authors concluded that women with three or more prior caesareans who attempt a subsequent vaginal delivery have similar rates of success and risk for maternal morbidity as those with one prior caesarean, and as those delivered by elective repeat caesarean [68]. A recent American College Practice Bulletin was published regarding patient selection for a trial of vaginal birth after cesarean. Although a goal of lowering rate of CDs is achieved by enabling vaginal deliveries in subsequent deliveries a point is made for suitable candidate selection [69].

The effect of different surgical techniques upon late complications is not agreed upon. (Some recommendations appear above in the section dealing with short term complications). In view of the evidence from several observational studies, single-layer uterine closure may be associated with increased risk of uterine rupture in subsequent pregnancies. There is some evidence that closure of the uterine incision in two layers rather than one will significantly reduce the frequency of scar dehiscence in a subsequent pregnancy [25]. A case can be made for use of double-layer uterine closure pending results from RCTs, particularly in resource-poor settings where women may not have access to CS facilities in subsequent pregnancies [23]. A multicenter, factorial, randomized trial (CORONIS) is recruiting in 6 countries. 5 separate technical aspects to cesarean section delivery will be studied, hopefully resolve unanswered issues.

Placental Complications

A delivery by CD may have some influence over several future issues not usually considered when consulting a patient towards elective CD or while contemplating the preferred mode of delivery. Family size may be limited by the increasing risks of repetitive CDs. Risk for antenatal stillbirth may be increased in women with a prior CD when compared with women with prior vaginal births [70]. Perhaps the greatest risk to future pregnancies is an increase in disorders caused by abnormal placentation, including placenta accreta and cesarean section scar ectopic pregnancies. In the process of placentation beginning at day 13-15 after ovulation, local oxygen levels have an important role in regulating differentiation and proliferation of the trophoblast cells. The early embryo requires a hypoxic environment and therefore might preferentially implant into a cesarean section scar, which tends to be acellular and avascular. This tendency may explain the increased risk for placenta previa and accreta in individuals with an increasing number of cesarean sections [71]. Alternatively, the placenta may preferentially develop in a hypoxic scar, not involuting over this area, as it would in an unscarred uterus. Trophoblast implanting over an avascular scar may invade more deeply into the uterine wall. Placenta accreta occurs when the placenta becomes abnormally adherent to the myometrium rather than the uterine decidua. If the placenta invades into the myometrium, it is termed increta. A placenta percreta invades to the level of the serosa or continues into adjacent organs. Approximately 50% of pregnancies complicated by accreta are preceded by a CD in a prior pregnancy [72]. The Maternal-Fetal Medicine Units Network evaluated the risk of placenta accreta with increasing numbers of cesarean sections. They found that the risk for placenta accreta was 0.24%, 0.32%, 0.57%, 2.13%, 2.33%, and 6.74% in women undergoing their first, second, third, fourth, fifth, and sixth or more cesarean delivery, respectively [71]. An increased risk of placenta accrete exists when a placenta previa is present. This risk increases with repeated CD. The risk for placenta previa-accreta is 3%, 11%, 39% and 60% in women undergoing their first, second, third and fourth CD, respectively [73]. Traditional teaching has been that, with each CD the endometrium underlying the implantation site is damaged and becomes unsuitable for subsequent placentation. Subsequent pregnancies are more likely to become implanted in the lower uterine segment by a process of elimination. An alternative hypothesis is that with each successive CD, the uterine scar becomes more accessible to the implanting embryo because successive incisions are created higher in the uterine wall to avoid bladder injury from adhesions or because elective repeat surgeries occur without labor.

Women who undergo a CD during labor have an increased risk of having the uterine incision preformed at the cervix level and not in the body of the uterus. This is detected by sonographic evaluation during subsequent pregnancy, and is correlated with increased risk of abnormal placentation. When abnormal placentation occurs, significant hemorrhage and severe maternal morbidity at the time of delivery are common. Infection, bladder injury, ureteral ligation or fistula formation, and spontaneous uterine rupture are well-known accompanying complications. The management of abnormal placentation deliveries whether detected prior to delivery (reported half of cases) or encountered during labor or subsequent CD consist of a surgical approach through a vertical skin incision, participation of an expert pelvic surgeon, often a gynecologic oncologist, preparation of adequate volumes of blood products (cell saver technology is frequently employed). In select cases of placenta percreta, interventional radiology for prophylactic arterial embolization may be applied. Topical hemostatic agents and activated factor VII may be employed to treat postpartum hemorrhage [74].

An important yet rare complication is of an ectopic pregnancy implanted within the uterine scar. The frequency of this condition is uncertain and depends on several factors, including the use of routine first-trimester ultrasound. An estimated incidence of approximately 1 in 2000 pregnancies was published. The common approach is termination of pregnancy, reports of conservative management show spontaneous abortion by 17 weeks [75]. Severe maternal morbidity may be associated with this condition including maternal death from internal hemorrhage. Surgical or medical treatment is applied. Both systemic and local administrations of Methotrixate have been reported as successful, as well as other drugs.

It is not known whether CD surgical technique may alter the risk of abnormal placentation or uterine scar ectopic pregnancy, some suggest meticulous repair of the uterine incision, though data is limited in this subject [74].

Abnormal placentation increases the risk for other CD complications. A retrospective study of Obstetrical Hysterectomies, a total of 42.1% of the cases had abnormal placentation with 21% experiencing placenta accreta, 15.8% with placenta previa, and 5.3% with placental abruption. A variety of complications arose including fever (52.6%) and blood transfusion CD in the current pregnancy and history of CD were strong (84.2%) [76].

Since future rates of cesarean have great impact upon health economy and women's health, some have targeted this issue by building a predictive model. If CD rates will increase as they have in recent years, by 2020 the cesarean delivery rate will be 56.2%, and there will be an additional 6236 women with placenta previa, 4504 with placenta accreta, and 130 maternal deaths annually [77].

Urinary Complications

Most urinary complications are of short term nature, and resolve spontaneously or require early surgical intervention. Vesicouterine fistula is a rare complication of CD, resulting from a communication between scar tissue of the uterine incision to the bladder. The fistula may become evident with the Youssef classical triad: cyclical hematuria (menouria), amenorrhea and urinary incontinence or present with total urinary incontinence with normal menstruation. Diagnosis may be confirmed by hysterogram and both were managed by transperitoneal surgical repair [78]. There may be a potential role for cesarean in preventing urinary incontinence resulting from pelvic floor dysfunction. The main benefit of planned cesareans is upon short-term stress urinary incontinence. However, this benefit appears to be eliminated in older, parous, and obese patients. Cesarean delivery is most protective for urinary incontinence in primipara women with no urinary incontinence before or during pregnancy [79].

Rare Long Term Complications

Uterine adherence to the anterior abdominal wall is not a frequently reported long-term complication after CD. A report of 13 women with history of CD who were investigated for pain or infertility, were diagnosed by ultrasound or by laparoscopy with uterine adherence to anterior abdominal wall. This complication may increase morbidity at future caesarean section and increase the need for hysterectomy [80].

Uterine artery pseudoaneurysm occurs rarely (nearly 60 cases published to date) and can develop after various gynecologic or obstetric procedures. The delayed diagnosis of this disease often results in life-threatening hemorrhage. Average interval to diagnosis was reported as two weeks after CD. Diagnosis by angiography and in recent years by color Doppler ultrasonography and contrast medium-enhanced computed tomography are possible. Management includes invasive radiology, with transcatheter arterial embolization. Consideration of uterine artery pseudoaneurysm in the differential diagnosis of a symptomatic patient following CD is crucial for proper treatment before rupture occurs and to preserve fertility [81]. Some advised routine postoperative evaluation following lateral extension of uterine incision during CD to detect a pseudoaneurysm. According to these publishers' experience, a routine postoperative evaluation with vaginal ultrasound on postpartum day 6 revealed a 49 mm parauterine mass with swirling flow. Selective angiography confirmed this mass as a uterine artery pseudoaneurysm. Uterine artery embolization was performed with success. Inadequate treatment may cause profuse life-threatening postpartum hemorrhage. Uterine artery pseudoaneurysm should be listed as a differential diagnosis of pelvic mass after CS [82].

The incidence of re-laparotomy after caesarean section is 0.12-0.70%. The most common indication for re-laparotomy is intra-abdominal bleeding, uterine atony, eventration, haematoma in the muscle and intra-abdominal abscesses [83]. Cesarean scar endometriosis is expected to be encountered more frequently with further increase of CD rate. The author described excision biopsy as both diagnostic and therapeutic [84].

One study described a possible link between CD and subsequent post menstrual abnormal uterine bleeding (AUB). This symptom has been correlated to an anatomical defect on the anterior uterine wall. They found that after a mean of 6 years some women with previous CD who complain of AUB have a hysteroscopic finding of isthmocele [85].

The incidence of adnexal masses found during CD was reported in one study at 1/329. The most common histopathologic diagnoses were mature cystic teratoma (32%) and functional cysts (26%). Six cases (5%) were bilateral. The mean cyst size was 6.4 cm; two of the masses were malignant. The authors suggested that incidental masses detected during CD should be extirpated in order to exclude the possibility of malignancy and to avoid additional surgical procedures [86].

The removal of a uterine myoma is seldom attempted during CD. Risk factors for complications of myomectomy during CD were published. Compared to CD without myomectomy, a myomectomy during CD resulted in higher volume of blood transfusion, postoperative ileus, and two days longer than average hospitalization. An intramural myoma and a myoma larger than 10cm without secondary change were factors correlated with a higher complication rate. Performing myomectomy during CS is feasible, yet significant complications might arise in various cases [87].

Complications of Emergency Cesarean Sections

In a study designed to compare morbidity between elective, emergency and crash-emergency CS, the lowest complication rate was in elective CDs and the highest in crash-emergency CS. Complication rate depends on the degree of emergency and is increased with maternal obesity, older age and pre-eclampsia [88]. As mentioned above, planned CD is associated with a lower rate of PPH (2.1%) than emergency CD (3.3%) [8]. More benefits of a planned CD compared to emergency CD are lower rates of urinary stress incontinence, lower rates of surgical complications for planned (versus unplanned) cesarean deliveries, fewer birth injuries or lacerations, reduced neonatal asphyxia, intracranial hemorrhages, and newborn infections [89]. The indication for emergency surgery is usually not anticipated. Therefore no preoperative planning is performed prior to surgery. Previous abdominal operation as well as morbid obesity may complicate surgery and prolong time interval from anesthesia to delivery of the newborn. A prolonged interval may lead to fetal distress from hemodynamic changes or effect of anesthetic drugs. Several authors have suggested modified CD for better results as supra umbilical transverse incision in the morbidly obese [90].

Pelvic organ prolapse and subsequent symptoms have been described following vaginal delivery and emergency CD with preceding labor. There is little information in the literature on when damage to the pelvic floor actually occurs. Increasing parity has been identified as a risk factor. Damage has been described already during pregnancy, but injury also occurs during vaginal delivery because of denervation of the pelvic floor. Evidence as to whether cesarean section (without prior labor) offers some protection is conflicting. Denervation of the pelvic floor has been shown to be present in women who have had a cesarean section during labor but not in those who have had an elective cesarean section. Women already request a CD to protect the pelvic floor without evidence that it is protective, although in certain cases it may be. Pelvic organ prolapse is a multifactorial disease, even nulliparous women do occasionally develop pelvic organ prolapse. The benefits and potential risks of a cesarean section, with resultant uterine scar have to be weighed against the risk of developing pelvic organ prolapsed [91].

Emergency CD during the first stage and second stage of labor differ in the rate of complications. Second stage CD have longer operation time and increased need for blood transfusion, higher rates of wound infection, intraoperative complications, and higher rate of transfer to intensive care unit. Further discussion of increased neonatal complications of emergency CD [92] will be discussed in the appropriate chapter.

Complications of Repeated Cesarean Section

In order to assess the impact of repeated Cesarean surgery, comparison of women at forth or fifth CD (n=122) with women at second or third CD (n=146) was conducted. Women at their 4th and 5th CD had lower birth weights (p=0.026), lower Apgar scores at 1 minute (p=0.0001) and 5 minutes (p=0.042), higher numbers of fetal death (p=0.03), higher rate of Omentum adhesions (p =0.0001) and peritoneal adhesions (p=0.008), increased risk of cesarean hysterectomy (p = 0.014), increased need for transfusion (p = 0.018), and an increase in hospitalization days (p=0.005). Multiple repeated CDs increase the risks for operative complications and poor perinatal outcomes [93].

Timing of the repeated CD has been addressed in several studies. (This issue will be further handled in the chapter regarding neonatal complications). Elective repeat cesarean section during the 38th week of pregnancy is associated with higher neonatal morbidity compared to neonates born thereafter [94], yet fifth percent of CD are preformed prior to 39 wks. The early planned CD had a significantly higher overall risk of various poor neonatal outcome measures, including resuscitation, sepsis, respiratory morbidity and support, admission to the NICU, and prolonged hospitalization [95].

Intra-abdominal adhesion formation increases with number of CD. The important outcome of intra-abdominal adhesions is a technical difficulty during surgery in the subsequent CD, longer time interval from skin incision to delivery and higher risk of surgical site complications, specifically bladder, vascular and bowel injury. Post operative adhesions following gynecology surgical procedures increase risk of need for repeat surgery, possible future infertility, intestinal obstruction, and chronic pelvic pain. Lower rates of bowel obstruction following CD compared with general gynecology surgery, suggested lower intra-abdominal adhesion formation rate following CD [96]. The reported bowel obstruction after CD is 0.5 per 1000 and 9 per 1000 (after 3 CDs), respectively [97]. Tulandi et al described adhesion formation in 24.4% of women at second CD. More patients were found to have adhesions after 3 (42.8%; 95% CI, 0.84-0.99; *P* <.05), and_4 cesarean deliveries (47.9%; 95% CI, 0.91-0.98; *P* <.001) compared with first CD. Interval to delivery was significantly longer at each subsequent CD though complication rate was not increased. Similar adhesion density was found across repeat cesarean deliveries. However, the proportion of adhesion sites to number of patients and the proportion of dense adhesion sites increased steadily across second, third, and >4 cesarean deliveries, which implies that more adhesion sites and more dense adhesion sites are involved with each subsequent CD. Accordingly, operating time was longer for subsequent CD, yet merely by a few minutes [98]. Key steps to decrease adhesion formation were adopted from general gynecology surgery. Among these are meticulous surgical technique, gentle tissue handling, minimizing ischemia and desiccation, controlling blood loss, avoiding powdered gloves, and achieving peritoneal closure [99]. Specifically, according to a meta analysis, closure of the peritoneum in modified Stark's CD resulted in less adhesion formation and is recommended [100]. There is no single surgical method applied for repeated CDs. A comparison of the Pfannenstiel-Kerr method (PKM) or modified Misgav-Ladach method (MMLM) for a second CD, showed a shorter mean operative time (18.0 ± 3.5 vs. 23.5 ± 5.7 min; $p < 0.0001$) and mean extraction time (90.1 ± 41.2 vs. 208.1 ± 79.1 s; $p < 0.0001$) in the MMLM group compared to the PKM group. Postoperative recovery (mobilization, normalization of bowel function, need for analgesics, time to oral feeding, and intra-operative blood loss) was similar between the groups [101].

Repeated CD increase risk of placenta accreta with every CD, OR for life-threatening placenta accreta were 2.4 (1.3–4.3) for a third cesarean and 9.0 (4.8–16.7) for a fourth cesarean compared with a primary cesarean [102] (See above in section regarding late complications – placental complications.)

The cosmetic results of repeated CD are challenging. A weaker abdominal muscle tone and repeated scarring result in an increasing rate of patient request to combine abdominoplasty with CD. There are theoretical concerns of a suboptimal cosmetic result from intervention as early as during delivery. In a study a follow up of 50 women who underwent combined abdominoplasty with CD, 18% developed wound infection, 9% developed wound dehiscence. Six patients (12%) developed lower abdominal skin necrosis. Of these, half were treated conservatively and healed by secondary intention, while surgical debridement and secondary sutures were needed in the other three patients. Residual abdominal skin redundancy in 9 patients (18%), outward bulging of the abdomen and lack of waist definition in 16 patients (32%), and outward bulging of the umbilicus in 12 patients (24%) were the reported unaesthetic results. The results were compared with results of 80 abdominoplasties in nonpregnant women. The study concluded that abdominoplasty combined with Cesarean delivery carries a higher incidence of complications and does not give the desired aesthetic outcome [103].

Complications of Analgesia and Anesthesia during Cesarean Delivery

Most CDs are performed with neuroaxial anesthesia (regional/spinal), as opposed to past description of a majority of general anesthesia. In a recent study, an annual rate of CD of 23.65% to 31.51% of an annual total ranging from 8543 to 10091 deliveries, CDs performed under general anesthesia ranged from 0.5% to 1%. Of these, half were performed due to perceived lack of time for neuroaxial anesthesia. Maternal factors accounted for 11.1% to 42.9%. While failures of neuroaxial techniques accounted for less than 4% of the general anesthesia cases. The low and declining rate of general anesthesia and rise of neuroaxial techniques, particularly in parturients with co-existing morbidities, changes the pattern of anesthesia related complications [104].

Complications of regional anesthesia include failure of anesthesia as in difficulty placing regional anesthesia or insufficient duration of regional block followed by conversion to general anesthesia. Other complications are cephaled spread of regional block with possible need of mechanical ventilation and supervision in ICU. Severe hypotension, Postdural puncture headache, aspiration, cardiac arrest. Epidural abscess, a possible long term complication of neurologic sequelae was documented.

Hypotension as well as bradycardia following spinal anesthesia for CD are common and serious complications. Incidence of hypotension (systolic pressure decrease > 30% of baseline value) in 52.6% and bradycardia (heart rate < 60 bpm) in 2.5% were reported. Probability of hypotension increased with estimated blood loss 500-1000 mL and analgesia level > T4. Left uterine displacement did not prevent hypotension. Probability of bradycardia increased if intrathecal morphine 0.2 mg (0.2 mL) was added to local anesthetics [105]. Others found that a preoperative increase in blood pressure after position change (from the right lateral position to supine) may be a good variable to predict hypotension during spinal anesthesia for cesarean delivery [106]. A decrease in mean arterial blood pressure by >30% is documented in nearly half of women undergoing regional anesthesia. Hypotension results from temporary sympathectomy leading to reduced preload (increased venous capacitance and pooling of blood volume in the splanchnic bed and lower extremities) and reduced afterload (decreased systemic vascular resistance), causing lower maternal mean arterial blood pressure and reduced uteroplacental perfusion. The risk factors for hypotension include preoperative hypertension, older age, type of spinal anesthesia, and higher infant birth weight. The hypotension is well tolerated by term healthy babies and no short term perinatal complications are noted [107].

The rate of morbidly obese women among reproductive age women (pre pregnancy BMI >35kg/m^2) reached 8% during the last decade, this increase results in higher complication rates of general anesthesia, as well as regional anesthesia. The latter estimated at 8.4% in teaching medical centers in the US.

Conversion from regional to general anesthesia occurs in 0.8% of cesarean deliveries, obesity does not increase this risk, although conflicting data were published in this matter [108].

Cranial nerve palsy is an uncommon complication following spinal anesthesia. The reported incidence after spinal anesthesia varies from 1:300 to 1:8,000. There are reports in the literature of cranial nerve complications after spinal anesthesia, lumbar puncture, unintentional dural tap, and epidural anesthesia. Palsy of the abducens (VI) cranial nerve has been reported most frequently. The oculomotor (III), trochlear (IV), trigeminal (V), facial (VII), and auditory nerves (VIII) all have been involved, but less frequently. Cranial nerve palsy may be associated with altered CSF pressure, including decreased or elevated CSF pressure. Sudden alteration in intracranial pressure may have compromised blood supply to the cranial nerves. Cranial nerve palsy has been attributed to CSF depletion and intracranial hypotension following subarachoid block or unintentional dural puncture. It has been explained on the basis of CSF loss causing descent of the brain and stretching of the nerve. The majority of cases occurred from the third to the fifth postoperative days, with some cases occurring within hours. There have been reports of 5th and 7th nerve palsy after extradural blood patch that was attributed to increased CSF pressure [109].

Postoperative analgesia may contribute to post CD urinary retention. In a study comparing post CD analgesia methods, women treated with epidural bolus morphine had a higher rate of urinary retention (33.3%) compared to patient-controlled epidural analgesia with ropivacaine-fentanyl (15%), and intramuscular pethidine (16.7%) (P = 0.038). Bladder catheterization was required in 12% to resolve their urinary retention at 1 day postpartum but all achieved spontaneous micturition prior to hospital discharge. Catheterization rate was increased in the group with epidural bolus morphine (21.7%) in comparison with the other two groups (6.7% and 3.3%, respectively, P = 0.011). At 3-month follow up, obstructive voiding problems were found in 4% and a similar rate of irritating voiding problems existed. Epidural analgesia with morphine was significantly associated with post-cesarean urinary retention. Nonetheless, it was not detrimental to later urinary function [110].

Investigation of the trends in anesthesia-related maternal mortality over time recorded a 60% decrease between anesthesia related maternal mortality in 1979-1990 compared to 1991-2000. 1.6% of total pregnancy related deaths were attributed to anesthesia. An anesthesia related- mortality ratio of 1.2 per million live births was calculated for 1991-2002. Deaths mostly occurred among younger women, but the percentage of deaths among women aged 35-39 years increased substantially. Case-fatality rates for general anesthesia were 16.8 per million in 1991-1996 and 6.5 per million in 1997-2002, and for regional anesthesia were 2.5 and 3.8 per million, respectively. The resulting risk ratio between the two techniques for 1997-2002 was 1.7 (confidence interval 0.6-4.6, P=.2). Anesthetic-related maternal mortality decreased nearly 60% in this period, yet rates for regional anesthesia were on the rise [111]. Neonatal complications related to anesthesia or analgesia will be discussed in the appropriate chapter.

Maternal Mortality Related to Cesarean Delivery

Maternal mortality ratio is the number of maternal deaths that result from the reproductive process per 100,000 live births (hence should be termed "ratio" with a denominator that does not include the whole population). A range of conditions is represented in the mortality ratio affecting a specific subgroup (women of reproductive age). Since dying from the reproductive process is globally perceived as intolerable and frequently avoidable, world initiative was set to reduce mortality by launching global recognition and intervention programs largely based upon epidemiology reports. These reports are strongly limited. Divergence of death causes and risk factors among populations in different regions of the world (age distribution, parity, infectious disease prevalence) requires a population adjusted approach for reduction of mortality rather than a world wide strategy [112].

A global study found that for countries with overall cesarean rates below 15%, higher cesarean rates were correlated with lower neonatal and maternal mortality while for countries with national cesarean rates above 15% higher CD rates were correlated with higher neonatal and maternal mortality [113]. Repeated cesarean deliveries are associated with a significantly higher neonatal and maternal mortality compared with cesarean or vaginal deliveries for women who do not have a prior cesarean [114].

Important causes of maternal death past mid pregnancy are thromboembolism, Amniotic fluid embolism, hemorrhage, hypertension and infection. CD contributes to these causes.

Death during early pregnancy, miscarriage, induced abortion or ectopic pregnancy is prominently from hemorrhage and infection. Other important causes of maternal mortality are anesthetic complications and non obstetric infections. Indirect maternal deaths result from preexisting conditions that are exacerbated by the process of pregnancy, abortion or delivery. Special attention should be given to prevalent risk factors such as high parity which is associated with maternal mortality. Illegal status of abortion in some countries remains an important contributory factor to the abortion related deaths. The proportion of preventable deaths is a main interest of investigation, reported as high as 58% of recorded maternal deaths within hospitals [112]. However, some report a lower rate (28%) of preventable mortality [115]. Maternal death associated with pregnancy rarely occurs in modern medicine. Therefore, current studies lack adequate power to quantify a relationship between mortality and method of delivery. Studies on neonatal and maternal mortality lack statistical power and consistent methodologies to reliably assess the effect of the planned delivery route. Since maternal and neonatal mortality are rare events for low-risk women in developed countries, very large sample sizes often are needed to detect statistically significant differences [116].

In one of the many studies addressing the issue of intrinsic maternal mortality from CD a 3.01-fold increase in the risk of maternal mortality was found, compared with vaginal delivery after exclusion of obstetric and medical co-morbidities. The risk of planned, prior to labor CD differed from CD after initiation of labor (OR 1.73 vs OR 4.86). There was a significantly increased risk of maternal death from complications of anesthesia, puerperal infection and venous thromboembolism. The risk of death from postpartum hemorrhage did not differ significantly (95% CI 0.7-3.95). Although CD is increasingly perceived as a low-risk procedure, the present study clearly demonstrates that the risk of maternal death due to CD is significantly high, particularly when performed in labor [117]. In a study with maternal mortality ratio of 6.5 per 100,000 pregnancies, leading causes of death were complications of preeclampsia, pulmonary thromboembolism, amniotic fluid embolism, obstetric hemorrhage, and cardiac disease. Only 1 death was seen from placenta accreta. The rate of maternal death causally related to mode of delivery was 0.2 per 100,000 for vaginal birth and 2.2 per 100,000 for CD, suggesting that the number of annual deaths resulting causally from cesarean delivery in the United States is about 20 [115].

Conclusion

Addressing the issue of the rising rates of CD through the key hole of maternal request CDs, enables the adviser as well as the patient to better understand risks and benefits [118]. The literature suggests that the overall risks of maternal complications with planned CD are slightly lower than with a trial of a vaginal delivery. CD occurring during labor has an associated increased rate of complications. This stresses the importance of an intent-to-treat approach for future research. Abnormal placentation with future pregnancies should be emphasized, an individualized approach according to family size plan is important. Correcting misconceptions and alleviating irrational fears are important steps towards receiving an informed consent [3]. Concerns of how well one can counsel regarding the birth process and how well one can understand and incorporate future sequelae into the decision-making process can not alter the adviser's obligation to reach informed consent. Each individual is the best supporter for his or her own welfare and each expectant mother is the best advocate for the health of her unborn child [119]. It is our duty as healthcare providers to further pursue the data that will guide us all through decision making, and not to be steered by trend.

REFERENCES

[1] MacDorman MF, Menacker F, Declercq E. Cesarean Birth in the United States: Epidemiology, Trends, and Outcomes. *Clin. Perinatol.* 2008;293–307.

[2] Todman D. A history of caesarean section: from ancient world to the modern era. *Aust. N. Z. J. Obstet. Gynaecol.* 2007;47:357–61.

[3] Lee YM, D'Alton ME. Cesarean Delivery on Maternal Request: the Impact on Mother and Newborn. *Clin. Perinatol.* 2008;505–518.

[4] Lydon-Rochelle MT, Holt VL, Cárdenas V, Nelson JC, Easterling TR, Gardella C, Callaghan WM. The reporting of pre-existing maternal medical conditions and complications of pregnancy on birth certificates and in hospital discharge data. *Am. J. Obstet. Gynecol.*2005;193:125–34.

[5] Stafford I, Dildy GA, Clark SL. Belfort MA. Visually estimated and calculated blood loss in vaginal and cesarean delivery. *Am. J. Obstet. Gynecol.* 2008;199:519.e1-519.e7.

[6] Bonanno C, Gaddipati S. Mechanisms of Hemostasis at Cesarean Delivery. *Clin. Perinatol.*2008; 531–47.

[7] Ohel I, Holcberg G, Sheiner E. Chapter XVII: Epidemiology of Postpartum Hemorrhage. In: Sheiner E. editor, Epidemiological perspectives in Maternal Fetal medicine. 2011 Nova Science Publishers. ISBN: 978-1-60741-648.

[8] Kolås T; Øian P; Skjeldestad FE. Risks for peroperative excessive blood loss in cesarean delivery. *Acta Obstet. Gynecol. Scand.* 2010; 89(5): 658-63.

[9] DoÄŸanay M., Tonguc EA, Var T. Effects of method of uterine repair on surgical outcome of cesarean delivery. *Int. J. Gynaecol. Obstet.*2010; 111(2): 175-8.

[10] Walsh CA, Walsh SR. Extraabdominal vs intraabdominal uterine repair at cesarean delivery: a metaanalysis. *Am. J. Obstet. Gynecol.* 2009;200:625.e1-625.e8.

[11] Malvasi A; Tinelli A; Tinelli R; Serio G; Pellegrino M; Mettler L. Subfascial hematomas and hemoperitoneum after cesarean section: prevalence according to closure and non-closure of the parietal peritoneum. *Gynecol. Obstet. Invest.* 2008; 66(3): 162-8.

[12] Sekhavat L, Tabatabaii A, Dalili M, Farajkhoda T, Tafti AD. Efficacy of tranexamic acid in reducing blood loss after cesarean section. *J. Matern Fetal Neonatal Med.* 2009; 22(1): 72-5.

[13] Gedikbasi A; Akyol A; Asar E; Bingol B; Uncu R; Sargin A; Ceylan Y. Re-laparotomy after cesarean section: operative complications in surgical delivery. *Arch. Gynecol. Obstet.*2008; 278(5): 419-25.

[14] Imudia AN, Awonuga AO, Dbouk T, Kumar S, Cordoba MI, Diamond MP, Bahado-Singh RO. Incidence, trends, risk factors, indications for, and complications associated with cesarean hysterectomy: a 17-year experience from a single institution. *Arch. Gynecol. Obstet.* 2009; 280(4): 619-23.

[15] Marshall NB; Catling S. Cardiac arrest due to uterine inversion during caesarean section. *Int. J. Obstet. Anesth.* 2010; 19(2): 231-4.
[16] Haas DM, Pazouki F, Smith RR, Fry AM, Podzielinski I, Al-Darei SM, Golichowski AM.. Vaginal cleansing before cesarean delivery to reduce postoperative infectious morbidity: a randomized controlled trial. *Am. J. Obstet. Gynecol.*2010;202:310.e1-6.
[17] Schneid-Kofman N, Sheiner E, Levy A, Holcberg G. Risk Factors for Wound Infections following Cesarean Deliveries. *Int. J. Gynaecol. Obstet.* 2005;90(1):10-5.
[18] Cardoso Del Monte MC; Pinto Neto AM. Postdischarge surveillance following cesarean section: the incidence of surgical site infection and associated factors. *Am. J. Infect. Control.* 2010; 38(6): 467-72.
[19] Leth RA, Uldbjerg N, Nørgaard M, Møller JK, Thomsen RW. Obesity, diabetes, and the risk of infections diagnosed in hospital and post-discharge infections after cesarean section: a prospective cohort study. *Acta Obstet. Gynecol. Scand.* 2011; 90(5): 501-9.
[20] Olsen MA; Butler AM; Willers DM; Devkota P; Gross GA; Fraser VJ. Risk factors for surgical site infection after low transverse cesarean section. *Infect Control Hosp Epidemiol.*2008; 29(6): 477-84.
[21] Alanis MC, Villers MS, Law TL, Steadman EM, Robinson CJ. Complications of cesarean delivery in the massively obese parturient. *Am. J. Obstet. Gynecol.2010*;203:271.e1-7.
[22] De Vivo A, Mancuso A, Giacobbe A, Priolo AM, De Dominici R, Maggio Savasta L. Wound length and corticosteroid administration as risk factors for surgical-site complications following cesarean section. *Acta Obstet. Gynecol. Scand.* 2010; 89(3): 355-9.
[23] Hofmeyr JG, Novikova N, Mathai M, Shah A. Techniques for cesarean section. ***Am. J. Obstet. Gynecol.*** **2009;**Vol.201(5).
[24] Hofmeyr GJ; Mathai M; Shah A; Novikova N. Techniques for caesarean section. *Cochrane Database Syst. Rev.* 2008(1): CD004662.
[25] Duff P. A simple checklist for preventing major complications associated with cesarean delivery. *Obstet. Gynecol.* 2010; 116(6): 1393-6.
[26] Basha SL, Rochon ML, Quiñones JN, Coassolo KM, Rust OA, Smulian JC. Randomized controlled trial of wound complication rates of subcuticular suture vs staples for skin closure at cesarean delivery. *Am. J. Obstet. Gynecol.* 2010;203:285.e1-8.
[27] Clay FS, Walsh CA, Walsh SR. Staples vs subcuticular sutures for skin closure at cesarean delivery: a metaanalysis of randomized controlled trials. *Am. J. Obstet. Gynecol.* 2011; 204(5):378-83.
[28] Tuuli MG; Rampersad RM; Carbone JF; Stamilio D; Macones GA; Odibo AO. Staples compared with subcuticular suture for skin closure after cesarean delivery: a systematic review and meta-analysis. *Obstet. Gynecol.* 2011; 117(3): 682-90.
[29] Koifman A, Harlev A, Sheiner E, Press F, Wiznitzer A. Routine cervical dilatation during elective cesarean delivery - Is it really necessary? *J. Matern Fetal Neonatal Med.* 2009; 22(7): 608-11).
[30] Haas DM, Pazouki F, Smith RR, Fry AM, Podzielinski I, Al-Darei SM, Golichowski AM.. Vaginal cleansing before cesarean delivery to reduce postoperative infectious morbidity: a randomized controlled trial. *Am. J. Obstet. Gynecol.*2010;202:310.e1-6.

[31] Asghania M, Mirblouk F, Shakiba M, Faraji R. Preoperative vaginal preparation with povidone-iodine on post-caesarean infectious morbidity. *J. Obstet. Gynaecol.* 2011; 31(5):400-3.

[32] Haas DM, Morgan Al, Darei S, Contreras K. Vaginal preparation with antiseptic solution before cesarean section for preventing postoperative infections. *Cochrane Database Syst. Rev.* 2010(3): CD007892.

[33] Smaill FM, Gyte GM. Antibiotic prophylaxis versus no prophylaxis for preventing infection after cesarean section. *Cochrane Database Syst. Rev.* 2010(1): CD007482.

[34] Yildirim G, Gungorduk K, Guven HZ, Aslan H, Celikkol O, Sudolmus S, Ceylan Y. When should we perform prophylactic antibiotics in elective cesarean cases? *Arch. Gynecol. Obstet.* 2009; 280(1): 13-8.

[35] Committee opinion no. 465: antimicrobial prophylaxis for cesarean delivery: timing of administration. *Obstet. Gynecol.* 2010; 116(3): 791-2.

[36] Wong GY; Lam H. Subphrenic abscess after cesarean section in term pregnancy complicated by chorioamnionitis. *Surg. Infect. (Larchmt).* 2008; 9(3): 399-401.

[37] Yamaguchi M; Kikuchi A; Ohkusu K; Akashi M; Sasahara J; Takakuwa K; Tanaka K. Abscess formation due to Mycoplasma hominis infection after cesarean section. *J. Obstet. Gynaecol. Res.* 2009; 35(3): 593-6.

[38] Alvi AR; Shamsi G. Rhizopus necrotizing fasciitis of caesarean wound - a rare life threatening condition. *J. Coll Physicians Surg. Pak.* 2009; 19(9): 579-81.

[39] Rahman MS, Gasem T, Al Suleiman SA, Al Jama FE, Burshaid S, Rahman J. Bladder injuries during cesarean section in a University Hospital: a 25-year review. *Arch. Gynecol. Obstet.*2009; 279(3): 349-52.

[40] Gungorduk K, Asicioglu O, Celikkol O, Sudolmus S, Ark C. Iatrogenic bladder injuries during caesarean delivery: a case control study. *J. Obstet. Gynaecol.* 2010; 30(7): 667-70.

[41] Tinelli A, Malvasi A, Vittori G. Laparoscopic treatment of post-cesarean section bladder flap hematoma: A feasible and safe approach. *Minim Invasive Ther Allied Technol.* 2009; 18(6): 356-60.

[42] Van Nieuwkoop C, Tijsterman JD, Van Dissel JT. Gather ye buds. Fungus formation of the bladder after complicated cesarean section. *Am. J. Obstet. Gynecol.* 2008;199:207.e1-207.e2.

[43] Chertin B, Prat O. Iatrogenic bladder diverticula following caesarean section. *Int Urogynecol J. Pelvic Floor Dysfunct.* 2008; 19(12): 1707-9.

[44] Stewart D,Waxman K. Management of postoperative ileus. *Dis. Mon.* 2010; 56(4): 204-14.

[45] Shang H, Yang Y, Tong X, Zhang L, Fang A, Hong L. Gum chewing slightly enhances early recovery from postoperative ileus after cesarean section: results of a prospective, randomized, controlled trial. *Am. J. Perinatol.* 2010; 27(5): 387-91.

[46] Sia WW, Powrie RO, Cooper AB, Larson L, Phipps M, Spencer P, Sauve N, Rosene-Montella K. The incidence of deep vein thrombosis in women undergoing cesarean delivery. *Thromb Res.* 2009; 123(3): 550-5.

[47] Jacobsen AF, Skjeldestad FE, Sandset PM. Incidence and risk patterns of venous thromboembolism in pregnancy and puerperium--a register-based case-control study. *Am. J. Obstet. Gynecol.* 2008; 198(2): 233.e1-7.

[48] O'Connor DJ, Scher LA, Gargiulo NJ 3rd, Jang J, Suggs WD, Lipsitz EC. Incidence and characteristics of venous thromboembolic disease during pregnancy and the postnatal period: a contemporary series. *Ann. Vasc. Surg.* 2011; 25(1): 9-14.
[49] Thachil J, Toh CH. Disseminated intravascular coagulation in obstetric disorders and its acute haematological management. *Blood Rev.* 2009; 23(4): 167-76.
[50] Imudia AN; Awonuga AO; Dbouk T; Kumar S; Cordoba MI; Diamond MP; Bahado-Singh RO. Incidence, trends, risk factors, indications for, and complications associated with cesarean hysterectomy: a 17-year experience from a single institution. *Arch. Gynecol. Obstet.* 2009; 280(4): 619-23.
[51] Duhl AJ; Paidas MJ; Ural SH; Branch W; Casele H; Cox-Gill J; Hamersley SL; Hyers TM; Katz V; Kuhlmann R; Nutescu EA; Thorp JA; Zehnder JL. Antithrombotic therapy and pregnancy: consensus report and recommendations for prevention and treatment of venous thromboembolism and adverse pregnancy outcomes. *Am. J. Obstet. Gynecol.* 2007; 197(5): 457.e1-21.
[52] Blondon M. Thromboprophylaxis after cesarean section: decision analysis. *Thromb. Res.* 2011; 127 Suppl 3: S9-S12.
[53] Matsubara S. Usui R. Ohkuchi A. Okuno S. Izumi A. Watanabe T. Seo N. Suzuki M. Prolonged activated partial thromboplastin time in thromboprophylaxis with unfractionated heparin in patients undergoing cesarean section. *J. Obstet. Gynaecol. Res.* 2010; 36(1): 58-63.
[54] Ranasinghe JS. Kafi S. Oppenheimer J. Birnbach DJ. Hemorrhagic stroke following elective cesarean delivery. *Int. J. Obstet Anesth.* 2008; 17(3): 271-4.
[55] Ehler E; Kopal A; Mrklovský M; Kostál M. Cerebral venous thrombosis after a cesarean delivery. *Acta Medica (Hradec Kralove).* 2010; 53(2): 109-13.
[56] Thompson JS, Baxter BT, Allison JG, Johnson FE, Lee KK, Park WY. Temporal patterns of postoperative complications. *Arch. Surg.* 2003;138(6):596-602.
[57] Fawzy M; Zalata K. Late post-cesarean surgical complication. *J. Obstet. Gynaecol. Res.* 2010; 36(3): 544-9.
[58] Daltveit AK; Tollånes MC; Pihlstrøm H; Irgens LM. Cesarean delivery and subsequent pregnancies. *Obstet. Gynecol.* 2008; 111(6): 1327-34.
[59] Frick AC; Drey EA; Diedrich JT; Steinauer JE. Effect of prior cesarean delivery on risk of second-trimester surgical abortion complications. *Obstet. Gynecol.* 2010; 115(4): 760-4.
[60] Ben-Ami I, Schneider D, Svirsky R, Smorgick N, Pansky M, Halperin R. Safety of late second-trimester pregnancy termination by laminaria dilatation and evacuation in patients with previous multiple cesarean sections. *Am. J. Obstet. Gynecol.* 2009;201:154.e1-5.
[61] Fleisch MC, Lux J, Schoppe M, Grieshaber K, Hampl M. Placenta percreta leading to spontaneous complete uterine rupture in the second trimester. Example of a fatal complication of abnormal placentation following uterine scarring. *Gynecol. Obstet. Invest.* 2008; 65(2): 81-3.
[62] Landon MB. Predicting uterine rupture in women undergoing trial of labor after prior cesarean delivery. *Semin. Perinatol.* 2010; 34(4):267-71.
[63] Rossi AC, D'Addario V. Maternal morbidity following a trial of labor after cesarean section vs elective repeat cesarean delivery: a systematic review with metaanalysis. *Am. J. Obstet. Gynecol.* 2008;224-31.

[64] Gregory KD, Fridman M, Korst L. Trends and patterns of vaginal birth after cesarean availability in the United States. *Semin. Perinatol.* 2010; 34(4):237-43.

[65] Kugler E; Shoham-Vardi I; Burstien E; Mazor M; Hershkovitz R. The safety of a trial of labor after cesarean section in a grandmultiparous population. *Arch. Gynecol. Obstet.* 2008; 277(4): 339-44.

[66] Bashiri A, Burstein E, Rosen S, Smolin A, Sheiner E, Mazor M. Clinical significance of uterine scar dehiscence in women with previous cesarean delivery: prevalence and independent risk factors. *J. Reprod. Med.* 2008; 53(1): 8-14.

[67] Scifres CM, Rohn A, Odibo A, Stamilio D, Macones GA. Predicting significant maternal morbidity in women attempting vaginal birth after cesarean section. *Am. J. Perinatol.* 2011; 28(3):181-6.

[68] Cahill AG, Tuuli M, Odibo AO, Stamilio DM, Macones GA. Vaginal birth after caesarean for women with three or more prior caesareans: assessing safety and success. *BJOG.* 2010; 117(4): 422-7.

[69] American College of Obstetricians and Gynecologists. ACOG Practice bulletin no. 115: Vaginal birth after previous cesarean delivery. *Obstet. Gynecol.* 2010;116(2 Pt 1):450-63.

[70] Smith GC, Pell JP, Cameron AD, Dobbie R. Risk of perinatal death associated with labor after previous cesarean delivery in uncomplicated term pregnancies. *JAMA.* 2002; 287:2684–90.

[71] Silver RM, Landon MB, Rouse DJ, Leveno KJ, Spong CY, Thom EA, Moawad AH, Caritis SN, Harper M, Wapner RJ, Sorokin Y, Miodovnik M, Carpenter M, Peaceman AM, O'Sullivan MJ, Sibai B, Langer O, Thorp JM, Ramin SM, Mercer BM; National Institute of Child Health and Human Development Maternal-Fetal Medicine Units Network. Maternal morbidity associated with multiple repeat cesarean deliveries. *Obstet. Gynecol.*. 2006;107:1226-32.

[72] Wu S, Kocherginsky M, Hibbard JU. Abnormal placentation: twenty-year analysis. *Am. J. Obstet. Gynecol.* 2005;192:1458–61.

[73] Grobman WA, Gersnoviez R, Landon MB, Spong CY, Leveno KJ, Rouse DJ, Varner MW, Moawad AH, Caritis SN, Harper M, Wapner RJ, Sorokin Y, Miodovnik M, Carpenter M, O'Sullivan MJ, Sibai BM, Langer O, Thorp JM, Ramin SM, Mercer BM; National Institute of Child Health and Human Development (NICHD) Maternal-Fetal Medicine Units (MFMU) Network. Pregnancy outcomes for women with placenta previa in relation to the number of prior cesarean deliveries. *Obstet. Gynecol.* 2007;110:1249–55.

[74] Rosen T. Placenta Accreta and Cesarean Scar Pregnancy: Overlooked Costs of the Rising Cesarean Section Rate. *Clin. Perinatol.* 2008; 519–29.

[75] Jurkovic D, Hillaby K, Woelfer B, Lawrence A, Salim R, Elson CJ. First-trimester diagnosis and management of pregnancies implanted into the lower uterine segment cesarean section scar.Ultrasound *Obstet. Gynecol.*.2003;21:220–7.

[76] Dandolu V, Graul AB, Lyons A, Matteo D. Obstetrical Hysterectomy, cesarean delivery and abnormal placentation. *J. Matern Fetal Neonatal Med.* 2011 Apr 4. [Epub ahead of print].

[77] Solheim KN, Esakoff TF, Little SE, Cheng YW, Sparks TN, Caughey AB. The effect of cesarean delivery rates on the future incidence of placenta previa, placenta accreta, and maternal mortality. *J Matern Fetal Neonatal Med.* 2011 Mar 7. [Epub ahead of print].
[78] Ikechebelu JI, Ugboaja JO, Okeke CF. Post-cesarean vesicouterine fistula (Youssef syndrome): Report of two cases. *J. Obstet. Gynaecol. Res.* 2011;37(7):912-5.
[79] Nygaard I. Urinary incontinence: Is cesarean delivery protective? *Semin Perinatol.* 2006;30:267–71.
[80] Shawarby S, Salim R, Lavery S, Saridogan E. Uterine adherence to anterior abdominal wall after caesarean section. *BJOG.* 2011;118(9):1133-5.
[81] Isono W; Tsutsumi R; Wada-Hiraike O; Fujimoto A; Osuga Y; Yano T; Taketani Y. Uterine artery pseudoaneurysm after cesarean section: case report and literature review. *J. Minim Invasive Gynecol.* 2010; 17(6): 687-91.
[82] . Kuwata T; Matsubara S; Kaneko Y; Izumi A; Nakata M; Suzuki M. Asymptomatic uterine artery pseudoaneurysm after cesarean section. *J. Obstet. Gynaecol. Res.* 2010; 36(2): 405-10.
[83] Záhumenský J; Zmrhalová B; Sottner O; Maxová K; Brtnická H; Horák J; Binder T; Halaska M Adhesive bowel strangulation after caesarean section, the rare puerperal complication. *Prague Med. Rep.* 2010; 111(1): 65-8.
[84] Singh M; Sivanesan K; Ghani R; Granger K. Caesarean scar endometriosis. *Arch. Gynecol. Obstet.* 2009; 279(2): 217-9.
[85] Borges LM; Scapinelli A; de Baptista Depes D; Lippi UG; Coelho Lopes RG. Findings in patients with postmenstrual spotting with prior cesarean section. *J. Minim Invasive Gynecol.* 2010; 17(3): 361-4.
[86] Ulker V; Gedikbasi A; Numanoglu C; Saygi S; Aslan H; Gulkilik A. Incidental adnexal masses at cesarean section and review of the literature. *J. Obstet. Gynaecol. Res.* 2010; 36(3): 502-5.
[87] Kim YS; Choi SD; Bae DH. Risk factors for complications in patients undergoing myomectomy at the time of cesarean section. *J. Obstet. Gynaecol. Res.* 2010; 36(3): 550-4.
[88] Pallasmaa N, Ekblad U, Aitokallio-Tallberg A, Uotila J, Raudaskoski T, Ulander VM, Hurme S. Acta Cesarean delivery in Finland: maternal complications and obstetric risk factors. *Obstet. Gynecol. Scand.* 2010;89(7):896-902.
[89] Hamrick SEG. Cesarean Delivery and Its Impact on the Anomalous Infant. *Clin. Perinatol.* 2008;395–406.
[90] Tixier H, Thouvenot S, Coulange L, Peyronel C, Filipuzzi L, Sagot P, Douvier S. Cesarean section in morbidly obese women: supra or subumbilical transverse incision? *Acta Obstet. Gynecol. Scand.* 2009; 88(9): 1049-52.
[91] Larsson C, Källen K, and Andolf E. Cesarean section and risk of pelvic organ prolapse: a nested case-control study. *Am. J. Obstet. Gynecol.* 2009;200:243.e1-243.e4.
[92] Seal SL; Kamilya G; Mukherji J; Bhattacharyya SK; De A; Hazra A. Outcome in second- versus first-stage cesarean delivery in a teaching institution in eastern India. *Am. J. Perinatol.*2010; 27(6): 507-12.
[93] Gedikbasi A; Akyol A; Bingol B; Cakmak D; Sargin A; Uncu R; Ceylan Y. Multiple repeated cesarean deliveries: operative complications in the fourth and fifth surgeries in urgent and elective cases. *Taiwan J. Obstet. Gynecol.* 2010; 49(4): 425-31.

[94] Tita AT, Landon MB, Spong CY, Lai Y, Leveno KJ, Varner MW, Moawad AH, Caritis SN, Meis PJ, Wapner RJ, Sorokin Y, Miodovnik M, Carpenter M, Peaceman AM, O'Sullivan MJ, Sibai BM, Langer O, Thorp JM, Ramin SM, Mercer BM; Eunice Kennedy Shriver NICHD Maternal-Fetal Medicine Units Network. Timing of elective repeat cesarean delivery at term and neonatal outcomes. *N. Engl. J. Med.* 2009; 360:111-20.

[95] Wilmink FA, Hukkelhoven CWPM, Lunshof S, Mol BW, van der Post JA, Papatsonis DN. Neonatal outcome following elective cesarean section beyond 37 weeks of gestation: a 7- year retrospective analysis of a national registry. *Am. J. Obstet. Gynecol.* 2010;202:250.e1-8.

[96] Al-Took S, Platt R, Tulandi T. Adhesion-related small-bowel obstruction after gynecologic operations. *Am. J. Obstet. Gynecol.* 1999;180(2 Pt 1):313-5.

[97] Andolf E, Thorsell M, and Källén K. Cesarean delivery and risk for postoperative adhesions and intestinal obstruction: a nested case-control study of the Swedish Medical Birth Registry. *Am. J. Obstet. Gynecol.* 2010;203:406.e1-6.

[98] Tulandi T, Agdi M, Zarei A. Miner L. Sikirica V. Adhesion development and morbidity after repeat cesarean delivery. *Am. J. Obstet. Gynecol.* 2009;201:56.e1-6.

[99] Sbarra M. Boyd M. Dardarian TS. Complications due to adhesion formation following cesarean sections: a review of deliveries in three cases. *Fertil Steril.* 2009; 92(1): 394.e13-6.

[100] Shi Z; Ma L; Yang Y; Wang H; Schreiber A; Li X; Tai S; Zhao X; Teng J; Zhang L; Lu W; An Y; Alla NR; Cui T. Adhesion formation after previous caesarean section-a meta-analysis and systematic review. *BJOG.* 2011; 118(4): 410-22.

[101] Gedikbasi A, Akyol A, Ulker V, Yildirim D, Arslan O, Karaman E, Ceylan Y. Cesarean techniques in cases with one previous cesarean delivery: comparison of modified Misgav-Ladach and Pfannenstiel-Kerr. *Arch. Gynecol. Obstet.* 2011;283(4):711-6.

[102] American College of Obstetricians and Gynecologists, Committee on Obstetric Practice. Cesarean delivery on maternal request. ACOG Committee Opinion number 394, December 2007. *Obstet. Gynecol.* 2007;110:1501–4.

[103] Ali A, Essam A. Abdominoplasty combined with Cesarean delivery: evaluation of the practice. *Aesthetic Plast Surg.* 2011;35(1):80-6.

[104] Palanisamy A, Mitani AA, Tsen LC. General anesthesia for cesarean delivery at a tertiary care hospital from 2000 to 2005: a retrospective analysis and 10-year update. *Int. J. Obstet. Anesth.* 2011;20(1):10-6.

[105] Somboonviboon W. Kyokong O. Charuluxananan S. Narasethakamol A. Incidence and risk factors of hypotension and bradycardia after spinal anesthesia for cesarean section. *J. Med. Assoc. Thai.* 2008; 91(2): 181-7.

[106] Jeon YT; Hwang JW; Kim MH; Oh AY; Park KH; Park HP; Lee Y; Do SH. Positional blood pressure change and the risk of hypotension during spinal anesthesia for cesarean delivery: an observational study. *Anesth. Analg.* 2010; 111(3): 712-5.

[107] Maayan-Metzger A, Schushan-Eisen I, Todris L, Etchin A, Kulnt. J.. Maternal hypotension during elective cesarean section and short-term neonatal outcome. *Am. J. Obstet. Gynecol.* 2010;202:56.e1-5.

[108] Vricella LK, Louis JM, Mercer BM, Bolden N. Anesthesia complications during scheduled cesarean delivery for morbidly obese women. *Am. J. Obstet. Gynecol.* 2010;203:276.e1-5.

[109] Fang JY, Lin JW, Li Q, Jiang N, Gao Y. Trigeminal nerve and facial nerve palsy after combined spinal-epidural anesthesia for cesarean section. *Journal of Clinical Anesthesia*. 2010; 22, 56–58.
[110] Liang CC; Chang SD; Wong SY; Chang YL; Cheng PJ. Effects of postoperative analgesia on postpartum urinary retention in women undergoing cesarean delivery. *J. Obstet. Gynaecol. Res*. 2010; 36(5): 991-5.
[111] Hawkins JL, Chang J, Palmer SK, Gibbs CP, Callaghan WM. Anesthesia-related maternal mortality in the United States: 1979-2002. *Obstet. Gynecol.* 2011;117(1):69-74.
[112] Schneid Kofman N. Sheiner E. Chapter XXXII: Epidemiology of maternal mortality. In: Sheiner E, editor. Perinatal mortality. 2010 Nova Science Publishers. ISBN: 978-1-60741-648-7.
[113] Betran AP, Merialdi M, Lauer JA, Bing-Shun W, Thomas J, Van Look P, Wagner M. Rates of caesarean section: analysis of global, regional and national estimates. *Paediatr Perinat Epidemiol*. 2007;21:98–113.
[114] Kolas T, Saugstad OD, Daltveit AK, Nilsen ST, Øian P. Planned cesarean versus planned vaginal delivery at term: comparison of newborn infant outcomes. *Am. J. Obstet. Gynecol*. 2006;195:1538–43.
[115] Clark SL, Belfort MA, Dildy GA, Herbst ma, Meyers JA, Hankins GD. Maternal death in the 21st century: causes, prevention, and relationship to cesarean delivery. *Am. J. Obstet. Gynecol*. 2008;199:36.e1-36.e5.
[116] NIH State-of-the-Science Conference statement on cesarean delivery on maternal request. *NIH Consens State Sci statements*. 2006;23(1):1–29.
[117] Kamilya G; Seal SL; Mukherji J; Bhattacharyya SK; Hazra A. Maternal mortality and cesarean delivery: an analytical observational study. *J. Obstet. Gynaecol. Res*. 2010; 36(2): 248-53.
[118] Ecker JL. Once a pregnancy, always a cesarean? Rationale and feasibility of a randomized controlled trial. *Am. J. Obstet. Gynecol*. 2004;190(2):314–8.
[119] Williams HO. The Ethical Debate of Maternal Choice and Autonomy in Cesarean Delivery. *Clin. Perinatol*. 2008: 455–62.

In: Cesarean Section: Procedures, Complications and Recovery ISBN: 978-1-62081-214-3
Editor: Eyal Sheiner

Chapter XI

Long-Term Risks after Cesarean Section

Tomohito Tanaka*
Department of Obstetrics and Gynecology,
National Hospital Organization Osaka Minami Medical Center, Kawachinagano, Japan

Abstract

Cesarean delivery increases the risk of abnormal placentation such as placenta previa, placenta accreta and placental abruption in future pregnancy. Furthermore, unexplained stillbirth may occur. Uterine rupture in a subsequent pregnancy is well known, and rupture in term pregnancy with or without trial of labor is well documented as a severe complication with vaginal birth after cesarean section (VBAC). However, it may occur in preterm pregnancy. Today, we also know that complications may develop in the scars resulting from hysterotomy or abdominal incision. These complications occur as scar pregnancy, numbness or pain, and incision endometriosis. To date, there is no strong evidence of a causal relationship between cesarean delivery and subfertility. Abdominal surgery including cesarean section (CS) is associated with long-term risk from the development of clinically significant adhesions. Although these adhesions may be completely asymptomatic, they may cause injury during repeat abdominal surgery as well as bowel obstruction and infertility. This paper reviews the long-term complications after CS.

Introduction

Cesarean section (CS) may be performed because of maternal or fetal problems that arise during labor, or the procedure may be planned before the mother goes into labor. The cesarean delivery rate is currently rising in most countries. For example, from 1970 to 2007, the cesarean delivery rate in the United States rose from 4.5% of all deliveries to 31.8% [1]. It

* Corresponding author: Tomohito Tanaka, M.D., Department of Obstetrics and Gynecology, *Osaka Minami Medical Center*, 2-1, Kidohigashi-machi, Kawachinagano, Osaka 586-8521, Japan. Phone: +81(Japan)-721-53-5761; Fax: +81(Japan)-721-53-6191; E-mail: tomohito@ommc-hp.jp.

is important to recognize the various complications that can occur following this surgery. This chapter reviews the long-term complications after CS.

Abnormal Placentation

It has been reported that cesarean delivery was associated with increased risk of abnormal placentation such as placenta previa, placenta accrete, and placental abruption in future pregnancies. Placenta previa and accrete complicate approximately 1 in 200 and 1 in 533 deliveries, respectively [2,3]. Silver *et al.* described increased morbidity in a cohort of 30,132 women who had from one to six repeat cesarean deliveries. In this report, placenta previa was present in 1.33% of patients having their second and in 3.37% of those undergoing their sixth or greater cesarean delivery. Placenta accrete was also present in 0.24%, 0.31%, 0.57%, 2.13%, 2.33%, and 6.74% of women undergoing their first, second, third, fourth, fifth, and sixth or more cesarean deliveries, respectively; there is a dose-response pattern in the risk of placenta previa and accreta with increasing number of prior cesarean deliveries (Table 1). In women with placenta previa, the risk for placenta accrete also increases with the number of cesarean deliveries [4]. Placental abnormalities may necessitate cesarean hysterectomy. In the report described above, the risk of peripartum hysterectomy at the fourth cesarean delivery was 1 in 40, increasing to 1 in 11 at the sixth cesarean delivery. On the other hand, placental abruption complicates 1 in 100 pregnancies [5,6]. In several reports, a cesarean first birth was associated with an increased risk of placenta previa and abruption in subsequent pregnancies (Table 2) [7-10]. However, the risk of placental abruption does not appear to increase with an increasing number of prior cesarean deliveries.

Table 1. The rate of placenta previa and placenta accrete in women who had cesarean deliveries

	First CD	Second CD	Third CD	Fourth CD	Fifth CD	≥ 6 CD
Placenta previa	6.42	1.33	1.14	2.27	2.33	5.74
Placenta accreta	0.24	0.31	0.57	2.13	2.33	6.74

CD, cesarean delivery.
Data are presented as n%.
From Silver and colleagues [4].

Table 2. The association of placental abruption and placenta previa in second pregnancies after previous cesarean delivery

	Yang *et al.* [9]	Getahun *et al.* [10]	Lydon-Rochelle *et al.* [11]	Kennare *et al.* [12]
Placental abruption	1.40 (1.37-1.45)	1.3 (1.2-1.5)	1.3 (1.1-1.5)	1.22 (0.90-1.64)
Placenta previa	1.47 (1.41-1.52)	1.5 (1.3-1.8)	1.4 (1.1-1.6)	1.66 (1.30-2.11)

Data are shown as the odds ratio or relative risk (95% CI).

It is biologically plausible that prior cesarean delivery may affect abnormal placentation in future pregnancies. For example, it is likely that a uterine low segment scar impairs placental attachment [9,11]. Ligation of uterine vessels at the time of CS may further increase the risk of damage to the endometrial and myometrial uterine lining, or both, which can predispose a woman to a low implantation of placenta in the uterus in a subsequent pregnancy [12]. The uterine muscle section may interfere with physiological stretching, and prevent or restrict the placenta from moving away to the upper uterine segment in a subsequent pregnancy [13]. It is important to consider not only the morbidity from the initial cesarean delivery, but that from subsequent pregnancies as well.

Unexplained Stillbirth

Stillbirth is one of the important problems in perinatal care. In 2005, the stillbirth rate in the United States was 6.2/1000 live births and fetal deaths (total births) [14]. Many risk factors for antepartum stillbirth have been identified, including fetal structural and/or chromosomal abnormalities, hypertensive disorders of pregnancy, infection, inherited thrombophilias, antiphospholipid antibody syndrome, Rh isoimmunization, cholestasis of pregnancy, maternal hypotension and diabetes mellitus, and other underlying maternal disorders such as chronic renal disease, cyanotic heart disease, connective tissue disorders, and vascular disease. The World Health Organization defines stillbirth as a "fetal death late in pregnancy" and allows each country to define the gestational age at which a fetal death is considered a stillbirth for reporting purposes [15]. In most studies, the cause of antepartum stillbirth is classified according to the Wigglesworth classification [16], which classifies stillbirths according to a hierarchy of direct obstetric causes: toxemia, hemorrhage, mechanical, maternal, miscellaneous, and unexplained. However, there is no universally accepted method for determining the precise cause of stillbirth; the definition of "unexplained" stillbirth could vary significantly among studies. Furthermore, many factors have been consistently associated with stillbirth, such as maternal age, smoking during pregnancy, and obesity. For these reasons, it is still unknown whether an independent association exists between cesarean delivery and subsequent risk of stillbirth.

In 2003, Smith *et al.* demonstrated an increased risk of unexplained antepartum stillbirth in second pregnancies in 17,754 Scottish women with a prior cesarean delivery [17]. This paper attracted widespread attention to the possibility of an increased risk of stillbirth in women with a prior cesarean delivery. However, Salihu *et al.* did not find an increased risk of stillbirth in 71,950 women with a prior cesarean delivery, although in subgroup analysis they did find an increased risk in African-American women [18]. The largest study to date was reported by Bahtiyar *et al.* In a study of 983,395 women with prior cesarean delivery, they concluded that a prior cesarean delivery was not associated with an increased risk of stillbirth in a subsequent pregnancy [19]. Kennare *et al.* reported the risks of adverse outcome in the next birth after a first cesarean delivery. In 8,725 women with prior cesarean delivery, the total risk of stillbirth was increased and was statistically significant after adjusted analysis. The risk of unexplained stillbirth was apparent in both crude and adjusted analysis [10]. Gray *et al.* reported an increased risk of explained stillbirth but no statistically significant increase in the risk of total or unexplained stillbirth in 5,839 women with prior cesarean delivery [20].

In a recent study reported by Wood *et al.*, among 30,110 Canadian women with prior cesarean delivery, the association between previous cesarean delivery and total or unexplained stillbirth was not consistently observed [21]. These data (Table 3) suggest that prior cesarean delivery is not associated with an increased risk of stillbirth in a subsequent pregnancy.

Table 3. The risk of unexplained stillbirth in second pregnancies following CS in the first pregnancy

	Number of patients	Risk of unexplained stillbirth
Smith *et at.* [17]	17,754	2.23 (1.48-3.36)
Salihu *et at.* [18]	71,950	1.1 (1.0-1.3)
Bahtiyar *et al.* [19]	983,395	0.9 (0.76-1.06)
Kennare *et al.* [10]	8,725	2.34 (1.26-4.37)
Gray *et al.* [20]	5,839	1.24 (0.60-2.56)
Wood *et al.* [21]	30,110	1.27 (0.92-1.77)

Data are shown as the odds ratio or relative risk (95% CI).

Uterine Rupture

Uterine rupture may occur as a result of anomaly or preexisting injury such as CS (Figure 1). It may be associated with trauma or even with labor in a previously unscarred uterus. The incidence of spontaneous uterine rupture is only 1 in 15,000 deliveries [22]. This type of rupture is more likely in women of high parity [23]. Uterotonic agents, including oxytocin and prostaglandin, used to stimulate labor have been commonly associated with uterine rupture, especially in women of high parity. Numerous reports about the risk of uterine rupture after cesarean delivery have been published. Uterine rupture is typically classified as "complete" or "incomplete". Complete rupture is defined as a disruption or tear of the uterine muscle and visceral peritoneum or a separation of the uterine muscle with extension to the bladder or broad ligament. Incomplete rupture, also called uterine dehiscence, is defined as a disruption of the uterine muscle with intact serosa. Women with a transverse scar confined to the lower uterine segment have the lowest risk of symptomatic scar separation during a subsequent pregnancy.

Chauhan *et al.* described women with uterine ruptures who had prior cesarean deliveries with classical scars. In a review of 157 women with a classical cesarean delivery, one woman had a complete uterine rupture prior to the onset of labor, while 15 (9%) others had an incomplete uterine rupture; rupture may occur several weeks before term. [24]. Spong *et al.* analyzed the risk of uterine rupture in 39,117 women with a term singleton gestation and prior cesarean delivery in five groups: trial of labor, elective repeat with no labor, elective repeat with labor, indicated repeat with labor, and indicated repeat without labor.

The most common indications for indicated repeat cesarean deliveries were unknown prior incision and noncephalic presentation. The overall risk for uterine rupture was 0.32% (125/39,117).

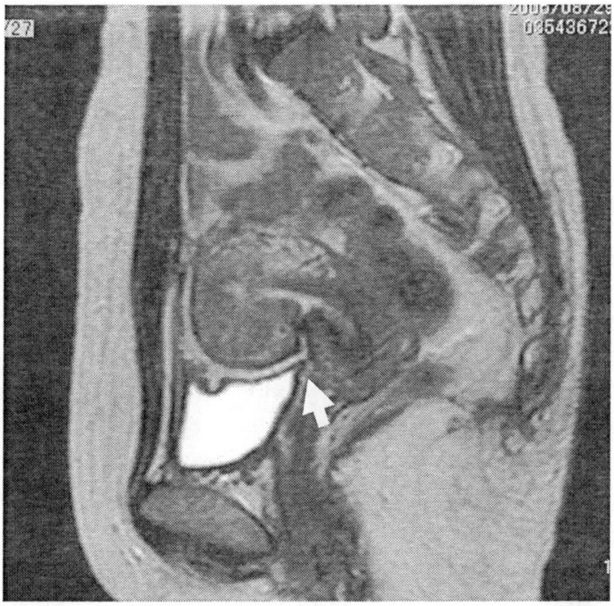

Figure 1. This case was a 32-year-old female (gravida 1, para 1) who had undergone CS 2 years earlier because of intrauterine fetal death with placental abruption at gestation 36 weeks. MRI revealed thinned uterine myometrium (arrows). Two years later, she was delivered of an infant in good condition by elective CS at gestation 36 weeks. At the CS, although there was no myometrium on the uterine scare, the scar was covered with intact serosa; she had uterine dehiscence.

Table 4. The risk of uterine rupture in women with a history of cesarean delivery

	Trial of labor	Elective repeat cesarean section	
		Without labor	With labor
Spong *et al.* [25]	0.74% (114/15,323)	0% (0/14,993)	0.15% (4/2,721)
Landon *et al.* [26]	0.7% (124/17,898)	0% (0/15,801)	

Uterine rupture was present in 0.74% (114/15,323), 0% (0/14,993), 0.15% (4/2,721), 0.08% (4/5,002), and 0.28% (3/1,078) of women undergoing trial of labor, elective repeat with no labor, elective repeat with labor, indicated without labor, and indicated repeat with labor, respectively; the highest rate of uterine rupture occurred in women undergoing trial of labor, and no woman had rupture in the elective repeat with no labor group [25].

Landon *et al.* reported the risk of uterine rupture in 33,699 women with prior cesarean delivery. The analysis was from two groups: trial of labor and repeated cesarean delivery without labor. Uterine rupture occurred in 0.7% (124/17,898) and 0% (0/15,801) of women undergoing trial of labor and repeated cesarean delivery, respectively. Uterine dehiscence was identified in 2.1% (100/4759) and 0.5% (76/15,801) of women with failed vaginal delivery and elective cesarean delivery, respectively [26]. Chauhan *et al.* reviewed uterine rupture described in 72 reports. In 142,075 women with prior cesarean delivery, a 6.2 per 1000 trial of labor rate of uterine rupture was determined [27]. These data (Table 4) suggested that a trial of labor after cesarean delivery is associated with a greater risk of uterine rupture than is elective repeated cesarean delivery without labor, although the risk is low regardless of mode of delivery.

SCAR PREGNANCY

Cesarean scar pregnancy, which refers to embryo implantation in a previous cesarean scar, is a rare form of ectopic pregnancy, with an incidence estimated at 1:1800-1:2216 pregnancies, and accounts for 6.1% of ectopic pregnancies among women with prior cesarean deliveries [28,29]. The gestational age at diagnosis ranged from 5 + 0 to 12 + 4 weeks (mean 7.5 ± 2.5 weeks), and the time interval between the last cesarean delivery and the cesarean scar pregnancy was 6 months to 12 years in the case series [29]. Although the mechanism of embryo implantation in a cesarean scar is still not understood, it is believed to occur through a microscopic dehiscence or a defect in the scar secondary to poor vascularization of the lower uterine segment with fibrosis and incomplete healing [28]. Such a phenomenon can occur as a result of the trauma from other uterine manipulation, such as curettage, myomectomy, hysteroscopy, metroplasty and manual removal of placenta [30]. It is biologically plausible that patients with a greater number of prior cesarean deliveries have a higher risk of scar pregnancy. However, it is uncertain whether the risk of scar pregnancy is related to the number of previous cesarean deliveries. In the published literature, the rate of scar pregnancy among women after two or more prior cesarean deliveries was 48-72% [28,31,32]. Some authors considered multiple cesarean deliveries as a risk factor, while other authors felt that the number of cesarean deliveries had no impact.

Making an appropriate diagnosis is important, because a ruptured scar pregnancy may cause life-threatening hemorrhage. Clinical manifestations may be helpful in differentiating from other pregnancy failure. Painless vaginal bleeding is the most common symptom, occurring in 38.6% of women with scar pregnancy. Compared to that, 15.8% of women with scar pregnancy had vaginal bleeding with mild to moderate abdominal pain, and 8.8% complained of only abdominal pain. The remaining 36.8% of women with scar pregnancy were asymptomatic [32]. Several types of imaging technology, such as transvaginal ultrasound and magnetic resonance imaging (MRI), have been used to make a diagnosis of scar pregnancy. Transvaginal ultrasound examination, the most common method used for these diagnoses, has a diagnostic sensibility of 86.4% (95% CI 0.763-0.905) [32]. The following ultrasound criteria have been proposed [33-35]: 1) The trophoblast is located between the bladder and the anterior wall of the uterus; 2) fetal parts are not present in the uterine cavity; 3) on a sagittal uterine view that runs through the amniotic sac, no myometrium is seen between the gestational sac and the urinary bladder, as illustrated by the lack of continuity of the anterior uterine wall. Color flow Doppler can be useful to get additional diagnostic information; Doppler evidence of perfusion of the trophoblastic vasculature can help delineate the scar pregnancy sac with location of the placenta in relation to the scar and proximity to the bladder [28,36]. Although MRI (Figure 2) and hysteroscopy have been useful methods for gathering additional information, many authors do not routinely recommend their use for this purpose [37,38].

Because of its rarity, no consensus treatment for scar pregnancy has yet been established. Generally, treatment selection is based on the severity of symptoms, desire for future fertility, serum human-chorionic-gonadotropin (HCG) level, hemodynamic stability, size and gestational age of the pregnancy, fetal viability, and surgical experience.

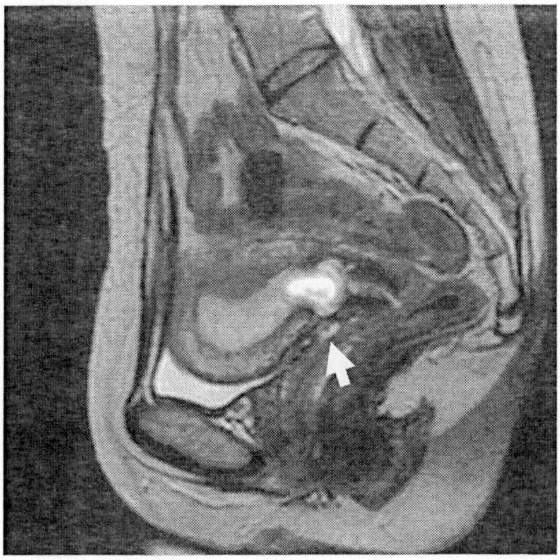

Figure 2. This case was a 35-year-old female (gravida 1, para 1) who had cesarean scar pregnancy. MRI revealed a gestational sac in the uterine scar. No myometrium was seen between the sac and urinary bladder (arrows). The serum HCG level was 32,451 IU/L. She underwent medical treatment with methotrexate. Two years later, she was delivered of an infant in good condition by elective CS at gestation 36 weeks. At the CS, no thinned myometrium was seen on the scar.

Expectant management of scar pregnancy has proven to be unacceptable. Of 7 patients with scar pregnancy observed expectantly, 4 had uterine rupture with massive bleeding and disseminated intravascular coagulation, which mandated hysterectomy [28,38-40]; termination of pregnancy in the first trimester is strongly recommended. Cesarean scar pregnancy can be treated either surgically or medically, mainly by administration of methotrexate (MTX). MTX, which is injected systemically or locally, has been used for ectopic pregnancies for two decades. The two most commonly used protocols for systemic MTX administration are a single dose (50 mg/m^2) and multiple doses (1 mg/kg per day on days 1, 3, 5, and 7). In the reviewed literature, 16 cases of scar pregnancy treated only by systemic intramuscular MTX were reported. Five women, whose serum HCG levels were less than 5,000 mIU/mL, were led to a complete resolution without complications within a few months after receiving single-dose MTX. Treatment was successful in 3 of another group of 5 women who received multiple doses of intramuscular MTX, while in the other 2 women of this group, treatment was complicated by hemorrhage that was managed by laparotomy and wedge resection in one and hysterectomy in the other. The remaining 6 women, whose serum hCG levels were from 6,000 to 48,000 mIU/mL, needed additional interventions [32]. Direct intragestational injection of MTX is also described in this case series. In another study, 8 of 15 women with scar pregnancy, whose serum hCG levels were from 14,086 to 93,000 mIU/mL, were treated successfully without additional interventions, while the remaining 7 patients required additional MTX [32]. Local injection with other drugs such as potassium chloride [41,42], hyperosmolar glucose [43], and crystalline trichosanthin [44] may also be performed. Surgical treatment involves either wedge resection of the gestational sac with laparoscopy or open surgery. The authors of one study reported that 8 of the 9 women with scar pregnancy who underwent a wedge resection of the gestational mass had no sequelae, while the treatment resulted in severe endometritis in one woman [32]. The follow-up period for surgical treatment was shorter than that with medical treatment. This procedure could be performed laparoscopically. Hysteroscopy may be used as the minimally invasive procedure for treatment of scar pregnancy [45]. Uterine curettage is not recommended, because the gestational sac of the scar pregnancy is not within the uterine cavity and the chorionic villi implant into the CS scar of the lower segment; the trophoblastic tissue is unreachable and massive hemorrhage caused by rupture of the uterine scar may occur. In a study cited above, only 5 of the 21 women with scar pregnancy treated by uterine curettage were uncomplicated and required no further treatment; the remaining 16 cases required additional treatment such as hysterectomy or MTX [32]. The reproductive outcomes following appropriate treatment of scar pregnancies are favorable. In a report of women with scar pregnancy whose uterus was conserved, 24 out of 29 (83%) women attempted to become pregnant again. Twenty out of 24 (83%) subsequent pregnancies were intrauterine, and one women had recurrent scar pregnancy. Of these intrauterine pregnancies, 13 out of 20 (65%) appeared normal on first trimester scan, whereas 7 out of the 20 (35%) ended in spontaneous abortion. Nine out of 13 (69%) were delivered by CS. The final outcomes of the remaining 4 cases were unknown [46]. These data suggest that if the uterus is successfully conserved following the treatment of scar pregnancy, women have a chance to try for another pregnancy.

Incision Endometriosis

Abdominal wall endometriosis is rare and its diagnosis is difficult. The overall incidence of abdominal wall endometriosis associated with a CS incision has been reported. Endometriosis is characterized by the presence of endometrial glands and stroma outside the uterine cavity. It occurs in 8-15% of women of reproductive age, with prevalence as much as 35% among infertile women [47]. The most common sites of the endometriosis are the ovaries followed by the pelvic peritoneum, the cul de sac of Douglas and the uterine ligament. Rarely, it may present on the abdominal wall. Abdominal wall endometriosis may be found near the umbilicus, inguinal ligament or in or near a surgical scar or at the site of the needle passage for amniocentesis. It is most frequently found in or near the scar from a prior abdominal surgery as a result of implants from the procedure. The overall incidence of abdominal wall endometriosis associated with a CS incision has been reported to be 0.03-1.0% [48-52]. There are several theories as to what may cause endometriosis [53]. One of these theories involves vascular or iatrogenic dissemination in the anterior abdominal wall. Another theory involves metaplasia of the cells in the abdominal wall into the endometrial tissue. This metaplasia may be induced by imitative metaplasia or hormonal manipulation [54]. The mechanism of abdominal wall endometriosis may be associated with a combination of these processes. Making a diagnosis is always difficult. The differential diagnosis for abdominal wall endometriosis is quite large. The differential diagnosis includes focal fibrosis, desmoid tumor, hernia, abscess, lipoma, neuroma, fat necrosis, hematoma, nodular and proliferative fascitis, suture granuloma and carcinoma. There have recently been reports of the malignant transformation of endometriosis which affects 0.7% and 0.8% of patients suffering from endometriosis [55,56]. Imaging (Figure 3) does not enable a diagnosis of malignant transformation. MRI could therefore be the best way to demonstrate the fast growth of an endometrioma, or to investigate any suspicious lesions such as a tumor measuring more than 10 cm in size, with a solid or mixed component [57]. Sonographically guided fine needle aspiration cytology (FNAC) is a rapid and accurate diagnostic procedure in women with abdominal wall endometriosis, enabling malignancy to be excluded and a definitive treatment to be defined [58]. FNAC showed most previously mentioned lesions to have well-defined cytological features: markedly cellular, with a hemorrhagic background, and 2 distinct cellular populations (Figure 4A). The epithelial component consists of large, monolayer sheets of small to medium columnar cells having scant cytoplasm and uniform, round to oval nuclei with inconspicuous nucleoli (Figure 4B). The stromal component consists of fibrous tissue fragments containing stromal spindle cells with ovoid or elongated nuclei and moderate cytoplasm (Figure 4A).

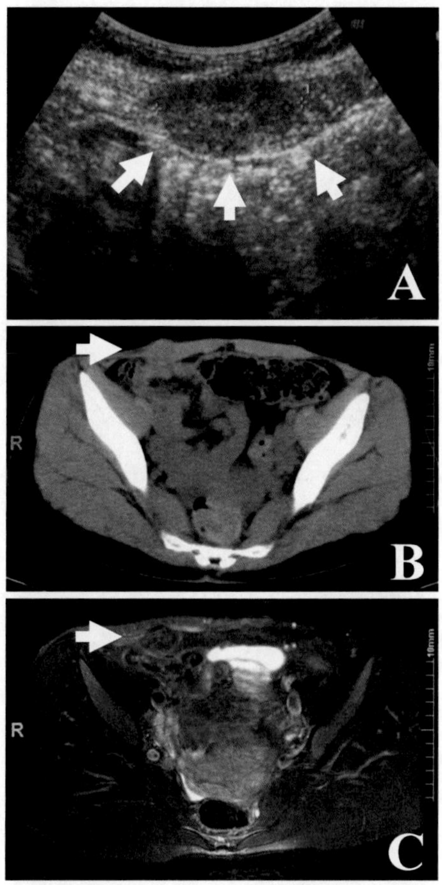

Figure 3. This case was a 26-year-old female who had undergone a CS after complaining of pain and variations in the abdominal mass associated with her menstrual periods. A: A transabdominal US scan shows a hypoechoic solid 3-cm mass. The mass is confined to the rectus abdominis sheath. B: Unenhanced CT shows the lesion in the right rectus sheath to be slightly less dense than muscular tissue. C: Axial T2-weighted fat-saturated fast-spin MR image depicts the lesion as a heterogeneous high-signal-intensity mass. A: On palpation, there was a 15×3×3 cm hard mass in her surgical scar. B: The mass was within the rectus abdominis muscle, freely mobile in relation to the skin and the fascia. C: The mass was resected with wide radicality.

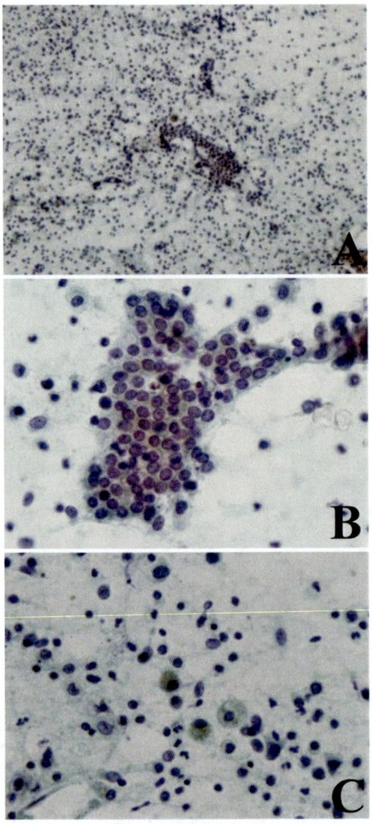

Figure 4. Cytological findings on FNAC in the case shown in Figure 3. A: FNAC shows a large sheet of benign epithelial cells forming a tubular structure. Spindle-shaped stromal cells are dispersed in the background. (Papanicolaou ×10) B: Large sheet of benign epithelial cells. (Papanicolaou ×20) C: Dispersed inflammatory cells, naked stromal nuclei, and pigment-laden histiocytes were frequently identified in the background. (Papanicolaou ×40).

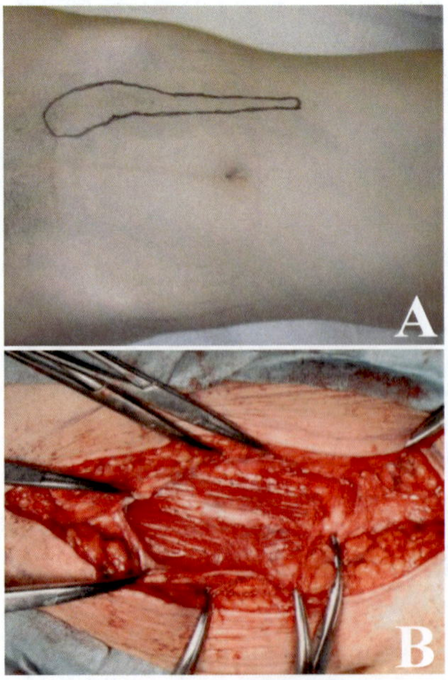

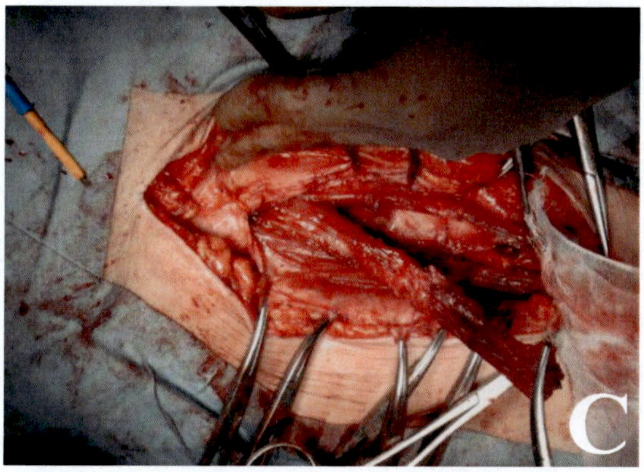

Figure 5. Surgical removal in the case shown in Figure 3. A: On palpation, there was a 15×3×3 cm hard mass in the patient's surgical scar. B: The mass was within the rectus abdominis muscle, freely mobile in relation to the skin and the fascia. C: The mass was resected with wide radicality.

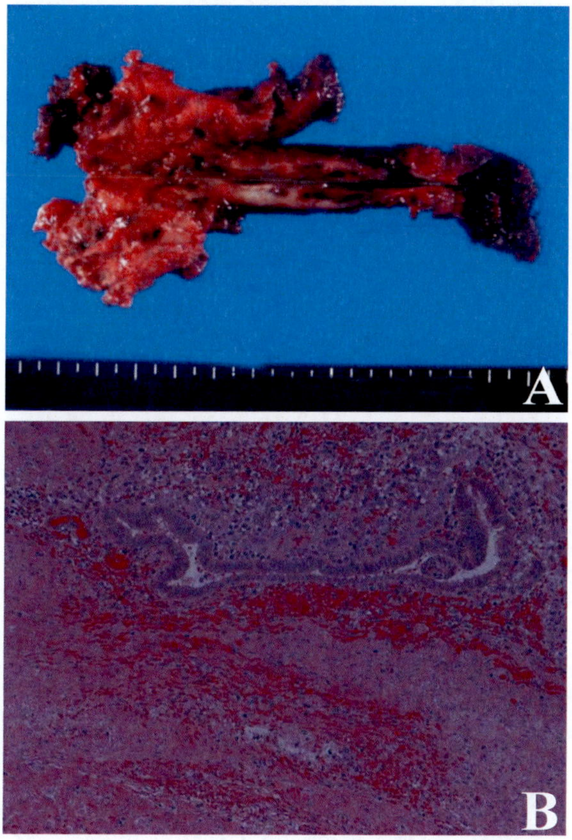

Figure 6. Surgical specimen in the case shown in Figure 3. A: Macroscopic appearance of the excised lesion. There was a 15×3×3 cm hard mass, immobile, which was firm on palpation at a right angle to the surgical scar along the rectus abdominis muscle to the umbilicus level. B: Microscopic appearance shows endometriotic glands and stroma surrounded by fibrosis as well as degraded blood products and inflammatory cells. (Hematoxylin-Eosin ×10).

The hemorrhagic background contains dispersed inflammatory cells, naked stromal nuclei, and pigment-laden histiocytes (Figure 4C). In past reports, the mean diameter of the removed abdominal wall lesions was 2.7-3.1 cm (1-15 cm) [59,60].

The treatment is chosen based on the severity of patient's symptom. Medical treatment may be effective. Medical agents that have been used in the past include oral contraceptives, danazol, progestogen and a GnRH analog may contribute to reducing the mass of an endometriotic lesion, pain and fibrous adhesions associated with periodic bleeding. However, some investigators reported that patients failed to respond medical treatment of abdominal wall endometriosis.

Those not responding to medical treatment were treated successfully using surgery (Figure 5,6) [61]. Abdominal wall endometriosis should be included in the differential diagnosis of women who present with a surgical scar and complaints related to cyclic pain associated with menses.

SUBFERTILITY

Several studies have demonstrated that women who delivered by CS in their first pregnancy are less likely to have further pregnancies than are women who delivered vaginally. Furthermore, when they have a further pregnancy, they are more likely to have a prolonged interpregnancy interval [62,63]. An association between CS and future conception is biologically plausible; the process of incision and repair of the uterus may affect future conception. However, the relationship is complex, involving pathological and psychological factors such as age, height, smoking, status, and history of primary subfertility [64,65]. Recent reports suggest that the association between cesarean birth and subsequent subfertility is likely to be caused by confounding than by a causal relationship; there is no strong evidence of a causal relationship between cesarean delivery and subfertility [66-68].

ADHESION

Gynecologic surgery including CS frequently causes intra-abdominal adhesions. Such adhesions may increase operative time, blood loss, and the risk of injury to surrounding organs during subsequent surgery. Furthermore, adhesion-related pelvic pain and intestinal obstruction may occur [69]. In the published literature, 50-75% of all small bowel obstructions were related to postoperative adhesions [70-72]. In the gynecologic surgery, the rate of adhesion-related bowel obstruction after surgery for benign disease is 8/1,000, with total abdominal hysterectomy leading at 13.6/1000 [73]. The rates of bowel obstruction subsequent to vaginal and cesarean delivery are 1.2 and 2.2 per 1,000, respectively [74]. Morales *et al.* reported encountering adhesions in 46% of second, 76% of third, and 83% of fourth or subsequent cesarean deliveries [75].

Several reports about peritoneal adhesion prevention at CS have been published. Most of them described the advantage of closure or non-closure of the peritoneum, the comparison of surgical procedures, and the effectiveness of an absorbable adhesion barrier at cesarean delivery. Many obstetricians have believed that non-closure of the peritoneum has more advantages and should be recommended [76]. Some studies showed that peritoneal healing occurs by simultaneous multi-site repair as the result of migrating mesothelial cells with mesothelial matrix formation without the need for repositioning of the perioneum; in these cases, peritoneal closure would lead to foreign body reactions to the suture material, ischaemia, tissue necrosis, and inflammation, and there would be less adhesion formation without closure of the peritoneum [77,78]. However, non-closure of the peritoneum does not restore the integrity of the abdominal anatomy. On the other hand, two meta-analyses compared adhesions after closure or non-closure of the peritoneum during the previous CS [79,80]. The authors concluded that closure of the peritoneum had the advantage of reduced adhesion formation. Concerning modifications of techniques in CS procedures, it is difficult to differentiate groups only by closure and non-closure of the peritoneum, because other parameters, such as operation time spent pushing down the bladder from its attachment position on the uterus, may contribute to adhesion formation.

Recently, different synthetic adhesion barriers have been heavily marketed as a means of reducing adhesion formation. Chapa *et al.* evaluated the effectiveness of an absorbable adhesion barrier utilized at cesarean delivery. Of the 262 primary cesareans performed, 43% had repeat CS. With use of the barrier material, 74% had no adhesion at repeat surgery, versus 22% in the no barrier group [81]. Although these adhesion barriers can reduce intra-abdominal adhesions, in the cost-effectiveness analysis of adhesion barriers to date, their use in CS is ill advised, because our health care system is already financially overburdened [82].

REFERENCES

[1] Births: Rreliminary Data for 2007. *National Center for Health Statistics*. Retrieved 2006-11-23.

[2] Faiz AS, Ananth CV. Etiology and risk factors for placenta previa: an overview and meta-analysis of observational studies. *J. Matern Fetal Neonatal Med.* 2003;13:175-90.

[3] Ananth CV, Demissie K, Smulian JC, Vintzileos AM. Placenta previa in singleton and twin births in the United States, 1989 through 1998: a comparison of risk factor profiles and associated conditions. *Am. J. Obstet. Gynecol.* 2003;188:275-81.

[4] Silver RM, Landon MB, Rouse DJ, Leveno KJ, Spong CY, Thom EA, Moawad AH, Caritis SN, Harper M, Wapner RJ, Sorokin Y, Miodovnik M, Carpenter M, Peaceman AM, O'Sullivan MJ, Sibai B, Langer O, Thorp JM, Ramin SM, Mercer BM; National Institute of Child Health and Human Development Maternal-Fetal Medicine Units Network. Maternal morbidity associated with multiple repeat cesarean deliveries. *Obstet. Gynecol.* 2006;107:1226-32.

[5] Ananth CV, Savitz DA, Williams MA. Placental abruption and its association with hypertension and prolonged rupture of membranes: a methodologic review and meta-analysis. *Obstet. Gynecol.* 1996;88:309-18.

[6] Ananth CV, Berkowitz GS, Savitz DA, Lapinski RH. Placental abruption and adverse perinatal outcomes. *JAMA.* 1999;282:1646-51.

[7] Yang Q, Wen SW, Oppenheimer L, Chen XK, Black D, Gao J, Walker MC. Association of caesarean delivery for first birth with placenta praevia and placental abruption in second pregnancy. *BJOG.* 2007;114:609-13.

[8] Getahun D, Oyelese Y, Salihu HM, Ananth CV. Previous cesarean delivery and risks of placenta previa and placental abruption. *Obstet. Gynecol.* 2006;107:771-8.

[9] Lydon-Rochelle M, Holt VL, Easterling TR, Martin DP. First-birth cesarean and placental abruption or previa at second birth(1). *Obstet. Gynecol.* 2001;97:765-9.

[10] Kennare R, Tucker G, Heard A, Chan A. Risks of adverse outcomes in the next birth after a first cesarean delivery. *Obstet. Gynecol.* 2007;109:270-6.

[11] Rasmussen S, Irgens LM, Dalaker K. A history of placental dysfunction and risk of placental abruption. *Paediatr Perinat Epidemiol.* 1999;13:9-21.

[12] Taylor VM, Kramer MD, Vaughan TL, Peacock S. Placenta previa and prior cesarean delivery: how strong is the association? *Obstet. Gynecol.* 1994;84:55-7.

[13] Hershkowitz R, Fraser D, Mazor M, Leiberman JR. One or multiple previous cesarean sections are associated with similar increased frequency of placenta previa. *Eur. J. Obstet. Gynecol Reprod. Biol.* 1995;62:185-8.

[14] MacDorman MF, Kirmeyer S. Fetal and perinatal mortality, United States, 2005. Natl Vital Stat Rep. 2009;57:1.

[15] World Health Organization. *Definitions and indicators in Family Planning Maternal and Child Health and Reproductive Health.* Geneva: WHO Press, 2001.

[16] Keeling JW, MacGillivray I, Golding J, Wigglesworth J, Berry J, Dunn PM. Classification of perinatal death. *Arch. Dis. Child.* 1989;64:1345-51.

[17] Smith GC, Pell JP, Dobbie R. Caesarean section and risk of unexplained stillbirth in subsequent pregnancy. *Lancet.* 2003;362:1779-84.

[18] Salihu HM, Sharma PP, Kristensen S, Blot C, Alio AP, Ananth CV, Kirby RS. Risk of stillbirth following a cesarean delivery: black-white disparity. *Obstet. Gynecol.* 2006;107:383-90.

[19] Bahtiyar MO, Julien S, Robinson JN, Lumey L, Zybert P, Copel JA, Lockwood CJ, Norwitz ER. Prior cesarean delivery is not associated with an increased risk of stillbirth in a subsequent pregnancy: analysis of U.S. perinatal mortality data, 1995-1997. *Am. J. Obstet. Gynecol.* 2006;195:1373-8.

[20] Gray R, Quigley MA, Hockley C, Kurinczuk JJ, Goldacre M, Brocklehurst P. Caesarean delivery and risk of stillbirth in subsequent pregnancy: a retrospective cohort study in an English population. *BJOG.* 2007;114:264-70.

[21] Wood SL, Chen S, Ross S, Sauve R. The risk of unexplained antepartum stillbirth in second pregnancies following caesarean section in the first pregnancy. *BJOG.* 2008;115:726-31.

[22] Miller DA, Paul RH. Rupture of the unscarred uterus. *Am. J. Obstet. Gynecol.* 1996;174:345.

[23] Miller DA, Goodwin TM, Gherman RB, Intrapartum rupture of the unscarred uterus. *Obstet. Gynecol.* 1997;89:671.

[24] Chauhan SP, Magann EF, Wiggs CD, Barrilleaux PS, Martin JN Jr. Pregnancy after classic cesarean delivery. *Obstet. Gynecol.* 2002;100:946-50.

[25] Spong CY, Landon MB, Gilbert S, Rouse DJ, Leveno KJ, Varner MW, Moawad AH, Simhan HN, Harper M, Wapner RJ, Sorokin Y, Miodovnik M, Carpenter M, Peaceman AM, O'Sullivan MJ, Sibai BM, Langer O, Thorp JM, Ramin SM, Mercer BM; National Institute of Child Health and Human Development (NICHD) Maternal-Fetal Medicine Units (MFMU) Network. Risk of uterine rupture and adverse perinatal outcome at term after cesarean delivery. *Obstet. Gynecol.* 2007;110:801-7.

[26] Landon MB, Hauth JC, Leveno KJ, Spong CY, Leindecker S, Varner MW, Moawad AH, Caritis SN, Harper M, Wapner RJ, Sorokin Y, Miodovnik M, Carpenter M, Peaceman AM, O'Sullivan MJ, Sibai B, Langer O, Thorp JM, Ramin SM, Mercer BM, Gabbe SG; National Institute of Child Health and Human Development Maternal-Fetal Medicine Units Network. Maternal and perinatal outcomes associated with a trial of labor after prior cesarean delivery. *N. Engl. J. Med.* 2004;351:2581-9.

[27] Chauhan SP, Martin JN Jr, Henrichs CE, Morrison JC, Magann EF. Maternal and perinatal complications with uterine rupture in 142,075 patients who attempted vaginal birth after cesarean delivery: a review of the literature. *Am. J. Obstet. Gynecol.* 2003;189:408-17.

[28] Jurkovic D, Hillaby K, Woelfer B, Lawrence A, Salim R, Elson CJ. First-trimester diagnosis and management of pregnancies implanted into the lower uterine segment Cesarean section scar. *Ultrasound Obstet. Gynecol.* 2003;21:220-7.

[29] Seow KM, Huang LW, Lin YH, Lin MY, Tsai YL, Hwang JL. Cesarean scar pregnancy: issues in management. *Ultrasound Obstet. Gynecol.* 2004;23:247-53.

[30] Fait G, Goyert G, Sundareson A, Pickens A Jr. Intramural pregnancy with fetal survival: case history and discussion of etiologic factors. *Obstet. Gynecol.* 1987;70:472-4.

[31] Maymon R, Halperin R, Mendlovic S, Schneider D, Vaknin Z, Herman A, Pansky M. Ectopic pregnancies in Caesarean section scars: the 8 year experience of one medical centre. *Hum. Reprod.* 2004;19:278-84.

[32] Rotas MA, Haberman S, Levgur M. Cesarean scar ectopic pregnancies: etiology, diagnosis, and management. *Obstet. Gynecol.* 2006;107:1373-81.

[33] Fylstra DL. Ectopic pregnancy within a cesarean scar: a review. *Obstet. Gynecol. Surv.* 2002;57:537-43.

[34] Vial Y, Petignat P, Hohlfeld P. Pregnancy in a cesarean scar. *Ultrasound Obstet. Gynecol.* 2000;16:592-3.

[35] Godin PA, Bassil S, Donnez J. An ectopic pregnancy developing in a previous caesarian section scar. *Fertil Steril.* 1997;67:398-400..

[36] Seow KM, Cheng WC, Chuang J, Lee C, Tsai YL, Hwang JL. Methotrexate for cesarean scar pregnancy after in vitro fertilization and embryo transfer. A case report. *J. Reprod. Med.* 2000;45:754-7.

[37] Maymon R, Halperin R, Mendlovic S, Schneider D, Herman A. Ectopic pregnancies in a Caesarean scar: review of the medical approach to an iatrogenic complication. *Hum. Reprod.* Update 2004;10:515-23.

[38] Smith A, Ash A, Maxwell D. Sonographic diagnosis of cesarean scar pregnancy at 16 weeks. *J. Clin. Ultrasound.* 2007;35:212-5.

[39] Herman A, Weinraub Z, Avrech O, Maymon R, Ron-El R, Bukovsky Y. Follow up and outcome of isthmic pregnancy located in a previous caesarean section scar. *Br. J. Obstet. Gynaecol.* 1995;102:839-41.

[40] Einenkel J, Stumpp P, Kösling S, Horn LC, Höckel M. A misdiagnosed case of caesarean scar pregnancy. *Arch. Gynecol. Obstet.* 2005;271:178-81.

[41] Godin PA, Bassil S, Donnez J. An ectopic pregnancy developing in a previous caesarian section scar. *Fertil Steril.* 1997;67:398-400.

[42] Hartung J, Meckies J. Management of a case of uterine scar pregnancy by transabdominal potassium chloride injection. *Ultrasound Obstet. Gynecol.* 2003;21:94-5.

[43] Roberts H, Kohlenber C, Lanzarone V, Murray H. Ectopic pregnancy in lower segment uterine scar. *Aust. N. Z. J. Obstet. Gynaecol.* 1998;38:114-6.

[44] Weimin W, Wenqing L. Effect of early pregnancy on a previous lower segment cesarean section scar. *Int. J. Gynaecol. Obstet.* 2002;77:201-7.

[45] Wang CJ, Yuen LT, Chao AS, Lee CL, Yen CF, Soong YK. Caesarean scar pregnancy successfully treated by operative hysteroscopy and suction curettage. *BJOG.* 2005;112:839-40.

[46] Ben Nagi J, Helmy S, Ofili-Yebovi D, Yazbek J, Sawyer E, Jurkovic D. Reproductive outcomes of women with a previous history of Caesarean scar ectopic pregnancies. *Hum. Reprod.* 2007;22:2012-5.

[47] . Mitchell, G..W. Extrapelvic endometriosis. In Endometriosis: *Contemporary Concept in Clinical Management*, 1989:307-328.

[48] Roncoroni, L., Costi, R., Violi, V., Nunziata, R. Endometriosis on laparotomy scar: A three-case report. *Arch. Gynecol. Obstet.* 2001;265: 165-167.

[49] Singh, K.K., Lessel, A.M., Adam, D.J., Jordan, C., Miles, W.F., Macintyre, I.M., et al. Presentation of endometriosis to general surgeon: a 10 years experience. *Br. Surg. 1995*;82:1349-51.

[50] Blanco, R.G., Parithivel, V.S., Shah, A.K., Gumbs, M.A., Schein, M., Gerst, P.H. Abdominal wall endometriomas. *Am. J. Surg.* 2003;185:596-8.

[51] Dwivedi, A.J., Agrawal, S.N., Silva, Y.J. Abdominal wall endometriomas. *Dig. Dis. Sci.* 2002;47:456-61.

[52] Hensen, J.H., Van, Breda, Vriesman A.C., Puylaert, J.B. Abdominal wall endometriosis: clinical presentation and imaging features with emphasis on sonography. *Am. J. Roentgenol.* 2006;186:616-20.

[53] Basu, P.A., Kesani, A.K., Stacy, G.S., Peabody, T.D. Endometriosis of the vastus lateralis muscle. *Skeletal Radiol.* 2006;35: 595-598.

[54] Steck, W.D., Helwig, E.B. Cutaneous endometriosis. *Clin. Obstet. Gynecol.* 1966;9:373-83.

[55] Nishida, M., Watanabe, K., Sato, N., Ichikawa, Y. Malignant transformation of ovarian endometriosis. *Gynecol. Obstet. Invest.* 2000;50:18-25.

[56] Scully, R.E., Richardson, G.S., Barlow, J.F. The development of malignancy in endometriosis. *Clin. Obstet. Gynecol.* 1966;9:381-414.

[57] Benoit, L., Arnould, L., Cheynel, N., Diane, B., Causeret, S., Machado, A., et al. Malignant extraovarian endometriosis: a review. *Eur. J. Surg. Oncol.* 2006;32:6-11.

[58] Simsir, A., Thorner, K., Waisman, J., Cangiarella, J. Endometriosis in abdominal scars: a report of three cases diagnosed by FNA biopsy. *Am. Surg.* 2001;67:984-986.

[59] Zhao, X., Lang, J., Leng J., Liu, Z., Sun, D., Zhu, L. Abdominal wall endometriomas. *Int. J. Gynecol. Obstet.* 2005;90:218-22.

[60] Horton, J.D., DeZee, K.J., Ahnfeldt, E.P., Wagner, M. Abdominal wall endometriosis: a surgeon's perspective and review of 445 cases. *Am. J. Surg.* 2008;196:207-212.

[61] Chatterjee, S.K. Scar endometriosis: a clinicopathologic study of 17 cases. *Obstet. Gynecol.* 1980;56:81-4.

[62] Hemminki E. Impact of caesarean section on future pregnancy--a review of cohort studies. *Paediatr Perinat Epidemiol*. 1996;10:366-79.
[63] Porter M, Bhattacharya S, van Teijlingen E, Templeton A; Reproductive Outcome Following Caesarean Section (ROCS) Collaborative Group. Does Caesarean section cause infertility? *Hum. Reprod*. 2003;18:1983-6.
[64] Pandian Z, Bhattacharya S, Templeton A. Review of unexplained infertility and obstetric outcome: a 10 year review. *Hum. Reprod*. 2001;16:2593-7.
[65] Smith GC, Pell JP, Dobbie R. Caesarean section and risk of unexplained stillbirth in subsequent pregnancy. *Lancet*. 2003;362:1779-84.
[66] Smith GC, Wood AM, Pell JP, Dobbie R. First cesarean birth and subsequent fertility. *Fertil Steril*. 2006;85:90-5.
[67] Collin SM, Marshall T, Filippi V. Caesarean section and subsequent fertility in sub-Saharan Africa. *BJOG*.. 2006;113:276-83.
[68] Eijsink JJ, van der Leeuw-Harmsen L, van der Linden PJ. Pregnancy after Caesarean section: fewer or later? *Hum. Reprod*. 2008;23:543-7.
[69] Practice Committee of American Society for Reproductive Medicine in collaboration with Society of Reproductive Surgeons. Pathogenesis, consequences, and control of peritoneal adhesions in gynecologic surgery. *Fertil Steril*. 2008;90:144-9.
[70] Ray NF, Denton WG, Thamer M, Henderson SC, Perry S. Abdominal adhesiolysis: inpatient care and expenditures in the United States in 1994. *J. Am. Coll Surg*. 1998;186:1-9.
[71] Fevang BT, Fevang J, Lie SA, Søreide O, Svanes K, Viste A. Long-term prognosis after operation for adhesive small bowel obstruction. *Ann. Surg*. 2004;240:193-201.
[72] Foster NM, McGory ML, Zingmond DS, Ko CY. Small bowel obstruction: a population-based appraisal. *J. Am. Coll Surg*. 2006;203:170-6.
[73] Al-Sunaidi M, Tulandi T. Adhesion-related bowel obstruction after hysterectomy for benign conditions. *Obstet. Gynecol*. 2006;108:1162-6.
[74] Andolf E, Thorsell M, Källén K. Cesarean delivery and risk for postoperative adhesions and intestinal obstruction: a nested case-control study of the Swedish Medical Birth Registry. *Am. J. Obstet. Gynecol*. 2010;203:406.
[75] Morales KJ, Gordon MC, Bates GW Jr. Postcesarean delivery adhesions associated with delayed delivery of infant. *Am. J. Obstet. Gynecol*. 2007;196:461.
[76] Hofmeyr GJ, Mathai M, Shah A, Novikova N. Techniques for caesarean section. *Cochrane Database Syst. Rev*. 2008; 1:CD004662.
[77] Montz FJ, Shimanuki T, Dezerega GS. Postsurgical mesothelial reepithelialization. In: DeCherney AG Polan ML, editors. Reproductive Surgery. Chicago: Yearbook Medical Publisher, 1987. pp.31-48.
[78] Hubbard TB Jr, Khan MZ, Carag VR Jr, Albites VE, Hricko GM. The pathology of peritoneal repair: its relation to the formation of adhesions. *Ann. Surg*. 1967;165:908-16.
[79] Cheong YC, Premkumar G, Metwally M, Peacock JL, Li TC. To close or not to close? A systematic review and a meta-analysis of peritoneal non-closure and adhesion formation after caesarean section. *Eur. J.* Obstet. *Gynecol. Reprod. Biol*. 2009;147:3-8.
[80] Shi Z, Ma L, Yang Y, Wang H, Schreiber A, Li X, Tai S, Zhao X, Teng J, Zhang L, Lu W, An Y, Alla NR, Cui T. Adhesion formation after previous caesarean section-a meta-analysis and systematic review. *BJOG*. 2011;118:410-22.

[81] Chapa HO, Venegas G, Vanduyne CP, Antonetti AG, Sandate JP, Silver L. Peritoneal adhesion prevention at cesarean section: an analysis of the effectiveness of an absorbable adhesion barrier. *J. Reprod. Med.* 2011;56:103-9.
[82] Albright CM, Rouse DJ. Adhesion barriers at cesarean delivery: advertising compared with the evidence. *Obstet. Gynecol.* 2011;118:157-60.

In: Cesarean Section: Procedures, Complications and Recovery ISBN: 978-1-62081-214-3
Editor: Eyal Sheiner

Chapter XII

NEONATAL COMPLICATIONS OF CESAREAN DELIVERY

Naomi Schneid-Kofman*[*,1] and Eyal Sheiner[2]
[1]Outpatient Obstetrics and Gynecology, Meuhedet Health Services. Israel
[2]Department of Obstetrics and Gynecology, Faculty of Health Sciences, Soroka University Medical Center, Ben-Gurion University of the Negev, Beer-Sheva, Israel

INTRODUCTION

The comprehensive discussion of cesarean delivery (CD) complications must include fetal- neonatal issues. This unique surgical intervention targets two patients. One is operated upon sometimes for the mere chance of sparing morbidity from the other. Furthermore, maternal and fetal interests may contradict at times. The decision to perform a CD at times of contradiction between fetus and mother may require ethical principals and in extreme occurrences involve legal intervention. The majority of CD indications are fetal indications. Yet the mainstay of informed consent consists of maternal morbidity issues [1], rarely are fetal complications discussed as main issues to consider. An exception to this practice is the issue of prematurity, especially if iatrogenic (as a result from the elected timing of the cesarean surgery).

In this chapter, a detailed discussion of the fetal aspects of maternal CD will be illuminated.

NEONATAL INJURIES DURING CESAREAN DELIVERY

The fetus is protected during pregnancy and delivery by the medium of the surrounding amniotic fluid. The various techniques of uterine wall incision are designed to prevent fetal

* Corresponding author: Naomi Schneid Kofman. Address: Sansana, D.N. Negev 3, 85334, Phone and Fax: 972-8-6519325, Email: shir2k@zahav.net.il.

injury (An initial sharp incision followed by blunt extension of the opening). Albeit the precautions fetal laceration is a recognized complication of CD, yet major injuries are rare. Various case reports of specific fetal injuries were published, as an injury to the extensor pollicis longus tendon during CD followed by surgical repair of the tendon at age six days with good recovery of function, published lately [2]. Bilateral femoral fracture as a result of birth trauma is extremely rare but has been reported during CD [3] as well as other iatrogenic fractures.

Neonatal morbidity identified following a CD intervention may not arise from surgery. Although sometimes not diagnosed prior to surgery, pre labor insult might be responsible for the morbidity, as well as genetic or developmental illness.

Some fetal anomalies are considered an indication for CD. The surgical mode of delivery is thought to prevent possible dystocia during vaginal delivery or birth trauma to exposed fetal tissue. Scarce data exist supporting the benefit of this mode of delivery for most anomalies. Furthermore, the preoperative compromised fetal condition and unfavorable outcome can falsely be attributed to CD complication. While fetal morbidity might promote CD in light of potential maternal complications, it is important to assess fetal viability, and avoid cesarean maternal complications when no fetal benefit is expected [4].

Neonatal Respiratory and Infectious Disease Related to Cesarean Delivery

Evidence suggests increased early neonatal respiratory complications from planned CD compared with those from vaginal delivery such as respiratory distress syndrome secondary to transient tachypnea of the newborn, surfactant deficiency, and pulmonary hypertension. In infants who develop respiratory distress after planned CD, the need for mechanical ventilation is dramatically higher [5]. Furthermore, longstanding evidence demonstrates that a significant number of infants will progress to severe respiratory failure and require prolonged hospitalization, and are at increased risk for chronic lung disease and death [6]. On the other hand, the same elective cesarean delivery reduces the occurrence of birth asphyxia, trauma, and meconium aspiration.

Physiologic changes during the last few weeks of pregnancy coupled with the onset of spontaneous labor are accompanied by changes in the hormonal milieu of the fetus and its mother, resulting in preparation of the fetus for the dramatic neonatal transition. Rapid clearance of fetal lung fluid is a key part of these changes, transepithelial sodium re-absorption through amiloride-sensitive sodium channels in the alveolar epithelial cells play a major roll, with only a limited contribution from mechanical factors and Starling forces, contrary to past understanding [7].

Timing of planned CD within the range of term weeks of pregnancy (37-42 weeks of pregnancy) alters the risk of neonatal respiratory complications. The adjusted risk of neonatal respiratory morbidity associated with prelabor cesarean birth at 37 weeks is four times higher than in intended vaginal birth after 37 weeks. The authors conclude that prelabor cesarean delivery should be performed after at least 38 weeks' of gestation in order to minimize neonatal respiratory morbidity [8]. Recent research supports a later stage for planned CD and discourages planned CD before 39 weeks of gestation unless there is evidence of fetal lung maturity. Compared with births at 39 weeks, births at 37 weeks and at 38 weeks were associated with an increased risk of neonatal death (aOR for births at 37 weeks gestation, 2.1; 95% CI, 1.7 to 2.5; aOR for births at 38 weeks gestation, 1.5; 95% CI, 1.3 to 1.7; P for trend <0.001). The rates of adverse respiratory outcomes, mechanical ventilation, newborn sepsis, hypoglycemia, admission to the neonatal ICU, and hospitalization for 5 days or more were increased by a factor of 1.8 to 4.2 for births at 37 weeks and 1.3 to 2.1 for births at 38 weeks [9]. Apart from delaying the planned CD to 39 weeks, administration of a single course of antenatal betamethazone at term, 48 hours prior to surgery has been suggested. A significant decrease in admissions due to respiratory distress was noted (5.1% in the control group versus 2.4% in the treatment group; RR 0.46, 95% CI 0.23–0.93) [10]. Delivery before 39 weeks was not associated with a decrease in severe maternal morbidity when compared with delivery at 39 weeks (adjusted odds ratio 1.16; 95% confidence interval 1.00-1.34). Early delivery was associated with increased maternal hospitalization of 5 days or more, but not with a composite of death or hysterectomy or with individual maternal morbidities. The authors concluded that elective repeat cesarean delivery at 37 or 38 weeks is not associated with decreased maternal morbidity [11].

In the view of these developments, the question of women with planned CD at 39 weeks who will go into labor prior to their planned date and therefore will have urgent cesareans rather than planned CD was addressed. Furthermore, the issue of high order repeat CD (4th or 5th cesarean) has not been addressed in these studies, it is yet to be determined whether it is safe to delay repeated CD to 39 weeks gestation.

In an attempt to define predictive factors of post CD neonatal respiratory complications, preoperative maternal pulse oxymeter perfusion index was studied along with placental evidence of chorioamnionitis. Further research is required to determine whether maternal oxygenation and placental subclinical chorioamnionitis are predictors of neonatal outcome rather than CD [12]. Planned CD is associated with reduced risk for neonatal encephalopathy.

In a study that compared infants born by elective repeat cesarean section to those born vaginally, a statistically significant increase in suspected sepsis was noted in infants delivered vaginally [13]. A lower rate of sepsis evaluation in neonates born to mothers after a planned CD compared to those born after a trial of vaginal delivery was also reported [14]. There are relatively few indications for performing cesarean delivery to avoid transmission of infectious agents to the neonate, active genital disease of Herpes simplex virus and HIV infection are considered indications for CD, yet some evidence promotes antepartum medical treatment to prevent vertical transmission. Perhaps in the future this line of therapy will eliminate the need for surgery in an otherwise morbid population [15].

No difference in infectious neonatal morbidity following timing of administration of prophylactic antibiotics (before skin incision or after cord clamping) was found [16]. Although a meta-analysis suggests that neonates delivered by cesarean are less likely to initiate breast-feeding, there does not appear to be any difference at 3 or 24 months [17].

PREMATURITY

CD of premature or very low birth weight infants has been suggested to increase survival, and provide no additional risk. Overall mortality during the first year of life is decreased after

CD compared to vaginal delivery. An important ethical issue is parental informed consent in light of fetal increased survival with poor neurodevelopmental outcome. The effect of CD upon other premature neonatal complications has been investigated. Respiratory distress syndrome (RDS) is reported to be moderately increased among very preterm infants delivered by cesarean section. A small metaanalysis of 122 women found no increased risk of RDS in planned CD for preterm deliveries [18]. Conflicting data exist, and some have found that primary CD may pose an increased risk of neonatal mortality and morbidity for low-risk preterm infants at 32 to 36 weeks' gestation [19].

Scarce data exist regarding rate of intraventricular hemorrhage (IVH) in premature deliveries by CD, although expected to provide a less traumatic mode of delivery IVH rates are not decreased. Rate of asphyxia determined by cord blood base deficit measurements > 12 mmol/L, are lower among infants 22 to 25 weeks' gestation delivered by CD. There is lack of evidence on rate of necrotizing enterocolitis following CD [20]. Neonatal complications of emergency CD are increased along with the reported increase of maternal complication rate outlined in the chapter regarding maternal complications. Higher rate of low Apgar score at 5 minutes were reported, as well as increased neonatal death, admission to neonatal intensive care unit, increased need for intubation, higher rate of septicemia, neonatal seizures, and fetal injury (all having $P < 0.05$) [21]. In order to assess the impact of repeated CDs, comparison of outcome in women at forth or fifth CD (n=122) with outcome of women at second or third CD (n=146) was conducted. Women at their 4th and 5th CD had lower birth weights (p=0.026), lower Apgar scores at 1 minute (p=0.0001) and 5 minutes (p=0.042), higher numbers of fetal death (p=0.03). Multiple repeated CDs increase the risks for operative complications and poor perinatal outcomes [22]. Timing of the repeated CD has been addressed in several studies. Elective repeat cesarean section during the 38th week of pregnancy is associated with higher neonatal morbidity compared to neonates born thereafter [9], yet fifth percent of CDs are preformed prior to 39 wks. This was not examined in the sub population of high order repeated CD as previously noted. The early planned CD had a significantly higher overall risk of various poor neonatal outcome measures, including resuscitation, sepsis, respiratory morbidity and support, admission to the NICU, and prolonged hospitalization [23].

Long Term Neonatal Complications

A previous CD has an impact upon neonatal complications in subsequent delivery. A comparison of maternal and neonatal outcome of the following delivery found an increased risk if the prior delivery was by CD; 17,406 births were examined prospectively. Prior CD patients without trial of labor (TOL) required more blood transfusions, intensive care unit admissions and hospital readmissions than women with a prior vaginal delivery. Prior CD patients with TOL required more aminoglycosides for postpartum infection. Term neonates of CD mothers without a TOL were more likely to have prolonged hospitalization and require ventilation support. The authors concluded that in their subsequent delivery, women with a prior CD are at significant risks for postpartum maternal and neonatal morbidities compared with parous patients who experienced a prior vaginal delivery [24]. Among children with Crohn's disease or ulcerative colitis CD rate was similar to that of control subjects. In children with celiac disease, a significantly enhanced likelihood of being born by cesarean delivery was found compared with control subjects (odds ratio: 1.8 [95% CI. 1.13-2.88]; P = .014). The authors concluded that mode of delivery and associated alterations in the development of the enteric homeostasis during the neonatal period might influence the incidence of celiac disease [25].

As an anecdote, while investigating the risk factors for post CD complication a study examined the possible connection between medical staff change of shift and complications. No association was found with physician shift. However, cesarean delivery during nursing change of shift was associated with increased risk of neonatal facial nerve palsy (5 vs 0) as were hysterectomies (33 [0.24%] vs 23[0.53%]; $P = .007$). The authors could not explain this impact, speculating a type I error or an impact upon the physicians to attempt and fail more aggressive forceps delivery or definite treatment as hysterectomy. Further investigation was recommended [26].

Neonatal Complications of Anesthesia

Awareness to the impact of anesthesia upon the neonate is not common. In the past most CDs were performed with conduction general anesthesia, while currently most CDs are performed with neuroaxial anesthesia (regional/spinal).

A decrease in mean arterial blood pressure by >30% is documented in nearly half of women undergoing regional anesthesia. The reduced afterload (decreased systemic vascular resistance), causes lower maternal mean arterial blood pressure and reduced uteroplacental perfusion. The risk factors for hypotension include preoperative hypertension, maternal older age, type of spinal anesthesia, and higher infant birth weight. The hypotension is well tolerated by term healthy babies and no short term perinatal complications are noted [27].

Some investigators found fetal exposure to general anesthesia a risk factor for learning disabilities and long term behavioral abnormalities, while others have not found such a connection. Lowest rates of learning disabilities were found among children who delivered by CD with regional anesthesia compared to general anesthesia or vaginal delivery [28].

In urgent or emergent CD surgeons' common practice is to shorten the time interval from the beginning of anesthesia to delivery of the fetus. In elective antepartum CD, the same approach is commonly practiced. Yet there are studies that found no association between skin incision-to-delivery interval and neonatal wellbeing in elective CD. A longer skin incision-to-delivery interval does not seem to compromise neonatal acid-base balance [29].

Neonatal Mortality Related to Cesarean Delivery

Several studies have found increased neonatal mortality following CD after exclusion of congenital anomalies and low Apgar scores (<4) and adjusting for social demographic and medical risk factors (OR 2.02 (1.60-2.55) [30]. A Nigerian report from recent years (2006-2007) stated perinatal mortality rate was 43.7 per 1000 live births. CD rate of merely 8.4% resulted in 11.1% perinatal deaths. Perinatal mortality from CD accounted for 21.4% of the total deaths. Emergency CD accounted for three times more perinatal death than elective CD

(12% vs 4%). Severe birth asphyxia was responsible for most perinatal deaths (70.8%). The main indications for cesarean section were cephalopelvic disproportion, previous CD plus an obstetric abnormality and prolonged obstructed labor [31].

A global study found that for countries with overall cesarean rates below 15%, higher cesarean rates were correlated with lower neonatal and maternal mortality while for countries with national cesarean rates above 15% higher CD rates were correlated with higher neonatal and maternal mortality [32]. Repeated cesarean deliveries are associated with a significantly higher neonatal and maternal mortality compared with cesarean or vaginal deliveries for women who do not have a prior cesarean [33].

Regarding the increased risk for stillbirth in infants born after a trial of labor [34], and the 1.5 fold increase in neonatal mortality in infants born by cesarean section, regardless of previous trial of labor [35], some conclude overall perinatal mortality is decreased for planned cesarean deliveries [36].

Conclusion

In a comprehensive review of the latest literature, it is evident that several aspects of cesarean delivery may generate neonatal complications. Choice of CD as the mode of delivery whether for maternal or fetal indication or due to maternal request only should be preceded by maternal comprehension of fetal complications as well as maternal complications. Let as hope the above words will have a small contribution to the knowledge and understanding of the neonatal prospective.

References

[1] NIH State-of-the-Science Conference statement on cesarean delivery on maternal request. *NIH Consens State Sci. statements*. 2006;23(1):1–29.

[2] Rinker B. Extensor tendon injury during cesarean delivery. *J. Hand Surg. Am.* 2011; 36(1): 125-8.

[3] Cebesoy FB, Cebesoy O, Incebiyik A. Bilateral femur fracture in a newborn: an extreme complication of cesarean delivery. *Arch. Gynecol. Obstet.* 2009; 279(1):73-4.

[4] Hamrick SEG. Cesarean Delivery and Its Impact on the Anomalous Infant. *Clin. Perinatol.* 2008;395–406.

[5] Roth-Kleiner M, Wagner BP, Bachmann D, Pfenninger J. Respiratory distress syndrome in nearterm babies after caesarean section. *Swiss Med. Wkly.* 2003;133:283–8.

[6] Keszler M, Carbone MT, Cox C, Schumacher RE. Severe respiratory failure after elective repeat cesarean delivery: a potentially preventable condition leading to extracorporeal membrane oxygenation. *Pediatrics.* 1992;89:670–2.

[7] Ramachandrappa A, Jain L. Elective Cesarean Section: Its Impact on Neonatal Respiratory Outcome. *Clin. Perinatol.* 2008; 373–93.

[8] Farchi S; Di Lallo D; Franco F; Polo A; Lucchini R; Calzolari F; De Curtis M. Neonatal respiratory morbidity and mode of delivery in a population-based study of low-risk pregnancies. *Acta Obstet. Gynecol. Scand.* 2009; 88(6): 729-32.

[9] Tita AT, Landon MB, Spong CY, Lai Y, Leveno KJ, Varner MW, Moawad AH, Caritis SN, Meis PJ, Wapner RJ, Sorokin Y, Miodovnik M, Carpenter M, Peaceman AM, O'Sullivan MJ, Sibai BM, Langer O, Thorp JM, Ramin SM, Mercer BM; Eunice Kennedy Shriver NICHD Maternal-Fetal Medicine Units Network. Timing of elective repeat cesarean delivery at term and neonatal outcomes. *N. Engl. J. Med.* 2009; 360:111-20.

[10] Stutchfield P, Whitaker R, Russell I. Antenatal Steroids for Term Elective Caesarean Section (ASTECS) Research Team. Antenatal betamethasone and incidence of neonatal respiratory distress after elective caesarean section: pragmatic randomised trial. *BMJ.* 2005;331:662.

[11] Tita AT, Lai Y, Landon MB, Spong CY, Leveno KJ, Varner MW, Caritis SN, Meis PJ, Wapner RJ, Sorokin Y, Peaceman AM, O'Sullivan MJ, Sibai BM, Thorp JM, Ramin SM, Mercer BM. Timing of elective repeat cesarean delivery at term and maternal perioperative outcomes. *Obstet. Gynecol.* 2011;117(2 Pt 1):280-6.

[12] De Felice C, Leoni L, Tommasini E, Tonni G, Toti P, Del Vecchio A, Ladisa G, Latini G. Maternal pulse oximetry perfusion index as a predictor of early adverse respiratory neonatal outcome after elective cesarean delivery. *Pediatr Crit. Care Med.* 2008; 9:203–8.

[13] Hook B, Kiwi R, Amini SB, Fanaroff A, Hack M. Neonatal morbidity after elective repeat cesarean section and trial of labor. *Pediatrics.* 1997;100(3 Pt 1):348–53.

[14] Signore C, Hemachandra A, Klebanoff M. Neonatal mortality and morbidity after elective cesarean delivery versus routine expectant management: a decision analysis. *Semin. Perinatol.* 2006;30(5):288–95.

[15] Sharma D, Spearman P. The Impact of Cesarean Delivery on Transmission of Infectious Agents to the Neonate. *Clin Perinatol.* 2008;407–420.

[16] Yildirim G, Gungorduk K, Guven HZ, Aslan H, Celikkol O, Sudolmus S, Ceylan Y. When should we perform prophylactic antibiotics in elective cesarean cases? *Arch. Gynecol. Obstet.* 2009; 280(1): 13-8.

[17] Hannah ME, Hannah WJ, Hodnett ED, Chalmers B, Kung R, Willan A, Amankwah K, Cheng M, Helewa M, Hewson S, Saigal S, Whyte H, Gafni A; Term Breech Trial 3-Month Follow-up Collaborative Group. Outcomes at 3 months after planned cesarean vs. planned vaginal delivery for breech presentation at term: the international randomized Term Breech Trial. *J. Am. Med. Assoc.* 2002;287:1822–31.

[18] Grant A, Glazener CM. Elective caesarean section versus expectant management for delivery of the small baby. *Cochrane Database Syst. Rev.* 2001;(1):CD000078.

[19] Malloy MH. Impact of cesarean section on intermediate and late preterm births: United States, 2000-2003. *Birth.* 2009; 36(1): 26-33.

[20] Malloy MH, Doshi S. Cesarean Section and the Outcome of Very Preterm and Very Low-Birthweight Infants. *Clin. Perinatol.* 2008; 421–35.

[21] Seal SL; Kamilya G; Mukherji J; Bhattacharyya SK; De A; Hazra A. Outcome in second- versus first-stage cesarean delivery in a teaching institution in eastern India. *Am. J. Perinatol.*2010; 27(6): 507-12.

[22] Gedikbasi A; Akyol A; Bingol B; Cakmak D; Sargin A; Uncu R; Ceylan Y. Multiple repeated cesarean deliveries: operative complications in the fourth and fifth surgeries in urgent and elective cases. *Taiwan J. Obstet. Gynecol.* 2010; 49(4): 425-31.

[23] Wilmink FA, Hukkelhoven CWPM, Lunshof S, Mol BW, van der Post JA, Papatsonis DN. Neonatal outcome following elective cesarean section beyond 37 weeks of gestation: a 7- year retrospective analysis of a national registry. *Am. J. Obstet. Gynecol.* 2010;202:250.e1-8.

[24] Galyean AM; Lagrew DC; Bush MC; Kurtzman JT. Previous cesarean section and the risk of postpartum maternal complications and adverse neonatal outcomes in future pregnancies. *J. Perinatol.* 2009; 29(11): 726-30.

[25] Decker E, Engelmann G, Findeisen A, Gerner P, Laass M, Ney D, Posovszky C, Hoy L, Hornef MW. Cesarean delivery is associated with celiac disease but not inflammatory bowel disease in children. *Pediatrics*. 2010; 125(6): e1433-40.

[26] Bailit JL, Landon MB, Lai Y, Rouse DJ, Spong CY, Varner MW, Moawad AH, Simhan HN, Harper M, Wapner RJ, Sorokin Y, Miodovnik M, O'Sullivan MJ, Sibai BM, Langer O; National Institute of Child Health and Human Development Maternal-Fetal Medicine Units Network. Maternal-Fetal Medicine Units Network Cesarean Registry. Impact of shift change on cesarean complications. *Am. J. Obstet. Gynecol.* 2008;198:173.e1-173.e5.

[27] Maayan-Metzger A, Schushan-Eisen I, Todris L, Etchin A, Kuint J. Maternal hypotension during elective cesarean section and short-term neonatal outcome. *Am. J. Obstet. Gynecol.* 2010;202:56.e1-5.

[28] Sprung J, Flick RP, Wilder RT, Katusic SK, Pike TL, Dingli M, Gleich SJ, Schroeder DR, Barbaresi WJ, Hanson AC, Warner DO. Anesthesia for Cesarean Delivery and Learning Disabilities in a Population-based Birth Cohort. *Anesthesiology*. 2009; 111:302–10.

[29] Fontanarosa M, Fontanarosa N. Incision-to-delivery interval and neonatal wellbeing during cesarean section. *Minerva Ginecol.* 2008; 60(1): 23-7.

[30] MacDorman MF, Declercq E, Menacker F, Malloy MH. Infant and neonatal mortality for primary cesarean and vaginal births to women with ‘‘no indicated risk,’’ United States, 1998–2001 birth cohorts. *Birth*. 2006;33:175–82.

[31] Onankpa B; Ekele B. Fetal outcome following cesarean section in a university teaching hospital. *J. Natl. Med. Assoc.* 2009; 101(6): 578-81.

[32] Betran AP, Merialdi M, Lauer JA, Bing-Shun W, Thomas J, Van Look P, Wagner M. Rates of caesarean section: analysis of global, regional and national estimates. *Paediatr Perinat Epidemiol*. 2007;21:98–113.

[33] Kolas T, Saugstad OD, Daltveit AK, Nilsen ST, Øian P. Planned cesarean versus planned vaginal delivery at term: comparison of newborn infant outcomes. *Am. J. Obstet. Gynecol.* 2006;195:1538–43.

[34] Ecker JL. Once a pregnancy, always a cesarean? Rationale and feasibility of a randomized controlled trial. *Am. J. Obstet. Gynecol.* 2004;190(2):314–8.

[35] Signore C, Hemachandra A, Klebanoff M. Neonatal mortality and morbidity after elective cesarean delivery versus routine expectant management: a decision analysis. *Semin. Perinatol.* 2006;30(5):288–95.

[36] Williams HO. The Ethical Debate of Maternal Choice and Autonomy in Cesarean Delivery. *Clin. Perinatol.* 2008: 455–62.

In: Cesarean Section: Procedures, Complications and Recovery ISBN: 978-1-62081-214-3
Editor: Eyal Sheiner

Chapter XIII

CESAREAN HYSTERECTOMY

Jason D. Wright* and Patricia Devine
Department of Obstetrics and Gynecology
Columbia University College of Physicians and Surgeons, NY, US

INTRODUCTION

Postpartum hemorrhage is a leading cause of maternal mortality in the developed and developing world. [1-5] Peripartum hysterectomy, although typically performed as a last resort, is often a life saving procedure. When necessary, peripartum hysterectomy is performed emergently, often in the setting of heavy bleeding with poor visualization, and frequently in settings with less than optimal equipment and personal. As such, the procedure is associated with substantial morbidity and not insignificant mortality [6-14].

In the United States it is estimated that peripartum hysterectomy occurs in 0.77 per 1000 deliveries. [15] Compared to a primary vaginal delivery without a history of cesarean delivery the odds ratio for peripartum hysterectomy is 2.70 for vaginal birth after cesarean, 6.54 for primary cesarean delivery and 8.90 at the time of a repeat cesarean delivery. [15] In the U.S. the incidence of both postpartum hemorrhage and peripartum hysterectomy are increasing. [16-18] Population-based studies have demonstrated that postpartum hemorrhage increased 26% from 1994 to 2006 while peripartum hysterectomy increased 15% from 1994 to 2007. [16, 17] Much of the increase in the rates of postpartum hemorrhage and hysterectomy is due to the dramatically rising cesarean delivery rate. [19, 20].

Prior cesarean delivery is the most important risk factor associated with peripartum hysterectomy. [15, 21] The risk for peripartum hysterectomy increases with the number of prior cesarean deliveries [22].

* Corresponding Author: Jason D. Wright, M.D. Division of Gynecologic Oncology, Department of Obstetrics and Gynecology, Columbia University College of Physicians and Surgeons, 161 Fort Washington Ave, 8th Floor, New York, NY 10032, Telephone: (212) 305-3410, Fax: (212) 305-3412, Email: jw2459@columbia.edu.

INDICATIONS

Abnormal placentation and uterine atony are the most common indications for peripartum hysterectomy. [7, 8, 10, 11, 23-29] A survey of 229 maternity hospitals in the United Kingdom identified 315 women who required peripartum hysterectomy. Fifty three percent of the procedures were performed for uterine atony while 38% were due to placenta accreta or its variants. [9] In the U.S. uterine atony and abnormal placentation also appear to account for the majority of cases with a gradual shift towards a higher proportion of cases attributable to placenta accreta. [7, 8, 10, 11, 23] Other less frequent indications for peripartum hysterectomy include uterine rupture, infection, laceration of the genital tract, extension of the cesarean scar, leiomyomata, and cancer [9, 11].

SURGICAL TECHNIQUE

Emergent Peripartum Hysterectomy

Peripartum hysterectomy is generally performed in one of two scenarios: emergently in the setting of bleeding and in a somewhat more planned fashion for patients with placenta accreta. When obstetric hemorrhage requires hysterectomy it is a life-threatening emergency and mandates the rapid mobilization of the appropriate surgical team. Preoperative readiness and planning to deal with these emergent situations is essential to optimizing outcomes. Standardized protocols, the availability of equipment, and the readiness of trained operating room staff are essential. Instrument trays containing the necessary equipment to perform hysterectomy as well as self-retaining retractors should be available and sterilized in all labor and delivery operating rooms. When obstetric hemorrhage is encountered it should be immediately communicated to the anesthesia team and operating room staff. Blood products including packed red cells, fresh frozen plasma, and platelets should be called and additional staff mobilized. Patients under regional anesthesia may require conversion to general anesthesia for patient comfort and to facilitate packing of the abdominal contents. Additional vascular access possibly including the placement of a central line or arterial line should be obtained.

When peripartum hysterectomy is undertaken for obstetric hemorrhage the goal is to gain control of the uterine vessels as quickly as possible. In patients who underwent a vaginal delivery a midline laparotomy should be performed. For those who had a cesarean delivery the abdominal incision may need to be extended. After opening the abdomen the patient should be placed in Trendelenburg position, the abdominal contents packed with moist laparotomy sponges, and a self-retaining retractor placed. The cornua of the uterus is then clamped with large Kelly clamps and the uterus elevated and placed under traction. The peritoneum is then incised, typically at the round ligaments and the retroperitoneum opened widely. Ovarian preservation is essential. After identification of the ureters the utero-ovarian pedicles are clamped and divided and the ovaries moved out of the surgical field. The vesicouterine peritoneum is then opened and bladder flap gently retracted. In emergent situations we advocate a "clamp-cut-drop" technique to expedite control of the uterine arteries. In this technique the vascular pedicles of the uterus are clamped, the tissue divided and the clamps left in place. The surgeon then marches down the pedicles until the uterine vessels have been clamped and control of bleeding is obtained. Once the patient has been stabilized further attention can be turned to ligation of the previously divided pedicles.

After vascular control is obtained care should be taken to ensure that the ureters and bladder are safely away from the field of dissection. It is often difficult to identify the cervix during peripartum hysterectomy, particular in women who have labored. To facilitate identification of the cervix a ring forceps can be placed vaginally on the cervix. Alternatively, a sponge stick placed vaginally can facilitate the procedure especially in patients who have not labored. After the uterus has been removed all of the vascular pedicles as well as the ovarian pedicles should be reinspected. The integrity of the urinary tract is verified. Placement of an intraperitoneal drain (Jackson Pratt or similar) should be considered.

Peripartum Hysterectomy for Placenta Accreta

Both the operative technique and the preoperative preparation are different in patients at high-risk to require hysterectomy (i.e., placenta accreta). Unlike an emergent hysterectomy for uterine atony, these procedures can be undertaken in a more controlled fashion. Preoperative planning is essential. While imaging modalities are inaccurate in defining the extent of placental invasion, all preoperative imaging including magnetic resonance imaging and ultrasound should be reviewed prior to the procedure. Consideration can be given to placement of ureteral stents, and iliac catheters either for embolization or balloon occlusion as discussed below. Prior to beginning the procedure there should be verification that all required blood products are available. We place all patients in lithotomy position and enter the abdomen through a midline vertical incision.

After entry into the abdomen the uterus is inspected and any abnormal vascularity noted. Invasion of the placenta into the bladder anteriorly or the lateral parametria should be noted (Figure 1). Hysterotomy should be planned to avoid the placenta if possible. Given that the most common location for the placenta is anterior, fundal or posterior hysterotomy is often necessary. After delivery of the infant the placenta is inspected. If there is clear evidence of placenta accreta the placenta should not be interrupted and should be left in situ. Manual removal of the placenta in women with placenta accreta results in increased morbidity. [6] If the placenta is left in situ the uterus should be closed with a large running stitch and the hysterectomy begun.

Again, the hysterectomy is begun with division of the round ligaments and entry into the retroperitoneum. The retroperitoneum is then opened widely and the ureters identified. The utero-ovarian ligaments are then clamped and divided. The vesicouterine peritoneum is then opened and the bladder gently dissected. For women with placenta increta and percreta there is often visible placental tissue bulging into the parametria or towards the back wall of the bladder. Every attempt should be made to avoid disrupting the placenta. The lateral wall of the uterus is typically thin and attenuated making it difficult to place clamps along the uterus as is typically done for hysterectomy. We dissect the peritoneal attachments down to the uterine arteries and attempt to directly ligate the uterine arteries and their branches after identification of the ureter. After the large vessels of the uterine vasculature have been divided dissection of the cardinal ligament can be continued. Ideally this dissection is continued well below the placental tissue.

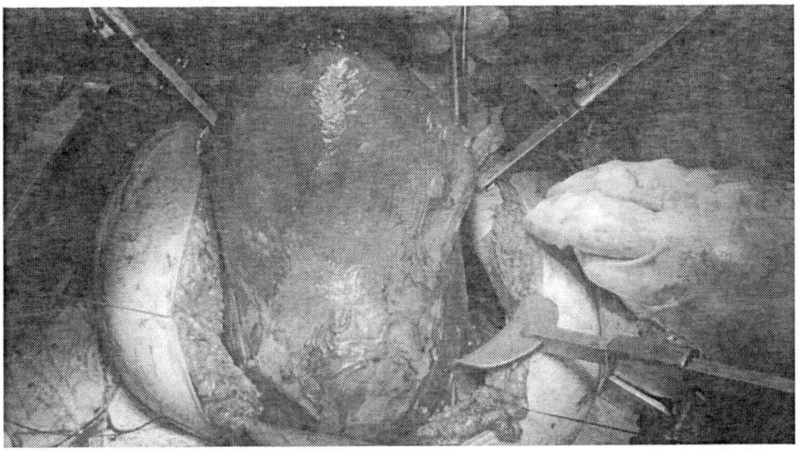

Figure 1. Intraoperative photograph of placenta accreta. The placenta is bulging into the anterior wall of the uterus.

For women with placenta percreta the plane between the bladder and uterus may be completely obliterated. Often an intentional cystotomy is required to identify the boundary between the placenta and bladder. Once below the placenta the uterus can be amputated. Placement of a sponge stick within the vagina will help to identify the cervix.

After removal of the uterus all of the vascular pedicles should be re-inspected. There are often many small perforating vessels along the wall of the bladder that require attention. It is critical that the integrity of the urinary tract is verified. If a cystotomy has been performed the ureteral orifices should be identify to ensure their patency. We have found that many available hemostatic agents facilitate controlling pelvic bleeding, particularly the bleeding that results from the raw surfaces along the bladder. Consideration can be given to placing an intraperitoneal drain prior to closure of the abdomen.

Perioperative Considerations

Interventional radiology techniques may be of assistance in women undergoing peripartum hysterectomy or in patients with suspected placenta accreta. The two most widely described procedures are selective arterial embolization and prophylactic intravascular balloon occlusion catheter placement. [25, 30-43] Which patients should undergo these procedures is an area of active debate.

Pelvic artery catheterization and embolization of the vascular supply to the uterus is the most frequently performed interventional radiologic procedure in this context. [25, 30-37] The procedure can be performed at the time of delivery in an attempt to decrease the chance of peripartum hysterectomy either after removal of the placenta or if the placenta is left in situ or used an adjuvant technique after hysterectomy to control residual bleeding. [25, 30-35, 37] Sivan and colleagues described a cohort of 30 women with suspected placenta accreta who underwent prophylactic catheterization of the internal iliac arteries prior to cesarean delivery. Embolization was performed in 77% of patients with 8% of the subjects requiring hysterectomy. The authors concluded that the technology was safe and decreased the likelihood of cesarean hysterectomy in women wishing to preserve fertility. [33]

Embolization may also be of value in patients who have undergone hysterectomy but have continued bleeding. In one series of seven patients with persistent bleeding after hysterectomy hemostasis was achieved in six with embolization. [34] Embolization is not without risk and has been associated with thrombotic complications and vaginal necrosis [34, 35].

A second approach is the placement of balloon occlusion catheters. [38-43] Occlusion catheters are placed in the interventional radiology suite preoperatively under fluoroscopic guidance. The catheter is typically placed either in the common femoral artery or the internal iliac artery. The balloons can be inflated either prophylactically or if heavy bleeding is encountered to reduce pulse pressure to the pelvis. [38-43] Like embolization, the reported efficacy of balloon occlusion catheters is variable and it remains unclear which patients are most likely to benefit from placement. A case-control study included 19 patients who had balloon catheters and hysterectomy and 50 patients who underwent hysterectomy alone noted no differences in blood loss, transfused products, operative time, or length of hospital stay. [38] Use of balloon occlusion catheters has been associated with substantial toxicity. In the study described 16% of patients had severe complications directly related to the catheters including an internal iliac thrombosis, a femoral artery thrombosis and dissection of the internal iliac artery [38].

Ureteral stents may aid in identification of the ureters at the time of hysterectomy in women with placenta accreta. [6, 11] Retrograde ureteral stents can be placed via cystoscopy prior to laparotomy. In one series of women who underwent hysterectomy for placenta accreta utilization of ureteral stents was associated with a reduction in the rate of ureteric injuries from 7% to 0% and a reduction in early morbidity. [6] In patients with placenta percreta and lateral invasion of the placenta ureteral stents may be particularly useful [12].

The choice between total and subtotal hysterectomy should be made on a case by case basis. Subtotal hysterectomy with retention of the cervix may be faster and potentially decrease the risk of bladder injury. However, the placenta is often adherent or invading the tissue of the lower uterine segment and removal of the lower portion of the uterus may be required to achieve hemostatsis. [7, 9, 27] In a case series Hoffman and colleagues noted that those three patients had an initial attempt at a supracervical hysterectomy. Substantial bleeding required removal of the cervix immediately in 2 patients and the third patient required removal of the cervix several hours later because of significant bleeding [7].

Blood Component Therapy and Hemostasis

The availability of large quantities of blood component therapy including packed red blood cells, fresh frozen plasma, and platelets is mandatory. While definitive guidelines are lacking, we often have 20 units of packed red blood cells (PRBC), 20 units of fresh frozen plasma (FFP) and 12 units of platelets cross matched preoperatively. Transfusion should be initiated early during the procedure as blood loss is often underestimated. Adequate communication with the operating room staff as well as anesthesia is essential.

Most traditional transfusion protocols utilize an FFP to PRBC ratio of 1:3 (that is one unit of FFP administered for every 3 units of PRBC) with 6 units of platelets after 10 units of PRBC's have been given. There is emerging evidence in the trauma surgery literature that utilization of a higher FFP to PRBC ratio and a higher platelet to PRBC ratio may be beneficial and associated with decreased coagulopathy and improved survival. [44-49]. An analysis of more than 450 civilian trauma patients noted that 30-day mortality was lover in patients who were treated with a higher FFP:PRBC ratio ($\geq$1:2) compared to those who received an FFP to PRBC ratio of <1:2.[44] Data in obstetrics to guide transfusion is largely lacking.

A large number of reports have now suggested that cell salvage is safe in obstetric cases. [50-54] Utilization of cell salvage technology with infusion of collected red cells offers a number of potential advantages in that it is associated with lower cost, decreased infectious risks and provides immediate access to blood. Potential theoretic concerns for use of cell salvage in obstetrics include the risk of reinfusion of fetal material as well as the potential for alloimmunization. [50-54] Commercially available cell salvage devices remove contaminants prior to infusion of red cells.

To aid with hemostasis a number of topical agents to facilitate coagulation are available. [55-59] These formulations are used in a number of surgical disciplines to facilitate hemostasis. As a last resort synthetic, recombinant activated factor VII (rFVIIa) can be considered. Recombinant factor VIIa promotes coagulation at sites of active bleeding in the presence of tissue factor. Recombinant factor VIIA is approved for bleeding associated with hemophilia A and in patients with inhibitors of coagulation. A number of reports of successful use of rFVIIa for postpartum hemorrhage have been described. [54, 60-65] Recombinant factor VIIA costs several thousand dollars and has been associated with thromboembolic complications. The drug should only be used for intractable hemorrhage.

Morbidity and Mortality

Peripartum hysterectomy is associated with substantial morbidity. [6-10, 13, 15, 22, 66, 67] Hysterectomy is associated with maternal mortality in 1-6% of cases. [9, 10, 26] A population-based analysis of women who underwent peripartum hysterectomy in the United States demonstrated a mortality rate of 1.0%. [68] The vast majority of women who undergo hysterectomy at the time of delivery require transfusion. [9, 11, 27, 69] A large series from the United Kingdom reported transfusion rates of 88% [26].

Transfusion requirements for women with placenta accreta are highly variable. [9, 10, 13] One report noted that the median blood loss after peripartum hysterectomy was 3000 cc while 13% of patients had a blood loss of greater than 10,000 cc. [13] The mean transfusion requirement for women who undergo peripartum hysterectomy is 5-10 units of packed red blood cells. [9, 13] Massive transfusion ($\geq$20 units of blood) is required in 16-38% of subjects [10, 13].

Both intraoperative and postoperative complications are frequent after peripartum hysterectomy (Table 1). The most frequent intraoperative complication is cystotomy which occurs in 6-29% of patients. [6, 8-10, 13, 15, 22, 66, 67] Ureteral injuries are less frequent but were still reported in nearly 7% of patients in one series. [6] Febrile morbidity and infections are the most common postoperative complications. Kastner and co-workers noted fevers in over a third of women who underwent peripartum hysterectomy [8].

Table 1. Morbidity and mortality associated with peripartum hysterectomy

	Wright (n=4967)[68]	Knight (n=315)[9]	Hoffman (n=29)[7]	Eller (n=76)[6]	Silver (n=216)[22]	Shellhaas (n=186)[11]
Death	1.0%	0.6%	0%	0%	0%	1.6%
Cystotomy	9.2%	12.2%	21.7%	28.9%	12.0%	NA
Ureteral injury	0.7%	4.5%	6.9%	6.6%	2.3%	3.0%
Oophorectomy	NA	5.8%	NA	NA	NA	NA
Reoperation	NA	19.6%	13.8%	7.9%	11.6%	3.8%
ICU admission	NA	84.0%	NA	27.6%	23.2%	NA
Mechanical ventilation	NA	7.2%	NA	NA	12.5%	NA
Thromboembolic events	1.0%	1.3%	10.3%	NA	1.9%	1.0%
Cardiac arrest	NA	1.9%	NA	NA	NA	NA
Febrile morbidity	NA	NA	0%	31.6%	NA	11.3%

NA-not available.

Surgical re-exploration is required in 4-33% of women who undergo peripartum hysterectomy. [6, 9-11] The most common indication for re-operation is for the control of bleeding, however a quarter of patients who require re-explore undergo the procedure to repair organ damage after the hysterectomy. [9].

Estimates of use of mechanical ventilation and intensive care unit services are highly variable. [6, 8-11, 22] The median hospital stay after peripartum hysterectomy ranges from 4-8 days [11, 13, 15].

Morbidity profiles differ somewhat based on the indication for hysterectomy.

Expectedly, women who undergo peripartum hysterectomy for placenta accreta are more likely to experience intraoperative complications than those who undergo the procedure for uterine atony. In one series bladder injuries were three times more common in patients who had a hysterectomy for placenta accreta than those who had the surgery for uterine atony. [13] In contrast, delayed postoperative bleeding and re-operation are more frequent in patients with uterine atony [13].

Systems Issues

Given the morbidity associated with peripartum hysterectomy there is an urgency to promote efforts to reduce the risk of adverse outcomes. One state-wide review noted that 90% of maternal deaths due to hemorrhage were preventable. [70] A range of patient safety initiatives to improve outcomes of women with postpartum hemorrhage have been proposed. Standardized protocols, obstetric rapid response teams, and simulations have all been suggested [71-76].

It is clear that management of these difficult cases requires a substantial amount of resources. [75-76] A number of institutions have now developed multidisciplinary teams consisting of physicians from maternal fetal medicine, gynecologic surgery, urology, vascular surgery, anesthesia, neonatology, and laboratory medicine. [67] Participation of a team from multiple disciplines allows coordination of all aspects of care and facilitates preoperative planning. In a review of women who underwent peripartum hysterectomy in Utah those women managed by a multidisciplinary team had lower transfusion requirements, were less likely to require reoperation and were less likely to have early morbidity. [67] Finally, there is emerging evidence that women with suspected placenta accreta have superior outcomes when treated at tertiary centers with experience in the management of the condition. A study of the influence of procedural volume for peripartum hysterectomy noted that patients treated at high volume centers had fewer perioperative surgical complications and a greater than 70% reduction in mortality. [77] Given the potential morbidity of peripartum hysterectomy further prospective studies to determine the ideal management of these women is clearly needed.

REFERENCES

[1] Brace V, Kernaghan D, Penney G. Learning from adverse clinical outcomes: major obstetric haemorrhage in Scotland, 2003-05. *Bjog* 2007;114:1388-96.

[2] Heron M, Hoyert DL, Murphy SL, Xu J, Kochanek KD, Tejada-Vera B. Deaths: final data for 2006. *Natl. Vital. Stat. Rep.* 2009;57:1-134.

[3] Khan KS, Wojdyla D, Say L, Gulmezoglu AM, Van Look PF. WHO analysis of causes of maternal death: a systematic review. *Lancet* 2006;367:1066-74.

[4] Wagaarachchi PT, Graham WJ, Penney GC, McCaw-Binns A, Yeboah Antwi K, Hall MH. Holding up a mirror: changing obstetric practice through criterion-based clinical audit in developing countries. *Int. J. Gynaecol. Obstet.* 2001;74:119-30; discussion 31.

[5] Weindling AM. The confidential enquiry into maternal and child health (CEMACH). *Arch. Dis. Child* 2003;88:1034-7.

[6] Eller AG, Porter TF, Soisson P, Silver RM. Optimal management strategies for placenta accreta. *Bjog* 2009;116:648-54.

[7] Hoffman MS, Karlnoski RA, Mangar D, et al. Morbidity associated with nonemergent hysterectomy for placenta accreta. *Am. J. Obstet. Gynecol.* 2010;202:628 e1-5.

[8] Kastner ES, Figueroa R, Garry D, Maulik D. Emergency peripartum hysterectomy: experience at a community teaching hospital. *Obstet. Gynecol.* 2002;99:971-5.

[9] Knight M. Peripartum hysterectomy in the UK: management and outcomes of the associated haemorrhage. *Bjog* 2007;114:1380-7.

[10] Kwee A, Bots ML, Visser GH, Bruinse HW. Emergency peripartum hysterectomy: A prospective study in The Netherlands. *Eur. J. Obstet. Gynecol. Reprod Biol* 2006;124:187-92.

[11] Shellhaas CS, Gilbert S, Landon MB, et al. The frequency and complication rates of hysterectomy accompanying cesarean delivery. *Obstet. Gynecol.* 2009;114:224-9.

[12] Wright JD, Bonanno C, Shah M, Gaddipati S, Devine P. Peripartum hysterectomy. *Obstet. Gynecol.* 2010;116:429-34.

[13] Wright JD, Pri-Paz S, Herzog TJ, et al. Predictors of massive blood loss in women with placenta accreta. *Am. J. Obstet. Gynecol.* 2011.

[14] Belfort MA. Placenta accreta. *Am. J. Obstet. Gynecol.* 2010;203:430-9.

[15] Whiteman MK, Kuklina E, Hillis SD, et al. Incidence and determinants of peripartum hysterectomy. *Obstet. Gynecol.* 2006;108:1486-92.

[16] Bateman BT, Mhyre JM, Callaghan WM, Kuklina EV. Peripartum hysterectomy in the United States: nationwide 14 year experience. *Am. J. Obstet. Gynecol.* 2011.

[17] Callaghan WM, Kuklina EV, Berg CJ. Trends in postpartum hemorrhage: United States, 1994-2006. *Am. J. Obstet. Gynecol.* 2010;202:353 e1-6.

[18] Bateman BT, Berman MF, Riley LE, Leffert LR. The epidemiology of postpartum hemorrhage in a large, nationwide sample of deliveries. *Anesth Analg.* 2010;110:1368-73.

[19] Martin JA, Hamilton BE, Sutton PD, et al. Births: final data for 2007. *Natl. Vital. Stat. Rep.* 2010;58:1-85.

[20] Martin JA, Hamilton BE, Sutton PD, et al. Births: final data for 2005. *Natl. Vital. Stat. Rep.* 2007;56:1-103.

[21] Bodelon C, Bernabe-Ortiz A, Schiff MA, Reed SD. Factors associated with peripartum hysterectomy. *Obstet. Gynecol.* 2009;114:115-23.

[22] Silver RM, Landon MB, Rouse DJ, et al. Maternal morbidity associated with multiple repeat cesarean deliveries. *Obstet. Gynecol.* 2006;107:1226-32.

[23] Glaze S, Ekwalanga P, Roberts G, et al. Peripartum hysterectomy: 1999 to 2006. *Obstet. Gynecol.* 2008;111:732-8.

[24] Chestnut DH, Eden RD, Gall SA, Parker RT. Peripartum hysterectomy: a review of cesarean and postpartum hysterectomy. *Obstet. Gynecol.* 1985;65:365-70.

[25] Yu PC, Ou HY, Tsang LL, Kung FT, Hsu TY, Cheng YF. Prophylactic intraoperative uterine artery embolization to control hemorrhage in abnormal placentation during late gestation. *Fertil Steril* 2009;91:1951-5.

[26] Yucel O, Ozdemir I, Yucel N, Somunkiran A. Emergency peripartum hysterectomy: a 9-year review. *Arch. Gynecol. Obstet.* 2006;274:84-7.

[27] Langdana F, Geary M, Haw W, Keane D. Peripartum hysterectomy in the 1990s: any new lessons? *J. Obstet. Gynaecol.* 2001;21:121-3.

[28] Clark SL, Yeh SY, Phelan JP, Bruce S, Paul RH. Emergency hysterectomy for obstetric hemorrhage. *Obstet. Gynecol.* 1984;64:376-80.

[29] Smith J, Mousa HA. Peripartum hysterectomy for primary postpartum haemorrhage: incidence and maternal morbidity. *J. Obstet. Gynaecol.* 2007;27:44-7.

[30] Alanis M, Hurst BS, Marshburn PB, Matthews ML. Conservative management of placenta increta with selective arterial embolization preserves future fertility and results in a favorable outcome in subsequent pregnancies. *Fertil Steril* 2006;86:1514 e3-7.

[31] La Folie T, Vidal V, Mehanna M, et al. Results of endovascular treatment in cases of abnormal placentation with post-partum hemorrhage. *J. Obstet. Gynaecol. Res.* 2007;33:624-30.

[32] Soyer P, Morel O, Fargeaudou Y, et al. Value of pelvic embolization in the management of severe postpartum hemorrhage due to placenta accreta, increta or percreta. *Eur. J. Radiol.* 2010.

[33] Sivan E, Spira M, Achiron R, et al. Prophylactic pelvic artery catheterization and embolization in women with placenta accreta: can it prevent cesarean hysterectomy? *Am. J. Perinatol.* 2010;27:455-61.

[34] Ojala K, Perala J, Kariniemi J, Ranta P, Raudaskoski T, Tekay A. Arterial embolization and prophylactic catheterization for the treatment for severe obstetric hemorrhage*. *Acta Obstet. Gynecol. Scand.* 2005;84:1075-80.

[35] Sewell MF, Rosenblum D, Ehrenberg H. Arterial embolus during common iliac balloon catheterization at cesarean hysterectomy. *Obstet. Gynecol.* 2006;108:746-8.

[36] Steinauer JE, Diedrich JT, Wilson MW, Darney PD, Vargas JE, Drey EA. Uterine artery embolization in postabortion hemorrhage. *Obstet. Gynecol.* 2008;111:881-9.
[37] Uchiyama D, Koganemaru M, Abe T, Hori D, Hayabuchi N. Arterial catheterization and embolization for management of emergent or anticipated massive obstetrical hemorrhage. *Radiat. Med. 2008*;26:188-97.
[38] Shrivastava V, Nageotte M, Major C, Haydon M, Wing D. Case-control comparison of cesarean hysterectomy with and without prophylactic placement of intravascular balloon catheters for placenta accreta. *Am. J. Obstet. Gynecol.* 2007;197:402 e1-5.
[39] Levine AB, Kuhlman K, Bonn J. Placenta accreta: comparison of cases managed with and without pelvic artery balloon catheters. *J. Matern Fetal Med.* 1999;8:173-6.
[40] Bodner LJ, Nosher JL, Gribbin C, Siegel RL, Beale S, Scorza W. Balloon-assisted occlusion of the internal iliac arteries in patients with placenta accreta/percreta. *Cardiovasc Intervent. Radiol.* 2006;29:354-61.
[41] Tan CH, Tay KH, Sheah K, et al. Perioperative endovascular internal iliac artery occlusion balloon placement in management of placenta accreta. *AJR Am. J. Roentgenol.* 2007;189:1158-63.
[42] Shih JC, Liu KL, Shyu MK. Temporary balloon occlusion of the common iliac artery: new approach to bleeding control during cesarean hysterectomy for placenta percreta. *Am. J. Obstet. Gynecol.* 2005;193:1756-8.
[43] Kidney DD, Nguyen AM, Ahdoot D, Bickmore D, Deutsch LS, Majors C. Prophylactic perioperative hypogastric artery balloon occlusion in abnormal placentation. *AJR Am. J. Roentgenol.* 2001;176:1521-4.
[44] Holcomb JB, Wade CE, Michalek JE, et al. Increased plasma and platelet to red blood cell ratios improves outcome in 466 massively transfused civilian trauma patients. *Ann. Surg.* 2008;248:447-58.
[45] Borgman MA, Spinella PC, Perkins JG, et al. The ratio of blood products transfused affects mortality in patients receiving massive transfusions at a combat support hospital. *J. Trauma* 2007;63:805-13.
[46] Gunter OL, Jr., Au BK, Isbell JM, Mowery NT, Young PP, Cotton BA. Optimizing outcomes in damage control resuscitation: identifying blood product ratios associated with improved survival. *J. Trauma* 2008;65:527-34.
[47] Holcomb JB, Zarzabal LA, Michalek JE, et al. Increased platelet:RBC ratios are associated with improved survival after massive transfusion. *J. Trauma* 2011;71:S318-28.
[48] Brown LM, Aro SO, Cohen MJ, et al. A high fresh frozen plasma: packed red blood cell transfusion ratio decreases mortality in all massively transfused trauma patients regardless of admission international normalized ratio. *J. Trauma* 2011;71:S358-63.
[49] Rowell SE, Barbosa RR, Diggs BS, et al. Effect of high product ratio massive transfusion on mortality in blunt and penetrating trauma patients. *J. Trauma* 2011;71:S353-7.
[50] Sullivan I, Faulds J, Ralph C. Contamination of salvaged maternal blood by amniotic fluid and fetal red cells during elective Caesarean section. *Br. J. Anaesth* 2008;101:225-9.
[51] Catling S, Joels L. Cell salvage in obstetrics: the time has come. *Bjog* 2005;112:131-2.
[52] Waters JH, Biscotti C, Potter PS, Phillipson E. Amniotic fluid removal during cell salvage in the cesarean section patient. *Anesthesiology* 2000;92:1531-6.

[53] Allam J, Cox M, Yentis SM. Cell salvage in obstetrics. *Int. J. Obstet. Anesth* 2008;17:37-45.

[54] Catling S. Blood conservation techniques in obstetrics: a UK perspective. *Int. J. Obstet. Anesth* 2007;16:241-9.

[55] Hong YM, Loughlin KR. The use of hemostatic agents and sealants in urology. *J. Urol.* 2006;176:2367-74.

[56] Pursifull NF, Morey AF. Tissue glues and nonsuturing techniques. *Curr. Opin. Urol.* 2007;17:396-401.

[57] Rousou J, Levitsky S, Gonzalez-Lavin L, et al. Randomized clinical trial of fibrin sealant in patients undergoing resternotomy or reoperation after cardiac operations. A multicenter study. *J. Thorac. Cardiovasc. Surg.* 1989;97:194-203.

[58] Oz MC, Cosgrove DM, 3rd, Badduke BR, et al. Controlled clinical trial of a novel hemostatic agent in cardiac surgery. The Fusion Matrix Study Group. *Ann. Thorac. Surg.* 2000;69:1376-82.

[59] Carless PA, Anthony DM, Henry DA. Systematic review of the use of fibrin sealant to minimize perioperative allogeneic blood transfusion. *Br. J. Surg.* 2002;89:695-703.

[60] Welsh A, McLintock C, Gatt S, Somerset D, Popham P, Ogle R. Guidelines for the use of recombinant activated factor VII in massive obstetric haemorrhage. *Aust. N. Z. J. Obstet. Gynaecol.* 2008;48:12-6.

[61] Franchini M, Franchi M, Bergamini V, Salvagno GL, Montagnana M, Lippi G. A critical review on the use of recombinant factor VIIa in life-threatening obstetric postpartum hemorrhage. *Semin. Thromb. Hemost.* 2008;34:104-12.

[62] Bouma LS, Bolte AC, van Geijn HP. Use of recombinant activated factor VII in massive postpartum haemorrhage. *Eur. J. Obstet. Gynecol. Reprod. Biol.* 2008;137:172-7.

[63] Alfirevic Z, Elbourne D, Pavord S, et al. Use of recombinant activated factor VII in primary postpartum hemorrhage: the Northern European registry 2000-2004. *Obstet. Gynecol.* 2007;110:1270-8.

[64] Phillips LE, McLintock C, Pollock W, et al. Recombinant activated factor VII in obstetric hemorrhage: experiences from the Australian and New Zealand Haemostasis Registry. *Anesth Analg.* 2009;109:1908-15.

[65] Wissa I, Ebeid E, El-Shawarby S, Chandakas S, Kamal T, Hill N. The role of recombinant activated Factor VII in major obstetric haemorrhage: the Farnborough experience. *J. Obstet. Gynaecol.* 2009;29:21-4.

[66] Awan N, Bennett MJ, Walters WA. Emergency peripartum hysterectomy: a 10-year review at the Royal Hospital for Women, Sydney. *Aust. N. Z. J. Obstet. Gynaecol.* 2011;51:210-5.

[67] Eller AG, Bennett MA, Sharshiner M, et al. Maternal morbidity in cases of placenta accreta managed by a multidisciplinary care team compared with standard obstetric care. *Obstet. Gynecol.* 2011;117:331-7.

[68] Wright JD, Devine P, Shah M, et al. Morbidity and mortality of peripartum hysterectomy. *Obstet. Gynecol.* 2010;115:1187-93.

[69] Zelop CM, Harlow BL, Frigoletto FD, Jr., Safon LE, Saltzman DH. Emergency peripartum hysterectomy. *Am. J. Obstet. Gynecol.* 1993;168:1443-8.

[70] Berg CJ, Harper MA, Atkinson SM, et al. Preventability of pregnancy-related deaths: results of a state-wide review. *Obstet. Gynecol.* 2005;106:1228-34.

[71] Skupski DW, Lowenwirt IP, Weinbaum FI, Brodsky D, Danek M, Eglinton GS. Improving hospital systems for the care of women with major obstetric hemorrhage. *Obstet. Gynecol.* 2006;107:977-83.

[72] Gosman GG, Baldisseri MR, Stein KL, et al. Introduction of an obstetric-specific medical emergency team for obstetric crises: implementation and experience. *Am. J. Obstet. Gynecol.* 2008;198:367 e1-7.

[73] Homer C, Clements V, McDonnell N, Peek M, Sullivan E. Maternal mortality: What can we learn from stories of postpartum haemorrhage? *Women Birth* 2009;22:97-104.

[74] Cameron CA, Roberts CL, Bell J, Fischer W. Getting an evidence-based post-partum haemorrhage policy into practice. *Aust. N. Z. J. Obstet. Gynaecol.* 2007;47:169-75.

[75] Sheiner E, Levy A, Katz M, Mazor M. Identifying risk factors for peripartum cesarean hysterectomy. A population-based study. J. Reprod. Med. 2003 Aug;48(8):622-6.

[76] Orbach A, Levy A, Wiznitzer A, Mazor M, Holcberg G, Sheiner E. Peripartum cesarean hysterectomy: critical analysis of risk factors and trends over the years. J. Matern Fetal Neonatal Med. 2011 Mar;24(3):480-4.

[77] Wright JD, Herzog TJ, Shah M, et al. Regionalization of care for obstetric hemorrhage and its effect on maternal mortality. *Obstet. Gynecol.* 2010;115:1194-200.

In: Cesarean Section: Procedures, Complications and Recovery ISBN: 978-1-62081-214-3
Editor: Eyal Sheiner

Chapter XIV

RECOVERY AFTER CESAREAN SECTION

Rachel Pope[1] and Eyal Sheiner[2]
[1]Case Western Reserve University Medical Center, MacDonald Women's Hospital, Department of Obstetrics and Gynecology, Cleveland, Ohio, US
[2]Department of Obstetrics and Gynecology, Faculty of Health Sciences, Soroka University Medical Center, Ben Gurion University of the Negev, Be'er Sheva, Israel

INTRODUCTION

Despite many international and institutional efforts to decrease the rise in cesarean sections, the rates continue to escalate, making it an increasingly common form of delivery. The Healthy People 2010 initiative set out to reduce cesarean delivery to 15% without success. [1] Current estimates reach near 32% of delivereies in the United States. [2] Concerns over this rise are multifactorial. Long-term sequelae of cesarean delivery demonstrate the need to avoid the procedure when possible. In this chapter, we examine three primary areas: recovery, early feeding, wound care, and mobilization to prevent thromboembolism. With increasing obesity in the general population, our attention should be drawn to the increased risk for complications including wound infections, and management thereof. Also, chronic pain due to incision wounds presumably increases medical consumption due to ongoing consultations and pain management needs beyond the postpartum hospital stay.

RECOVERY IN GENERAL

Although a common procedure, cesarean section (CS) is classified as a major abdominal surgery and carries with it extended recovery time and increased risks when compared to vaginal delivery. In general, women require at least two days of hospitalized recovery and most insurance plans will compensate up to four to five days total. Therefore, many institutions worldwide allow for three-four full postoperative days (depending on the obstetric history, number of previous CS and course of operation) for a patient to recover. This is primarily due to the need of analgesic administration, monitoring of vital signs, and reducing risk factors for complications. Pain management is of utmost importance in the first few days of recovery and both scheduled administration of analgesics and patient controlled infusion pumps are commonly used. An antiemetic is also usually administered as the procedure and analgesics can incite nausea and vomiting. [3] Several agents adequately alleviate pain, however morphine has been associated with higher rates of breast-feeding continuation and infant rooming-in, suggesting that women tend to feel well sooner when taking morphine. [4]

In terms of vital signs, in several institutions blood pressure, heart rate, respiration, temperature and urine output are monitored hourly for the first four hours and every subsequent four hours thereafter. [3] Any deviation should be evaluated for underlying cause and treated while in the hospital and followed up on an outpatient basis as deemed appropriate. Blood should be drawn to inspect hematocrit values the morning after the operation in order to assess patient's hemodynamic stability and need for supportive measures such as a blood transfusion and iron therapy.

WOUND CARE

Several studies have examined the type of surgical preparation used and correlation with wound infection. None have found remarkable results favoring one method over the other; however, the general practice is to clean before surgery with an antiseptic solution such as iodophor, chlorhexidine gluconate, or alcohol. Both solutions and adhesive films with solutions impregnanted are useful preparation agents. Due to the low virulence of epidermal commensals, no particular agent has stood above the others in reducing postoperative infection. However, organisms with higher virulence may be present in the case of a woman admitted to the hospital for several days before her cesarean section, as she is exposed to nosocomial pathogens, and is therefore at higher risk to suffer a wound infection. [5]

The incision wound should be inspected on a daily basis while the woman is in the hospital. Staples should be removed before discharge unless there is strong suspicion for wound separation. In these cases, found especially in obese patients, the sutures/staples may be left in up to ten days. [3] In several hospitals the staples are removed only after 5-7 days, at the out-patient clinic.

Wound infections after cesarean section have been reported from 2.5% to as high as 16%. [4, 6] Clinical presentation involves a low-grade fever between 99-100.4 degrees Fahrenheit (about 37.8-38.0 degrees Celsius), serosanguineous drainage from the wound, mild erythema of the edges of the wound, and elevating temperatures at night. [5] Special attention should be given to wounds in the presence of endometritis as signs and symptoms may be masked by antibiotic treatment. In addition, spiking fever above 101 degrees Fahrenheit (above 38.0 degrees Celsius) that do not resolve is more indicative of a wound abscess.The most common pathogen causing wound infection is *Ureaplasma urealyticum* and the majority of infections will manifest between postoperation day four to seven. Infections caused by group A and group B beta-hemolytic streptococci, however, are more likely to manifest in the first 24-48 hours. [5] As described by Cruse in 1973, the risk for wound infection postoperatively is directly related to the degree of intraoperative contamination. [7] The spectrum of contamination includes: clean, clean-contaminated, contaminated, and dirty (see Table 1).

Table 1. Contamination spectrum in context of labor [5]

Classification	Description
Clean	Closed cervix, intact membranes, sterile amniotic cavity
Clean-contaminated	Labor with ruptured chorioamnion
Contaminated	Chorioamnionitis
Dirty	Gross contamination from pus and necrotic tissue

Risk factors for wound complications after cesarean include, but are not limited to: maternal obesity, insulin-dependent diabetes mellitus, number of vaginal exams, use of internal fetal monitoring, duration of labor/membrane rupture, intrapartum chorioamnionitis, and postoperative endometritis. [5]

Treatment of Wound Infections

When a wound infection is diagnosed, treatment should involve opening the wound down to the fascia, cleansing with normal saline, and debriding any necrotic tissue. [5] Broad-spectrum antibiotics should be given intravenously and a new packing and dressing applied and changed twice daily until healed. One continuous packing gauze should be used so that nothing is left inadvertently between dressing changes. Proper treatment of simple wound infections prevents the development of serious complications such as necrotizing fasciitis and will allow for proper collagen deposition and remodeling.

Wound Pain

Although the Pfannenstiel incision is aesthetically advantageous and seems to result in fewer incisional hernias, [8] pain over the incision site is nevertheless a limiting factor. Up to one third of participants in Loos *et al.*'s study reported chronic pain at the incision site two years later. [9] For 8.9%, this pain impaired their daily functioning and was primarily due to nerve entrapment. The nerves most commonly entrapped include the iliohypogastric and ilioinguinal. [10]Neuropathic pain as described by Loos *et al.* is an activity-induced "sharp" pain at one or both lateral edges of the incision, radiating toward a labium and/or upper inner thigh. [9] Such pain can be elicited by flexion of the hip joint, which compresses the entrapped nerve. Administering 10 mL of 1% lidocaine to the trigger point of the pain should immediately relieve neuropathic pain.

In a recent prospective, double-blinded, placebo-controlled study, patients undergoing elective CS were randomly assigned to receive 1% lidocaine solution or placebo to the incision site, prior to the performance of a Pfannenstiel incision. [11] Pain intensity was evaluated for up to 48 hours after surgery and analgesic requirements of the patients were recorded. During the study period 153 patients were enrolled; 77 received preemptive analgesia with lidocaine, and 76 received a placebo. No significant differences were noted between the groups in respect to parity, previous CS, maternal age and gestational age. Pain scores or requirements of analgesia did not differ between the groups.

The authors concluded that preemptive analgesia with local incision-site injection with lidocaine does not seem beneficial in reducing post cesarean pain scores and analgesic requirements.

Chronic Pain

Chronic pain for a Pfannenstiel incision is qualified by pain beyond three months, after which the tissue is thought to have healed. [9] Multiple incisions increase the risk of chronic pain. In Loos *et al.*'s study, more than two Pfannenstiel incisions (OR 2.92; 95% CI 1.33-5.93) independently predicted chronic pain. [9] Chronic pain presumably increases medical consumption due to ongoing consultations and pain management needs. When cesarean section is medically necessary, intraoperative prevention of chronic pain could include limiting the length of incision to the lateral edges of the rectus sheath as to avoid damaging nerves. [12] Encouraging patients to attempt a trial of labor after cesarean section would also be theoretically beneficial in effort to decrease scarring and fibrosis.

Ambulation

Venous thromboembolism (VTE) is the number one cause of maternal deaths in developed countries. [13] Deep venous thrombosis (DVT) has been reported as up to four times as high in incidence compared to vaginal delivery. [14] A quarter of women who have DVT that are not treated develop into pulmonary embolism (PE). Therefore, the American College of Chest Physicians recommend early mobilization in women postpartum and prophylactic low molecular weight heparin or unfractionated heparin or mechanical prophylaxis for women with an additional risk factor such as a CS. [15] One popular form of mechanical prophylaxis of DVT is the intermittent pneumatic compression devices.

Traditionally, physicians have advised women to not exert themselves postoperatively, despite lack of evidence. Limitations are usually advised due to the thought that increased intra-abdominal pressure would interfere with wound and pelvic floor healing. [16] Weir *et al.* found that most physical activities women engage in postoperatively such as climbing stairs, getting out of a chair, lifting 8-13 pounds, and walking briskly do not increase abdominal pressures dangerously. [17] In addition, Minig found that a forceful cough raised intraabdominal pressure more than all of those things. [16] General consensus is that postoperatively one should not lift anything heavier than the baby. [16] In addition, ambulation after anesthesia has dissipated is thought to encourage the return of normal bowel function.

Obesity

Obesity tends to increase recovery disturbances in nearly all aspects. Obese and diabetic patients experience increased morbidity of cesarean sections as they tend to have large wound incisions and lack optimal healing. One study that examined nearly 20,000 deliveries for infection found that the following factors increased the risk of wound infection: obesity (OR= 2.2; 95% CI, 1.6–3.1), hypertensive disorders (OR=1.7; 95% CI, 1.4–2.1), and diabetes mellitus (OR=1.4; 95% CI, 1.1–1.7).[18] Furthermore, combined obesity and diabetes (both gestational and pregestational) increased the risk for wound infection 9.3-fold (95% CI, 4.5–19.2; $P<.001$). [18] Diabetes mellitus, hypertension, and obesity are all also risk factors for necrotizing fasciitis. [5] If staples have been used for wound closure, they may need to stay in place longer to assure adequate healing in a large wound disturbed by a large pannus. In addition, obese patients are at increased risk for thromboembolic events and should be especially encouraged to ambulate, use intermittent pneumatic compression devices, and be anticoagulated.

Early Feeding

Traditionally, clinicians have requested that women pass flatus before resuming regular diet for all types of deliveries. Although this has been largely left by the wayside for vaginal deliveries, many still recommend similar restrictions for women after CS. This limitation of food could potentially prevent a woman from eating in twenty-four hours after delivery if bowel sounds are not detected. Although the reasoning behind such practice are to prevent ileus and gastrointestinal disruption, the research comparing "early" feeding (within 8 hours based on the woman's request) versus "late" feeding (8-12 hours after bowel sounds were detected) have demonstrated no difference in complications between the groups. [19] In fact, women who ate per their request were overall more satisfied with their experience and tended to breastfeed earlier. [19] A gradual introduction of fluids followed by solid foods based on the woman's own comfort could be instated as a less harsh regimen.

Breast Care

Breastfeeding can be initiated in the first day of recovery if the woman wishes. The same risks of mastitis and engorgement exist for women after a cesarean as they do after vaginal delivery. However, a CS poses an obvious barrier to early breastfeeding due to maternal discomfort and need to recover from the major abdominal surgery. The woman can hold her infant on the side to minimize disturbance to the wound for increased comfort. [20]

After Leaving the Hospital

After discharge from the hospital, patients will still need pain relief and time to recover fully. Several issues may arise for which women and their families will request guidance, including when to resume daily activities such as driving. Controversy about when to safely resume driving a car postoperatively spans across surgical specialties. The patient should not drive if still taking opiate analgesics, which would interfere with cognitive abilities. [21]

However, once the patient is only taking nonsteroidal analgesics, some surgeons still fear that she would hesitate to slam on the brakes in an emergency situation due to the pain of the incision or fear that it would dehisce. Since there is no evidence for when exactly is safe, Nunez *et al.* recommend that patients first try the pedals and hand controls in a stationary car and resume driving when they feel comfortable. [22]

Postpartum depression may be more likely to affect women after a CS; therefore, mood should also be assessed at follow up visits. [23, 24] Unplanned cesarean sections have been found to leave women dissatisfied, angry, and even despondent with their newborns [25] indicating a need for physicians to tend to emotional and psychological needs of their patients as well.

CONCLUSION

Despite the undesired rise of cesarean sections and risks postpartum due to obesity and diabetes, it is necessary that we manage patients vigilantly in order to encourage speedy recoveries and to prevent complications. Recovery can be improved by monitoring vital signs, inspecting wounds for signs of infection in order to provide treatment as needed, providing adequate pain relief, allowing women to resume eating when they deem ready, helping them to bond with their infants, and by encouraging mobilization to prevent thromboembolism. All of these efforts will allow for a return to normal functioning as soon as possible and provide as pleasant an experience of birth as possible.

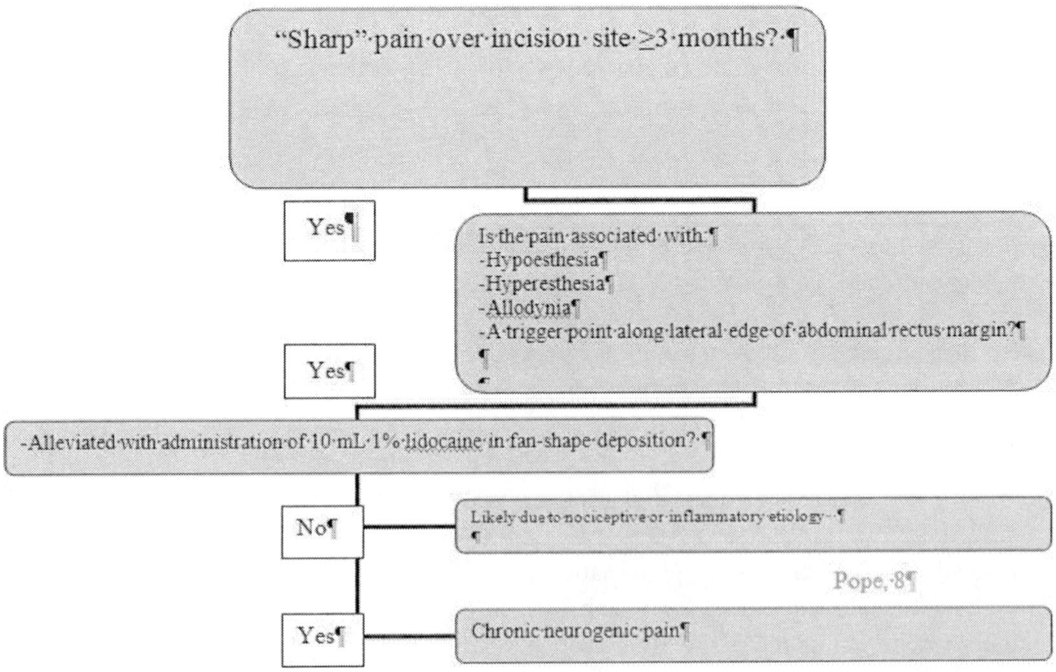

Figure 1. Incisional Pain [9].

References

[1] US Department of Health and Health Services. *Healthy People 2010: understanding and improving health.,* 2000.

[2] Queenan JT. How to stop the relentless rise in cesarean deliveries. *Obstet Gynecol*, 2011;118:199-200.

[3] Cunningham L, Bloom, Hauth, Rouse, and Spong. *Williams obstetrics.* New York, New York: McGraw-Hill, 2010.

[4] Yost NP, Bloom SL, Sibley MK, Lo JY, McIntire DD, Leveno KJ. A hospital-sponsored quality improvement study of pain management after cesarean delivery. *Am. J. Obstet. Gynecol.*, 2004;190:1341-6.

[5] Owen J, Andrews WW. Wound complications after cesarean sections. *Clin. Obstet. Gynecol.*, 1994;37:842-55.

[6] Webster J. Post-caesarean wound infection: a review of the risk factors. *Aust. NZJ Obstet. Gynaecol.*, 1988;28:201-7.

[7] Cruse PJ, Foord R. A five-year prospective study of 23,649 surgical wounds. *Arch. Surg.*, 1973;107:206-10.

[8] Kisielinski K, Conze J, Murken AH, Lenzen NN, Klinge U, Schumpelick V. The Pfannenstiel or so called "bikini cut": still effective more than 100 years after first description. *Hernia*, 2004;8:177-81.

[9] Loos MJ, Scheltinga MR, Mulders LG, Roumen RM. The Pfannenstiel incision as a source of chronic pain. *Obstet. Gynecol.*, 2008;111:839-46.

[10] Whiteside JL, Barber MD. Ilioinguinal/iliohypogastric neurectomy for management of intractable right lower quadrant pain after cesarean section: a case report. *J. Reprod. Med.*, 2005;50:857-9.

[11] Kessous R WA, Polachek H, Press F, Aricha-Tamir B, Leizerovich A, Pariente G, Weintraub AY, Sheiner E. The effect of preoperative analgesia with local lidocaine infiltration for post cesarean delivery pain management: A prospective double-blind randomized controlled study. *Am. J. Obstet. Gynecol.*, 2004;1.

[12] Luijendijk RW, Jeekel J, Storm RK, et al. The low transverse Pfannenstiel incision and the prevalence of incisional hernia and nerve entrapment. *Ann. Surg.*, 1997;225:365-9.

[13] Gates S, Brocklehurst P, Davis LJ. Prophylaxis for venous thromboembolic disease in pregnancy and the early postnatal period. Cochrane *Database Syst. Rev.*, 2002:CD001689.

[14] Simpson EL, Lawrenson RA, Nightingale AL, Farmer RD. Venous thromboembolism in pregnancy and the puerperium: incidence and additional risk factors from a London perinatal database. *BJOG,* 2001;108:56-60.

[15] Hirsh J, Guyatt G, Albers GW, Harrington R, Schünemann HJ, American College of Chest Physician. Antithrombotic and thrombolytic therapy: American College of Chest Physicians Evidence-Based Clinical Practice Guidelines (8th Edition). *Chest*, 2008;133:110S-12S.

[16] Minig L, Trimble EL, Sarsotti C, Sebastiani MM, Spong CY. Building the evidence base for postoperative and postpartum advice. *Obstet. Gynecol.*, 2009;114:892-900.

[17] Weir LF, Nygaard IE, Wilken J, Brandt D, Janz KF. Postoperative activity restrictions: any evidence? *Obstet Gynecol.*, 2006;107:305-9.

[18] Schneid-Kofman N, Sheiner E, Levy A, Holcberg G. Risk factors for wound infection following cesarean deliveries. *Int. J. Gynaecol. Obstet.*, 2005;90:10-5.

[19] Bar G, Sheiner E, Lezerovizt A, Lazer T, Hallak M. Early maternal feeding following caesarean delivery: a prospective randomised study. *Acta. Obstet. Gynecol. Scand.*, 2008;87:68-71.

[20] Berghella V. Cesarean delivery: Postoperative issues. www.uptodate.com: UpToDate, 2011.

[21] Giddins GE, Hammerton A. "Doctor, when can I drive?': a medical and legal view of the implications of advice on driving after injury or operation. *Injury*, 1996;27:495-7.

[22] Nuñez VA, Giddins GE. 'Doctor, when can I drive?': an update on the medico-legal aspects of driving following an injury or operation. *Injury*, 2004;35:888-90.

[23] Weisman O, Granat A, Gilboa-Schechtman E, et al. The experience of labor, maternal perception of the infant, and the mother's postpartum mood in a low-risk community cohort. *Arch. Womens Ment. Health*, 2010;13:505-13.

[24] Xie RH, Lei J, Wang S, Xie H, Walker M, Wen SW. Cesarean Section and Postpartum Depression in a Cohort of Chinese Women with a High Cesarean Delivery Rate. *J. Womens Health*, (Larchmt) 2011.

[25] Clement S. Psychological aspects of caesarean section. *Best Pract. Res. Clin. Obstet. Gynaecol.*, 2001;15:109-26.

In: Cesarean Section: Procedures, Complications and Recovery ISBN: 978-1-62081-214-3
Editor: Eyal Sheiner

Chapter XV

Timing of Elective Repeat Cesarean Section: Maternal and Neonatal Morbidity and Mortality

Tamar Tzur*, Adi Y. Weintraub, Gershon Holcberg, Moshe Mazor and Eyal Sheiner

Department of Obstetrics and Gynecology, Faculty of Health Sciences, Soroka University Medical Center, Ben-Gurion University of the Negev, Beer-Sheva, Israel

Abstract

Timing of elective repeat cesarean section should take into account both fetal and maternal considerations. The percentage of cesarean deliveries has dramatically increased during the last decades. It undoubtedly leads to an increase in the number of women having multiple cesarean sections. While maternal morbidity increases with increased number of cesarean sections, and the risk potential is elevated with gestational age, when compared with their term counterparts late preterm infants face increased morbidity. Establishing the optimal time of delivery for both mother and child is a major challenge faced by clinicians. The aim of this chapter is to better understand neonatal and maternal morbidity and mortality that are associated with elective repeat cesarean section, in order to provide an educated decision regarding the optimal timing for elective repeat cesarean section.

Introduction

The optimal timing for an elective repeat cesarean section (ERCS) is a critical obstetrical challenge. This decision should take into account both fetal and maternal considerations that may contradict one another. From the maternal point of view an earlier cesarean section (CS) could prevent an unscheduled, frequently emergent cesarean section (EmCS), which generally

* Corresponding author: Tamar Tzur, Department of Obstetrics and Gynecology, Soroka University Medical Center, Faculty of Health Sciences, Ben-Gurion University of the Negev, Beer-Sheva, Israel. Email: tzort@bgu.ac.il.

has a greater risk than that of an elective surgery1. For women who previously had multiple CS, the risk in EmCS is greatly increased due to potential complications being performed by a less skilled team. Delaying the delivery also increases the risk for complications such as antepartum bleeding, uterine rupture, contractions and labor in women that have contraindications for vaginal birth. From the fetal standpoint, delaying surgery can reduce adverse neonatal outcomes especially respiratory complications [2]. Recently, late preterm, or "minimally preterm", infants have received heightened attention as they too, face increased morbidity and even mortality when compared with their term counterparts [3-4]. On the other hand, delaying the timing of elective CS (ECS) may increase intrauterine fetal demise which has been shown to increase with increasing gestational age [5].

It is not possible to compare maternal and neonatal morbidities. In general maternal considerations prevail. Although neonatal morbidity may be complicated, maternal morbidity can be severe and may even lead to mortality which is unforgivable in modern obstetrics. As previously discussed in other chapters, the CS rate in the world has increased substantially (in the United States rates increased from 20.7% in 1996 to 31.1% in 20066-11. The decline in VBAC numbers has attracted attention and is the focus of an ongoing process to remedy the situation [12,13]. The increase in cesarean rate may also be explained by concerns from litigation, as well as improved techniques to control hemorrhage, infection, and thromboembolism which enhanced the safety of the procedure. Studies examining changes in the medical risk profile of mothers over time have found little evidence to suggest that the rising CS rates are due to such changes [14-16]. According to all these data, the number of women having multiple CS will increase, and hence the importance of understanding its implications [17-18].

This chapter aims to summarize neonatal and maternal morbidity and mortality that is associated with ERCS, and to explore factors and issues regarding the appropriate timing of ERCS.

Maternal Considerations

Obstetrical Complications

Delaying delivery until 39 weeks may increase the risk for pregnancy complications such as gestational hypertension, preeclampsia and eclampsia. The rates of these complications increase with gestational age from 37 to 43 weeks when calculated according to ongoing pregnancies [19].

Multiple Cesarean Sections

Although in developed countries many women have only one or two children, there are many countries and communities in which larger families are common. Implementation of the "once cesarean always cesarean" policy on such populations will obviously lead to an increase in the number of women having multiple CS. To date, only a limited number of studies specifically addressed the issue of maternal complications that are associated with multiple CS and they have conflicting results. Nisenblat et al. [20] in a retrospective cohort study assessed maternal complications after multiple CS. They observed that multiple CS are associated with an increased surgical difficulty and increased intrasugical blood loss compared with a second planned CS.

They found that the risk of major complications increased with the number of CS. Abnormal placentation seems to be the leading cause of major complications in women with multiple CS [20]. In another study which evaluated outcomes of high order (4–7) repeated CS, Juntunen et al. [21] found that a quarter of the women in the study group complained of low abdominal pain during late gestation. A thin or fenestrated isthmic myometrial layer was observed in 55% of surgeries. Abnormal placentation with an increased risk of major operative complications occurred more often in the study group. However, no differences in post-operative complications or perinatal outcomes were noted between the groups [21].

Emergency Cesarean Section (EmCS)

Delaying ECS until 39 completed gestational weeks in order to decrease neonatal respiratory morbidity would probably result in a higher EmCS rate and an increase in associated maternal morbidities. Ten to fourteen percent of ongoing pregnancies go into spontaneous labor between 38-39 weeks [22,23]. This means that over 10% of elective cesarean deliveries scheduled to 39 weeks will likely convert to non-elective ones between 38 to 39 weeks. It is well known that the risks of EmCS in general are much greater than those of elective surgery[1]. Severe maternal morbidities including deep vein thrombosis, pulmonary embolism, amniotic fluid embolism, puerperal infection, severe hemorrhage, uterine rupture or inversion and intestinal obstruction have been reported to be significantly more frequent in non-elective than in elective cesarean deliveries [24]. Operative interventions after delivery were also significantly more frequent after a non-elective cesarean delivery [24]. However, a retrospective study involving 258 planned ECS found an increased rate of EmCS, when the ECS delayed until 39 completed weeks. Nevertheless, this increase was not statistically significant. Similar rates of epidural/spinal anesthesia were noted among patients with a planned ECS and those who delivered by an EmCS. No difference in major complications was noted between the groups. The authors concluded that there is no evidence that delaying elective CS until 39 completed weeks gestation results in increased rates of adverse maternal outcomes [25]. In this study the indications for elective CS were: previous CS (40%), breech presentation (30%), placenta previa (13%); and other indications (25%). When the indication for ECS is multiple previous CS, surgery could be complicated; therefore, appropriate preparation is required. In those recurrent surgeries, emergency operations have been found to pose a specific risk for intraoperative complications [25,26]. The consequences of delaying these surgeries are not clear. Another study from Israel reporting deliveries that occurred between 1984 and 1992 compared maternal mortality among vaginal deliveries, emergency and elective cesarean deliveries. The authors reported maternal mortality rates of 2.8, 3.6, and 30 per 100,000 deliveries for elective cesarean delivery, vaginal delivery, and emergency cesarean delivery, respectively [27].

Scar tenderness in the third trimester is a common complaint in women after multiple (4-7) CS [21]. The presence of this complaint is a common cause for hospitalization and may result in a preterm EmCS. Delaying ECS due to previous multiple CS may increase the chance of spontaneous contractions and labor.

Vaginal Birth after Cesarean (VBAC)

The literature regarding vaginal birth after cesarean (VBAC), usually relates to one previous CS. Tahseen et al. in a systemic review, described the success rate and the adverse outcomes of vaginal birth after two cesarean sections. They observed a success rate of 71.1% and uterine rupture rate of 1.36% [28]. There is not enough data regarding the ramifications of spontaneous contractions and labor after multiple CS. There is no consensus regarding morbidity in VBAC versus ERCS. While some studies observed a higher incidence of uterine rupture/dehiscence in women planning VBAC compared with women electing an ERCS, others did not report a significant difference between the two modes of delivery [29]. Nevertheless, it seems that advanced gestational age is associated with a decreased rate of successful VBAC, and a higher rate of uterine rupture [30].

Uterine Rupture

The main risk in spontaneous contractions and labor in patients with multiple CS is uterine rupture. Uterine rupture is a life-threatening event resulting in serious complications, including hemorrhage, shock, peripartum hysterectomy and even maternal and perinatal mortality [31,32]. Uterine rupture occurs in 0.035% of deliveries [33]. Complete rupture involves the entire uterine wall and results in a direct connection between the peritoneal space and the uterine cavity. It is less common than an incomplete rupture (dehiscence), when there is disruption of the uterine musculature but the serosa, the visceral peritoneum or the broad ligament remain intact and cover the uterus [34]. Ruptures may develop spontaneously in grand multiparous parturient, in a congenitally abnormal uterus (eg, unicornuate or bicornuate) which lacks the normal uterine ability to expand, in a patient with a history of an invasive mole or because of abnormal placental implantation [35-38]. Uterine rupture most often involves a scarred uterus [39]. Uterine rupture occurs mostly during labor, however, gestational age was not found to be an independent risk factor for uterine rupture [32]. In contrast, Hammoud et al. showed that the risk of uterine rupture is significantly higher in patients with advanced gestational age [40].

Harper et al. recently published a large retrospective cohort study on the effect of gestational age at a prior CS on maternal morbidity in a subsequent VBAC attempt. They showed that a CS at or prior to 34 weeks' gestation did not increase maternal morbidity in the subsequent VBAC attempt. They also showed that all incidences of uterine rupture occurred in patients at 35 completed weeks of gestation or later. The gestational age at uterine rupture did not differ significantly between women with a prior CS after 34 completed weeks and women with a prior CS before 34 weeks [41].

The key to the prevention of uterine ruptures requires an understanding of the causative factors and high-risk clinical situations that predispose this complication such as: previous CS, uterine surgery, administration of agents for induction of labor, congenital uterine malformations, and trauma.

Uterine rupture is an unpredictable catastrophic event. Finding a predicting factor for uterine rupture could be useful to setting the optimal timing for an ERCS. Using a sonographic measurement of the lower uterine segment thickness in pregnant women with a previous CS as a predictor for the uterine rupture or dehiscence is controversial but probably lacking clinical significance. A prospective analysis used two- and three-dimensional transabdominal and transvaginal ultrasound to measure the thickness of the lower uterine segment (LUS) [42,43].

It was demonstrated that an ultrasonographic measurement of the LUS muscular thickness trans-vaginally was more reliable than the entire LUS thickness transabdominally. The use of three-dimensional ultrasound can also be considered to improve measurement reliability. Nonetheless, its clinical implication, hence the association between a thin LUS muscular thickness measurement obtained by ultrasound, and the risk of uterine rupture, still needs confirmation [42,43].

Ridgeway et al. showed that fetal bradycardia in the first and second stages of labor, was the only finding that differentiated between a delivery complicated by uterine rupture and a successful vaginal delivery. This suggests that the cardiotocograph may change only after a rupture has already occurred [44]. Likewise, Sheiner et al. found that severe fetal bradycardia was strongly associated with uterine rupture. In addition they found that uterine tachysystole and reduced baseline variability were independent patterns preceding uterine rupture in the first and second stages of labor [45].

Surgical Skills

A major limitation of emergency surgery is the inability to choose the appropriate surgical team for the procedure. The incidence of surgical complications associated with EmCS versus ECS was studied prospectively in 1319 patients undergoing CS [26].

The complication rate in emergency operations was significantly higher than in elective ones (18.9% vs. 4.2%; $p<0.05$). Among other risk factors, the surgeons' skill was found to be significantly associated with the occurrence of surgical complications during emergency CS, this was not so for elective surgeries.

The authors concluded that emergency CS requires great surgical skills, and should therefore not be entrusted to young, inexperienced obstetricians [26]. Rahman et al. reported in a retrospective cohort study that the operator experience and emergency nature of the CS were considered risk factors in a few cases of bladder injury [46]. In contrast, a retrospective study that was held in Copenhagen between 1995 and 1996 [47], assessed if a correlation exists between the incidences of intraoperative surgical complications and the surgeon's educational level.

The rate of complications in EmCS was 14.5% compared with 6.8% in the elective surgery group. The surgeon's educational level and a history of previous CS were not found to be significantly associated to intraoperative complications [47].

Nevertheless, elevated stress levels and sleep deprivation are known to be associated with poor job performance in medical residents [48]. Therefore, EmCS is a complicated surgery that should be performed electively when possible during the day time.

Anesthetic Complications

Failed intubation and pulmonary aspiration are the leading causes of anesthesia related maternal morbidity and mortality. Fasting for a period of six to eight hours is recommended before an elective cesarean delivery [49]. Women scheduled for an ECS and who go into spontaneous labor may present while not in the fasting state.

Performing an immediate operation because the woman is in labor may increase anesthesia related morbidity and mortality. Alternatively, delaying the procedure six to eight hours may increase the likelihood of progression into advanced labor which may further complicate the surgery. Anesthetic perspectives are discussed in a separate chapter in this book.

Advance Maternal Age

More women are postponing pregnancy into the fourth and fifth decades of life for a variety of reasons. Advanced maternal age, traditionally defined as over 35 years, has been associated with increased obstetric morbidity and higher rates of obstetrical interventions. Older women are more likely to have elective cesarean deliveries [50]. The risk for severe complications in nonelective cesarean deliveries is even higher among older women than in younger ones [24]. Furthermore, perinatal complications are reported to be higher among this population [51]. Intrauterine fetal death and perinatal mortality are significantly higher in older women even after excluding deaths due to congenital malformations and adjusting for existing illnesses or pregnancy complications [52]. A relatively high rate of stillbirth was reported among older women after 38 weeks of gestation [53].

Urinary Incontinence

Women with severe urinary incontinence have a marked deterioration in their quality of life, limited daily activities, and some older patients may become homebound, and urinary incontinence is the defining event that prompts admission to nursing home. In the United States each year, an estimated 135,000 women undergo surgery for urinary incontinence [54]. An estimate of direct costs for urinary incontinence in the United States has been reported to be $16 billion annually [55]. Given the substantial public health burden of pelvic floor disorders, much research has been focused on identifying risk factors, especially modifiable risk factors, for the development of pelvic floor disorders. Childbirth is a major risk factor for urinary incontinence in younger women [56].

Whether cesarean delivery may protect child-bearing women from developing urinary incontinence and to what degree, is an unresolved issue. Several prospective studies evaluated the risk of postpartum urinary incontinence by delivery type, grouping all cesarean deliveries together and reported inconsistent results. In one study, however, elective cesarean deliveries were compared with non-elective ones. Chin et al. assessed the impact of delivery on the pelvic floor and to what degree cesarean deliveries could prevent pelvic floor injury. Five hundred thirty nine women were divided into three groups according to the delivery method: elective cesarean delivery, non-elective cesarean delivery, and vaginal delivery. Only elective cesarean delivery was found to be protective against pelvic floor injury. They concluded that the key to optimal protection against postpartum urinary incontinence seems to lie in the timing of the cesarean delivery; that is, the cesarean delivery has to be performed before labor or uterine contractions have commenced [57].

NEONATAL CONSIDERATIONS

A Trend toward Earlier Deliveries

Recently, a significant trend toward earlier deliveries in the gestational age distribution for singleton births in the United States has raised concerns about its implications on infant health [58]. Increased obstetrical interventions to better manage high-risk pregnancies, including those occurring post-term, are partly responsible for this trend. Questions regarding iatrogenic preterm deliveries are more challenging to answer. Increases in medically indicated labor induction and CS in recent decades have resulted in increased rates of late preterm (34-36+6 weeks) births [58-60]. Such trends in obstetric practice are the paradox of modern obstetrics, since they are not consistent with traditional obstetric theory in which obstetric models of perinatal death demonstrate an exponential decrease in perinatal mortality rates as gestational age increases [61].

In the year 2004, the premature birth rate in the United States was 12.5%, representing a more than 30% increase since 1981 [62]. Although the number of infants born at less than 32 weeks has slightly declined since 1990, deliveries between 32 and 37 weeks have increased over time. In 1992, late preterm births in the United States accounted for 6.9% of singleton births and increased to 7.4% of singleton deliveries in 2002. Data from the US National Center for Health Statistics show that in 2002, 74% of preterm singleton deliveries occurred at 34-36 weeks gestation [58].

Short-Term Morbidity of Late Preterm Infants

Although late preterm infants have also been referred to as "near term" or "minimally preterm", these term may mislead by implying fetal maturity [63]. Numerous studies have shown that late preterm infants face increased morbidity when compared with their term counterparts. Although meconium aspiration syndrome is less common in late preterm infants than in term infants [64], all other forms of respiratory morbidity (including transient tachypnea of the newborn, respiratory distress syndrome, pneumonia, and pulmonary hypertension) affect late preterm infants at a higher rate than infants of a more advanced gestational age [65,66]. Hypothermia too, can complicate late preterm neonates and has been shown to bring about unnecessary sepsis investigations and more frequent neonatal intensive care unit (NICU) admissions in this population [67]. The suck-swallow reflex and intestinal motility could be immature in late preterm infants. This could lead to difficulty in breastfeeding and to a higher likelihood of poor weight gain and dehydration [68]. Among these infants, the incidence of hypoglycemia is significantly higher than demonstrated in term infants [67]. The relative immaturity of the livers of late preterm infants makes hyperbilirubinemia and its subsequent complications more common and more severe in these [69].

In addition to the increased morbidity rates in late preterm neonates, several studies have also demonstrated an increased risk of infant mortality among infants born between 34 and 37 weeks [64]. One study demonstrated a two to fivefold increased risk of infant death among late preterm infants and a twofold higher risk of sudden infant death as compared to term neonates [70].

Long-Term Morbidity of Late Preterm Infants

Although the majority of late preterm infants survive the neonatal period, recent evidence suggests that preterm and low birth weight infants suffer from long-term behavioral and developmental morbidities. A number of studies with long-term follow up of low-birth weight infants demonstrated clinically significant behavioral problems in almost 20% of patients. An 80% increased risk of childhood attention-deficit/hyperactivity disorder was noted in infants born between 34 and 37 weeks [71,72]. Because late preterm infants account for the majority of preterm infants in the United States and they experience increased morbidity compared with their term counterparts, late preterm births impose an enormous impact on the health care system. Late preterm infants accrue increased hospital expenses during their[73] and have a higher rate of rehospitalization than those of infants born after 37 weeks of gestation [74,75]. A population-based cohort study demonstrated a 4.8% rehospitalization rate among late preterm infants, even with no history of prior NICU admission, during the delivery hospitalization [74]. One estimate suggests that in the state of California alone over 49 million dollars could be saved if nonindicated deliveries were avoided for one year [76].

Timing of Elective CS

In a large retrospective multicenter study, Alan et al. investigated neonatal morbidity and mortality in elective CS based on gestational age at birth. The primary outcome was the composite of neonatal death and any of several adverse events, including respiratory complications, treated hypoglycemia, newborn sepsis, and admission to the NICU. They found that neonatal morbidity significantly decreased as gestational age at birth increased from 37 to 39 weeks. They concluded that ERCS before 39 weeks of gestation is common and is associated with respiratory and other adverse neonatal outcomes [77]. Tita et al. in a recent multicenter cohort study found similar results. They assessed neonatal outcomes of 24,077 repeat cesarean deliveries at term, of which 13,258 were performed electively. The primary outcome was the composite of neonatal death and any of several adverse events, including respiratory complications, treated hypoglycemia, newborn sepsis, and admission to the neonatal intensive care unit (ICU). Of repeat cesarean deliveries at term, 35.8% were performed before 39 completed weeks of gestation and 49.1% at 39 weeks of gestation. One neonatal death occurred. As compared with births at 39 weeks, births at 37 weeks and at 38 weeks were associated with an increased risk of the primary outcome. The rates of adverse respiratory outcomes, mechanical ventilation, newborn sepsis, hypoglycemia, admission to the neonatal ICU, and hospitalization for 5 days or more were increased by a factor of 1.8-4.2

for births at 37 weeks and 1.3-2.1 for births at 38 weeks. They concluded that elective repeat cesarean delivery before 39 weeks of gestation is common and is associated with respiratory and other adverse neonatal outcomes [78]. Hansen et al. reported that a significant reduction in neonatal respiratory morbidity may occur if elective caesarean delivery is postponed to 39 weeks. Carrying out elective cesarean deliveries at a later gestational age resulted in higher rates of laboring cesarean deliveries since some women went into spontaneous labor. In their cohort 25% of women entered labor before the 39th week. They also stated that compared with elective cesarean deliveries, laboring cesarean deliveries may carry an increased risk of complications such as uterine rupture, infections, or even maternal mortality [79].

A much earlier study, from 1995, showed that elective CS before 40 weeks' gestation was associated with increased neonatal admissions to the special care unit for respiratory distress (mainly for transient tachypnea of the newborn) [80]. In addition, at term, the incidence of respiratory distress in elective CS was higher than in vaginal delivery [80].

Neonatal Morbidities after Elective Cesarean Section (ECS)

De Luca et al. conducted a cohort study in order to evaluate the age-stratified risk of intrapartum and neonatal mortality as well as morbidities of clinical relevance after an ECS. They included over 56,500 women with late preterm and term deliveries, and compared ECS with planned vaginal deliveries and EmCS. Mortality and morbidities had a strong gestational age-related trend with the lowest incidences consistently found between 38 and 40 weeks of gestation independent of delivery mode.

They found that ECS is consistently associated with increased intrapartum and neonatal mortality, risk of admission to NICU, and respiratory morbidity compared with planned vaginal delivery and has no advantage over EmCS in terms of mortality. Neonatal morbidities are lower after ECS than EmCS only with term births. Their data provide evidence that ECS should not be performed [81].

Fetal Maturity and Steroid Administration before Elective Cesarean Section

In a randomized controlled trial, Stutchfield et al. confirmed that if women were given two intramuscular injections of 12 mg of betamethasone in the 48 hours before ECS admission rates to the special care unit for respiratory distress declined at 39 weeks' gestation, even more so at 38 weeks' gestation, and most profoundly at 37 weeks of gestation [82]. Their results also demonstrated that delaying non-urgent ECS until 39 weeks' gestation is more effective in avoiding neonatal admissions than steroid administration. For the 15% of women who will go into spontaneous labor between 37 and 39 weeks, the inconvenience of having their cesarean "out of hours" is likely to be less than that of having their newborn admitted to special care [82].

Because these late preterm births have significant morbidity, the American College of Obstetricians and Gynecologists (ACOG) cautions against elective induction and CS before 39 weeks without evidence of fetal lung maturity [83,84].

Neonatal Risks in Delaying ECS

Delaying ECS can theoretically expose fetuses to an elevated risk for intrauterine death [5,85], breech delivery [86], traumatic injury to the fetus/newborn [87] congenital infections [88], asphyxia and death due to uterine rupture [40].

Intrauterine fetal death: An increased risk of intrauterine fetal death has been reported with increasing gestational age. The timing of fetal death for stillborn infants born between 23 and 40 weeks is evenly distributed with nearly 5% of all stillbirths occurring during each week of [5]. This is important when considering all stillborn infants at 38 weeks and beyond, where significant complications of prematurity would be very rare if only these fetuses had simply been delivered earlier.

Furthermore, it has been reported that a fairly stable rate of fetal death of 0.6 per 1000 live births occurs from 33 weeks to 39 weeks of gestation. However, at 39 weeks, the rate increases significantly to 1.9 per 1000 live births [85]. De la Vega et al. in a mixed high risk population with unrestricted access to testing for fetal wellbeing and sonographic evaluations concluded that, despite intensive surveillance, they were still unable to reduce the rate of fetal death. The investigators suggested that this is probably due to the occurrence of acute placental and cord accidents that cannot be detected through antenatal fetal surveillance and are simply unavoidable [89]. The sudden death of a fetus in utero has medical, social and economic implications. It is particularly tragic when it occurs shortly before the expected date of delivery.

Breech presentation: In the term breech trial, 6% of women who were assigned to a planned cesarean delivery, delivered vaginally because cesarean delivery was not possible due to imminent vaginal [86]. Delaying an elective cesarean delivery scheduled for breech presentation may expose some of the fetuses to preventable morbidity and mortality associated with vaginal breech delivery in cases where vaginal delivery is imminent at admission.

Traumatic injury: The risk of traumatic injury to the fetus/newborn is increased in unscheduled CS [87]. The reported incidence of iatrogenic fetal trauma during cesarean delivery is 0.1% to 1.9% of births [90]. Several risk factors for fetal injury at the time of the cesarean delivery have been identified through various case reports.

These include lack of surgical experience, labor with thinning of the lower uterine segment exposing the fetus to injury with the scalpel, and a lack of amniotic fluid secondary to rupture of the membranes making the underlying fetal parts more accessible [91,92]. All these risks factors relate to EmCS. Although traumatic delivery is still associated with cesarean delivery, it is almost unheard of with elective cesarean delivery of the vertex fetus at term [87].

Congenital infections: In women whose indication for a cesarean delivery is human immunodeficiency virus infection or genital herpes, the risk of neonatal infection may increase if abdominal delivery is delayed [88].

Uterine rupture: The main risk in spontaneous contractions and labor in patients with multiple CS is uterine rupture. Uterine rupture is a life-threatening event resulting in serious complications, including perinatal mortality [31,11,93,94]. Hammoud et al. showed that the risk of uterine rupture is significantly higher in patients with advanced gestational age [40].

CONCLUSION

The percentage of cesarean deliveries, primary and repeated, has increased substantially in recent years. It leads to an increase in the number of women having multiple CS. Maternal morbidity increases with the number of CS. Abnormal placentation seems to be the leading cause of major complications in these women. Timing of ERCS should take in to account both fetal and maternal considerations. ERCS before 39 weeks is associated with adverse neonatal outcomes, especially respiratory morbidity. Late preterm infants face increased morbidity when compared with their term counterparts.

Antenatal betamethasone before ECS at term was suggested to reduce admissions to a special care unit due to respiratory distress, although further large prospective studies should examine such intervention.

The American College of Obstetricians and Gynecologists (ACOG) cautions against elective induction and CS before 39 weeks, without evidence of fetal lung maturity. Several authors believe that if dating is confirmed with an ultrasound study prior to 20 weeks of gestation, scheduling cesarean delivery to 38+0-6 weeks may be another reasonable and alternative option to 39 weeks. This is particularly true among a selected group of women, namely older women and in women where a complicated cesarean delivery is anticipated [22,95].

It is reasonable to inform women of the risks entailed with each of the above options. The benefits of reducing neonatal morbidity from 11% at 38 weeks to 8% at 39 weeks, as reported by Tita et al. [78], need to be weighed against the possible increase in the risks of severe maternal morbidity and perinatal mortality associated with delaying delivery [22,95]. Alan et al. in a reply to Salim et al. disagree to their suggestion that spontaneous labor preceding elective delivery is associated with severe maternal morbidity and perinatal mortality, which may outweigh the benefits that delaying delivery beyond 38 weeks of gestation holds. Women who have an otherwise elective (usually non-urgent) cesarean delivery after the onset of labor are commonly categorized as undergoing "emergency" cesarean deliveries, the vast majority of which are due to failed labor or potential fetal compromise.

Consequently, directly applying overall outcome estimates for this heterogeneous group to the small proportion of elective cesarean deliveries is inappropriate [96]. As compared with prelabor cesarean delivery, elective cesarean delivery after the onset of labor is associated with improved neonatal79.

The risk of severe adverse maternal outcomes is very low and is not associated with labor preceding elective cesarean delivery, especially with a prior transverse lower uterine incision [97]. Thus, since neonatal outcomes continue to improve and relatively few women deliver early because of spontaneous labor, planning elective cesarean delivery for 39 weeks of gestation is preferable. To date, there is no evidence of adverse maternal outcomes when delaying planned cesarean delivery to 39 weeks, except for cases with abnormal placentation. However, further investigations are needed to evaluate the significance of urgent ECS due to contractions or labor in women after multiple CS. Patients should be informed regarding the pros and cons of planning an earlier vs. a later elective CS, and the optimal timing of delivery should be tailored for each patient.

REFERENCES

[1] Enkin M. Labor and delivery following previous caesarean section. Childbirth p.1196-1215 Oxford University Press.

[2] Engle WA, Tomashek KM, Wallman C. ''Late-preterm'' infants: a population at risk. *Pediatrics*, 2007;120:1390–401.

[3] Escobar GJ, Clark RH, Greene JD. Short-term outcomes of infants born at 35 and 36 weeks gestation: we need to ask more questions. *Semin. Perinatol.*, 2006;30:28–33.

[4] Melamed N, Klinger G, Tenenbaum-Gavish K, Herscovici T, Linder N, Hod M, Yogev Y. Short-term neonatal outcome in low-risk, spontaneous, singleton, late preterm deliveries. *Obstet. Gynecol.*, 2009;114:253-60.

[5] Copper RL, Goldenberg RL, Dubard MB, and Davis RO: Risk factors for fetal death in white, black, and Hispanic women. Collaborative Group on Preterm Birth Prevention. *Obstet. Gynecol.*, 1994, 84:490-495.

[6] Hamilton BE, Martin JA, Ventura SJ. Births: preliminary data for 2005. *Natl. Vital. Stat. Rep.*, 2006;55:1-18.

[7] Hamilton BE, Martin JA, Ventura SJ, Sutton PD, Menacker F. Births: preliminary data for 2004. *Natl. Vital. Stat. Rep.*, 2005;54:1-17.

[8] Zhang J, Troendle J, Reddy UM. Contemporary cesarean delivery practice in the United States. *Am. J. Obstet. Gynecol.*, 2010;203(4):326.

[9] DeFrances CJ, Hall MJ. 2005 National Hospital Discharge Survey. *Advance data from vital and health statistics*; 2007 Jul 12;(385):1-19.

[10] MacDorman MF, Menacker F, Declercq E. Cesarean Birth in the United States: Epidemiology, Trends, and Outcomes. *Clin. Perinatol.,* 2008;35:293-307.

[11] Goetzinger KR, Macones GA. Operative vaginal delivery: current trends in obstetrics. *Women's Health* (Lond Engl) 2008;4(3):281–90.

[12] ACOG Practice bulletin no. 115: vaginal birth after previous cesarean delivery. *Obstet. Gynecol.*, 2010;116(2 Pt 1):450–63.

[13] National Institutes of Health Consensus Development conference statement: vaginal birth after cesarean: new insights March 8–10, 2010. *Obstet. Gynecol.*, 2010;115(6):1279–95.

[14] Menacker F, Declercq E, Macdorman MF. Cesarean delivery: background, trends, and epidemiology. *Semin. Perinatol.*, 2006;30:235-41.

[15] Reddy UM, Spong DY. Introduction. *Semin. Perinatol.*, 2006;30:233–4.

[16] Declercq E, Menacker F. MacDorman MF. Maternal risk profiles and the primary cesarean rate in the United States 1991–2002. *Am. J. Public Health*, 2006;96:867–72.

[17] Bulger T, Howden-Chapman P, Stone P. A cut above: the rising cesarean section rate in New Zealand. *N Z Med. J.,* 1998;11:30-3.

[18] Murray SF, Serani-Pradenas F. Cesarean birth trends in Chile, 1986 to 1994. *Birth* 1997; 24:258-63.

[19] Caughey AB, Stotland NE, Escobar GJ: What is the best measure of maternal complications of term pregnancy: ongoing pregnancies or pregnancies delivered? *Am. J. Obstet. Gynecol.,* 2003, 189:1047-1052.

[20] Nisenblat V, Barak S, Griness OB, Degani S, Ohel G, Gonen R. Maternal complications associated with multiple cesarean deliveries. *Obstet. Gynecol.*, 2006;108:21-6.
[21] Juntunen K, Mäkäräinen L, Kirkinen P. Outcome after a high number (4–7) of repeated caesarean sections. *BJOG*, 2004;111:561-3.
[22] Salim R, Shalev E. Health implications resulting from the timing of elective cesarean delivery. *Reprod. Biol. Endocrinol.*, 2010 Jun 21; 8:68.
[23] Thomas J, Callwood A, Brocklehurst P, Walker J. The national sentinel caesarean section audit report. London: *BJOG*. 2000 May;107(5):579-80.
[24] Pallasmaa N, Ekblad U, Gissler M: Severe maternal morbidity and the mode of delivery. *Acta. Obstet. Gynecol. Scand.,* 2008, 87:662-668.
[25] Jido. Delaying planned cesarean delivery. *Obstet. Gynaecol.*, 1999;19:142-5.
[26] Nielsen TF, Hokega°rd K. Caesarean section and intraoperative surgical complications. *Acta. Obstet. Gynecol. Scand.*, 1984;63:103–108.
[27] Yoles I, Maschiach S: Increased maternal mortality in cesarean delivery as compared to vaginal delivery? Time for re-evaluatio. *Am. J. Obstet.*, Gynecol 1998, 178:s78.
[28] Tahseen S, Griffiths M. Vaginal birth after two caesarean sections (VBAC-2)-a systematic review with meta-analysis of success rate and adverse outcomes of VBAC-2 versus VBAC-1 and repeat (third) caesarean sections. *BJOG*, 2010;117:5-19.
[29] Rossi AC, D'Addario V. Maternal morbidity following a trial of labor after cesarean section vs elective repeat cesarean delivery: a systematic review with metaanalysis. *Am. J. Obstet. Gynecol.*, 2008;199:224-31.
[30] Hammoud A, Hendler I, Gauthier RJ, Berman S, Sansregret A, Bujold E. The effect of gestational age on trial of labor after Cesarean section. *J. Matern. Fetal. Neonatal. Med.*, 2004;15:202-6.
[31] Yap OW, Kim ES, Laros RK Jr. Maternal and neonatal outcomes after uterine rupture in labor. *Am. J. Obstet. Gynecol.*, 2001;184:1576-81.
[32] Miles AL, Monga M, Waller DK, Dande D, Pschirrer ER. Risk factors for symptomatic uterine rupture during a trial of labor: the 1990s.*Am. J. Perinatol.*, 2000;17:385-9.
[33] Ofir K, Sheiner E, Levy A, Katz M, Mazor M. Uterine rupture: risk factors and pregnancy outcome. *Am. J. Obstet. Gynecol.*, 2003;189:1042-6.
[34] Cunningham FG, Gant NF, Leveno KJ, Gilstrap LC 3d, Hauth JC, Wenstrom KD. Williams' obstetrics. 21st ed. Philadelphia: *McGraw-Hill*; 2001. p. 646-7.
[35] Kore S, Pandole A, Akolekar R, Vaidya N, Ambiye VR. Rupture of left horn of bicornuate uterus at twenty weeks of gestation. *J. Postgrad. Med.*, 2000;46:39-40.
[36] LeMaire WJ, Louisy C, Dalessandri K, Muschenheim F. Placenta percreta with spontaneous rupture of an unscarred uterus in the second trimester. *Obstet. Gynecol.*, 2001;98:927-9.
[37] Nagy PS. Placenta percreta induced uterine rupture and resulted in intraabdominal abortion. *Am. J. Obstet. Gynecol.*, 1989;161:1185-6.
[38] Miller DA, Paul RH. Rupture of the unscarred uterus. *Am. J. Obstet. Gynecol.*, 1996;174:345.
[39] Ofir K, Sheiner E, Levy A, Katz M, Mazor M. Uterine rupture: Differences between a scarred and an unscarred uterus. *Am. J. Obstet. Gynecol.*, 2004;191:425-9.

[40] Hammoud A, Hendler I, Gauthier RJ, Berman S, Sansregret A, Bujold E. The effect of gestational age on trial of labor after cesarean section. *J. Matern. Fetal. Neonatal. Med.*, 2004;15:202–206.

[41] Harper LM, Cahill AG, Stamilio DM, Odibo AO, Peipert JF, Macones GA. Effect of gestational age at the prior cesarean delivery on maternal morbidity in subsequent VBAC attempt. *Am. J. Obstet. Gynecol.,* 2009;200:276.1-6.

[42] Cheung VY, Yang F, Leung KY. 2D versus 3D transabdominal sonography for the measurement of lower uterine segment thickness in women with previous cesarean delivery. *Int. J. Gynaecol. Obstet.*, 2011 Jul 1.

[43] Martins WP, Barra DA, Gallarreta FM, Nastri CO, Filho FM. Lower uterine segment thickness measurement in pregnant women with previous Cesarean section: reliability analysis using two- and three-dimensional transabdominal and transvaginal ultrasound. *Ultrasound. Obstet. Gynecol.*, 2009 Mar;33(3):301-6.

[44] Ridgeway JJ, Weyrich DL, Benedetti TJ. Fetal heart rate changes associated with uterine rupture. *Obstet. Gynecol.*, 2004;103:506–512.

[45] Sheiner E, Levy A, Ofir K, Hadar A, Shoham-Vardi I, Hallak M, Katz M, Mazor M. Changes in fetal heart rate and uterine patterns associated with uterine rupture. *J. Reprod. Med.*, 2004; 49:373–378.

[46] Rahman MS, Gasem T, Al Suleiman SA, Al Jama FE, Burshaid S, Rahman J: Bladder injuries during cesarean section in a University Hospital: a 25- year review. *Arch. Gynecol. Obstet.*, 2009, 279:349-352.

[47] Bergholt T, Stenderup JK, Vedsted-Jakobsen A, Helm P, Lenstrup C. Intraoperative surgical complication during cesarean section: an observational study of the incidence and risk factors. *Acta. Obstet. Gynecol. Scand.*, 2003;82:251-6.

[48] Feddock CA, Hoellein AR, Wilson JF, Caudill TS, Griffith CH.. Do pressure and fatigue influence resident job performance? *Med. Teach.*,2007;29:495-7.

[49] American College of Obstetrics and Gynecology: Obstetric analgesia and anesthesia. ACOG practice bulletin Number 36, July 2002. *Int. J. Gynaecol. Obstet.*, 2002, 78:321-335.

[50] Ecker JL, Chen KT, Cohen AP, Riley LE, Lieberman ES: Increased risk of cesarean delivery with advancing maternal age: indications and associated factors in nulliparous women. *Am. J. Obstet. Gynecol.*, 2001, 185:883-887.

[51] Usta IM, Nassar AH: Advanced maternal age. Part I: obstetric complications. *Am. J. Perinatol.*, 2008, 5:521-534.

[52] Jacobsson B, Ladfors L, Milsom I: Advanced maternal age and adverse perinatal outcome. *Obstet. Gynecol.*, 2004, 104:727-733.

[53] Smith GC: Life-table analysis of the risk of perinatal death at term and post term in singleton pregnancies. *Am. J. Obstet. Gynecol.*, 2001, 184:489-496.

[54] Waetjen LE, Subak LL, Shen H, Lin F, Wang TH, Vittinghoff E, Brown JS: Stress urinary incontinence surgery in the United States. *Obstet. Gynecol.*, 2003, 101:671-676.

[55] Wilson L, Brown JS, Shin GP, Luc K, Subak LL: Annual direct cost of urinary incontinence. *Obstet. Gynecol.*, 2001, 98:398-406.

[56] Hunskaar S, Burgio K, Clark A, Lapitan MC, Nelson R, Sillen U, Thom D: Epidemiology of urinary incontinence (UI) and faecal incontinence (FI) and pelvic organ prolapse (POP). In Incontinence. 3rd International Consultation on Incontinence Volume 1. 3rd edition. Edited by: Abrams P, Cardozo L, Khoury S, Wein A. Plymouth: *Health Publication Ltd*; 2005:255-313.

[57] Chin HY, Chen MC, Liu YH, Wang KH: Postpartum urinary incontinence: a comparison of vaginal delivery, elective, and emergent cesarean section. Int Urogynecol *J. Pelvic. Floor Dysfunct.*, 2006, 17:631-635.

[58] Davidoff MJ, Dias T, Damus K. Changes in the gestational age distribution among singleton births: impact on rates of late preterm birth, 1992 to 2002. Semin Perinatol. .2006

[59] MacDorman MF, Mathews TJ, Martin JA, Malloy MH. Trends and characteristics of induced labour in the United States, 1989–98. *Paediatr. Perinat. Epidemiol.*, 2002;16:263-73.

[60] Canadian Perinatal Surveillance System Steering Committee Members (2000). The State of Perinatal Health in Canada – *An. Overview*, 2000.

[61] Joseph KS: Incidence-based measures of birth, growth restriction and death can from erroneous concepts of risk. *J. Clin. Epidemiol.*, 2004, 57:889-97.

[62] Hoyert DL, Mathews TJ, Menacker F. Annual summary of vital statistics: 2004. *Pediatrics*, 2006;117:168–83.

[63] Engle WA. A recommendation for the definition of ''late preterm'' (near-term) and the birth weight - gestational age classification system. *Semin. Perinatol.*, 2006;30:2-7.

[64] Escobar GJ, Clark RH, Greene JD. Short-term outcomes of infants born at 35 and 36 weeks gestation: we need to ask more questions. *Semin. Perinatol.*, 2006;30:28–33.

[65] Clark RH. The epidemiology of respiratory failure in neonates born at an estimated gestational age of 34 weeks or more. *J. Perinatol.*, 2005;25:251–7.

[66] Stutchfield P, Whitaker R, Russell I. Antenatal betamethasone and incidence of neonatal respiratory distress after elective cesarean section: pragmatic randomized trial. *BMJ*, 2005;331:645-6.

[67] Laptook A, Jackson DL. Cold stress and hypoglycemia in the late preterm (''near-term'') infant: impact on nursery of admission. *Semin. Perinatol.*, 2006;30:77–80.

[68] Neu J. Gastrointestinal maturation and feeding. *Semin. Perinatol.*, 2006;30:24–7.

[69] Bhutani VK, Johnson L. Kernicterus in late preterm infants cared for as term healthy infants. *Semin. Perinatol.*, 2006;30:89–97.

[70] Kramer MS, Demissie K, Yang H, Platt RW, Sauvé R, Liston R. The contribution of mild and moderate preterm birth to infant mortality. Fetal and Infant Health Study Group of the Canadian Perinatal Surveillance System. *JAMA*, 2000;284:843–9.

[71] Gray RF, Indurkhya A, McCormick MC. Prevalence, stability, and predictors of clinically significant behavior problems in low birth weight children at 3, 5, and 8 years of age. *Pediatrics*, 2004;114:736–43.

[72] Linnet KM, Wisborg K, Agerbo E, Secher NJ, Thomsen PH, Henriksen TB. Gestational age, birth weight, and the risk of hyperkinetic disorder. *Arch. Dis. Child.*, 2006;91:655–60.

[73] Wang ML, Dorer DJ, Fleming MP, Catlin EA. Clinical outcomes of near-term infants. *Pediatrics*, 2004;114:372–6.

[74] Shapiro-Mendoza CK, Tomashek KM, Kotelchuck M, Barfield W, Weiss J, Evans S. Risk factors for neonatal morbidity and mortality among ''healthy,'' late preterm infants. *Semin. Perinatol.*, 2006;30:55–60.

[75] Tomashek KM, Shapiro-Mendoza CK, Weiss J, Kotelchuck M, Barfield W, Evans S, Naninni A, Declercq E. Early discharge among late preterm and term newborns and risk of neonatal morbidity. *Semin. Perinatol.*, 2006;30:61–8.

[76] Gilbert WM, Nesbitt TS, Danielson B. The cost of prematurity: quantification by gestational age. *Obstet. Gynecol.*, 2003;102:488–92.

[77] Alan T.N. Timing of Elective Repeat Cesarean Delivery at Term and Neonatal Outcomes. *N. Engl. J. Med.*, 2009;360:111-20.

[78] Tita AT, Landon MB, Spong CY, Lai Y, Leveno KJ, Varner MW, Moawad AH, Caritis SN, Meis PJ, Wapner RJ. Timing of elective repeat cesarean delivery at term and neonatal outcomes. *N. Engl. J. Med.,* 2009 Jan 8; 360(2):111-20.

[79] Hansen AK, Wisborg K, Uldbjerg N, Henriksen TB: Risk of respiratory morbidity in term infants delivered by elective cesarean section: cohort study. *BMJ*, 2008, 336:85-87.

[80] Morrison JJ, Rennie JM, Milton PJ. Neonatal respiratory morbidity and mode of delivery at term: influence of timing of elective caesarean section. *Br. J. Obstet. Gynaecol.*, 1995;102:101-6.

[81] De Luca R, Boulvain M, Irion O, Berner M, Pfister RE. Incidence of early neonatal mortality and morbidity after late-preterm and term cesarean delivery. *Pediatrics*, 2009 Jun;123(6):e1064-71.

[82] Stutchfield P, Whitaker R, Russell I. Antenatal betamethasone and incidence of neonatal respiratory distress after elective caesarean section: pragmatic randomized trial. *BMJ*, 2005;331:662-4.

[83] American College of Obstetricians and Gynecologists. ACOG Committee Opinion no. 394, December 2007: cesarean delivery on maternal request. *Obstet. Gynecol.,* 2007;110:1501-4.

[84] American College of Obstetricians and Gynecologists. ACOG Committee Opinion no.97 September 2008 Fetal Lung Maturity. *Obstet. Gynecol.*, 2008;112:717-26.

[85] Yudkin PL, Wood L, Redman CWG: Risk of unexplained stillbirth at different gestational ages. *Lancet*, 1987, 1:1192-1194.

[86] Hannah ME, Hannah WJ, Hewson SA, Hodnett ED, Saigal S, Willan AR: Planned caesarean section versus planned vaginal birth for breech presentation at term: a randomized multicentre trial. Term Breech Trial Collaborative Group. *Lancet*, 2000, 356:1375-1383.

[87] Hankins GD, Clark SM, Munn MB: Cesarean section on request at 39 weeks: impact on shoulder dystocia, fetal trauma, neonatal encephalopathy, and intrauterine fetal demise. *Semin. Perinatol.*, 2006, 30:276-287.

[88] D Sharma D, Spearman P. The impact of cesarean delivery on transmission of infectious agents to the neonate. *Clin. Perinatol.*, 2008 Jun;35(2):407-20.

[89] De la Vega A, Verdiales M: Failure of intensive fetal monitoring and ultrasound in reducing the stillbirth rate. P R *Health Sci. J.,* 2002, 21:123-125.

[90] Aburezq H, Chakrabarty KH, Zuker RM: Iatrogenic fetal injury. *Obstet. Gynecol.*, 2005, 106:1172-1174.

[91] Puza S, Roth N, Macones GA, Mennuti MT, Morgan MA: Does cesarean section decrease the incidence of major birth trauma? *J. Perinatol.*, 1998, 18:9-12.

[92] Haas DM, Ayres AW: Laceration at cesarean section. *J. Matern. Fetal. Neonatal. Med.*, 2002, 11:196-198.

[93] Brailovschi Y, Sheiner E, Wiznitzer A, Shahaf P, Levy A. Risk factors for intrapartum fetal death and trends over the years. *Arch. Gynecol. Obstet.*, 2011 Jul 7.

[94] Ronel D, Wiznitzer A, Sergienko R, Zlotnik A, Sheiner E. Trends, risk factors and pregnancy outcome in women with uterine rupture. *Arch. Gynecol. Obstet.*, 2011 Jul 7.

[95] Salim R, Zafran N, Shalev Timing of elective repeat cesarean delivery at term. E. N Engl J Med. 2009 Apr 9;360(15):1570; author reply, 1570-1.

[96] Thomas J, Paranjothy S. Obstetricians and Gynaecologists Clinical Effectiveness Support Unit. The national sentinel caesarean section audit report. London: RCOG Press, 2001.

[97] Spong CY, Landon MB, Gilbert S. Risk of uterine rupture and adverse perinatal outcome at term after cesarean delivery. *Obstet. Gynecol.,* 2007;110:801-7.

In: Cesarean Section: Procedures, Complications and Recovery ISBN: 978-1-62081-214-3
Editor: Eyal Sheiner

Chapter XVI

VAGINAL BIRTH AFTER CESAREAN DELIVERY

Asnat Walfisch*
Department of Obstetrics and Gynecology,
Hillel Yaffe Medical Center, Hadera, Israel

INTRODUCTION

This century has set record rates of cesarean deliveries. It is the most common surgical procedure for women in the United States (US) with nearly 1.5 million cesarean surgeries performed every year. When the US national rate of cesarean delivery was first measured in 1965, it was 4.5%. [1] Between 1970 and 2007, the cesarean delivery rate in the US increased dramatically to more than 31%. [2,3] In 2007, 19% of women in Israel, and 32.8% of women in the US were delivered by a cesarean section. [4]

Among 26 industrialized countries that provided data to the Organization for Economic Cooperation and Development, cesarean rates ranged from a low of 14% for the Netherlands to a high of 40% for Italy in 2007. [5] Three countries had rates that were even higher than the US rate (Korea, Turkey and Italy). This worldwide increase in cesarean rates is a result of tremendous changes in the clinical environment, including the introduction of electronic fetal monitoring, and the decrease in vaginal breech deliveries and forceps deliveries. [6-8]

As the 21st century approached, there emerged a demand for elective primary cesarean delivery on maternal request, without any medical indication. Patient autonomy, safety of the neonate and the perceived safety of the mother, fear of pain, avoidance of pelvic floor damage and esthetics, all may have contributed to this request. Presently, approximately 15% of cesarean deliveries are attributed to elective, non-medical, maternal request. [9]

Unfortunately, the dramatic rise in cesarean rates worldwide has not resulted in significant improvement in neonatal or maternal health. Although primary cesarean delivery accounts for the largest number of cesarean deliveries, the largest *single* indication for a cesarean is a prior cesarean. Thus, safety and success rates of trial of labor after a cesarean delivery (TOLAC) remain extremely relevant. [10]

---

* Email: asnatwalfisch@yahoo.com.

The degree to which cesarean deliveries and vaginal births after cesareans (VBACs) are affecting health remains a subject of continued controversy and uncertainty. This chapter discusses different aspects relating to TOLAC. The chapter includes benefits, risks and success rates of vaginal birth after a cesarean section, patient eligibility issues, appropriate counseling, and factors affecting maternal decision-making. Delivery process considerations and management are discussed as well.

History and Trends

Prior to 1980, the rule "once a cesarean, always a cesarean" was common practice. A series of studies by Flamm and colleagues [11-12] in the 1980s provided some of the early support for attempting trials of labor for women with prior cesareans. Other initial reports supported the relative safety of a "scar labor."

Vaginal birth after cesarean delivery emerged from the 1980 National Institutes of Health (NIH) Consensus Conference as a mechanism to safely reduce the cesarean delivery rates. [13] The NIH consensus report questioned the necessity of a routine repeat cesarean delivery and encouraged attempts to increase TOLAC rates.

The American College of Obstetricians and Gynecologists (ACOG) issued guidelines encouraging VBAC in the 1980s likely contributing to the rising rate seen in the early 1990s. [14] Indeed, VBAC proved to be an effective method to reduce cesarean delivery rates through the early 1990s. VBAC rates were 3.4% in 1980, 5% in 1985, 20% in 1990, and a peak rate of 28.3% in 1996. [15,16] The cesarean rate declined, in parallel, to 20.7% in 1996. [16] As the number of women and physicians perusing TOLAC/VBAC increased, reports of associated maternal and perinatal morbidity started to accumulate. [17-21] The major shift in trend occurred in 1996 following the New England Journal of Medicine publication by McMahon and colleagues. [20] The authors found higher rates of hysterectomy and uterine rupture in the trial of labor group compared with elective repeat cesarean in their Nova Scotia database. In October 1998, the ACOG issued new guidelines on VBAC that included a section based on level C evidence (expert opinion) calling for VBACs only "in institutions equipped to respond to emergencies with physicians readily available." [22] Soon after (July 1999), the ACOG re-issued the guidelines changing the word "readily," to "immediately". [23] Following these publications, trends in cesarean section and VBAC rates started to reverse. Since 1996, VBAC rates have declined sharply. In July 2001, Lydon-Rochelle and colleagues [21] published an article on the use of labor induction in trials of labor, accompanied by an editorial by Greene [24] that concluded that elective repeat cesareans were "unequivocally" safer for infants. In June 2001, the month before their publication, the national VBAC rate was 17.6%. By August 2001, the rate was down to 14.9%, a 15% decline in only 2 months, and by December, it had fallen to 13.4%, a 24% drop in 6 months. Later, VBAC rates have continued to decline, with a rate of 9.2% in 2004 and a low of 8.3% in 2007. [25-27] Concerns about medical liability claims as well as fear from catastrophic complications have probably contributed to this sharp decline in VBAC rates [28-30] to the point where, again, over 90 percent of women with a prior cesarean are delivered by a repeat cesarean. In some hospitals, TOLAC is no longer offered.

As opposed to the 70s, both primary and repeat cesarean deliveries have become more common, and the percentage of women with a prior cesarean delivery has substantially increased. In 2007, 21.3% of women with a prior live birth in the US had had a previous cesarean delivery, which suggests that further increases in the cesarean rate are likely. [4]

Nevertheless, in the past decade, reassuring publications on VBAC safety and success rates (in appropriate settings) continued to accumulate. [31-32] In December 2004, a study by Landon and colleagues, [31] the largest multicenter study of trial of labor compared with an elective cesarean, was published in the New England Journal of Medicine. The investigators found low rates of symptomatic uterine rupture (0.7%), and low absolute risks for poor outcomes associated with VBACs. There is little evidence, however, that this reassuring article by Landon and colleagues had any effect on VBAC rates.

In 2010, the National Institute of Child Health and Human Development (NICHD) and the Office of Medical Application and Research of the NIH published a report summarizing trends and the state-of-knowledge on risks and benefits of TOLAC versus elective repeat cesarean delivery (ERCD). [33] The NIH panel recognized that TOLAC was a reasonable option for many women with a prior cesarean delivery and called on organizations to facilitate access to TOLAC. Additionally, the panel recognized that liability concerns have a major impact on the providers' willingness to offer a trial of labor after TOLAC. [33]

Although controversy over the ideal CS rate continues, [34] an international study published in 2007 found a decrease in maternal mortality associated with cesarean rates of up to 15%. For countries with cesarean rates greater than 15%, higher cesarean rates were correlated with higher maternal mortality rates. [35].

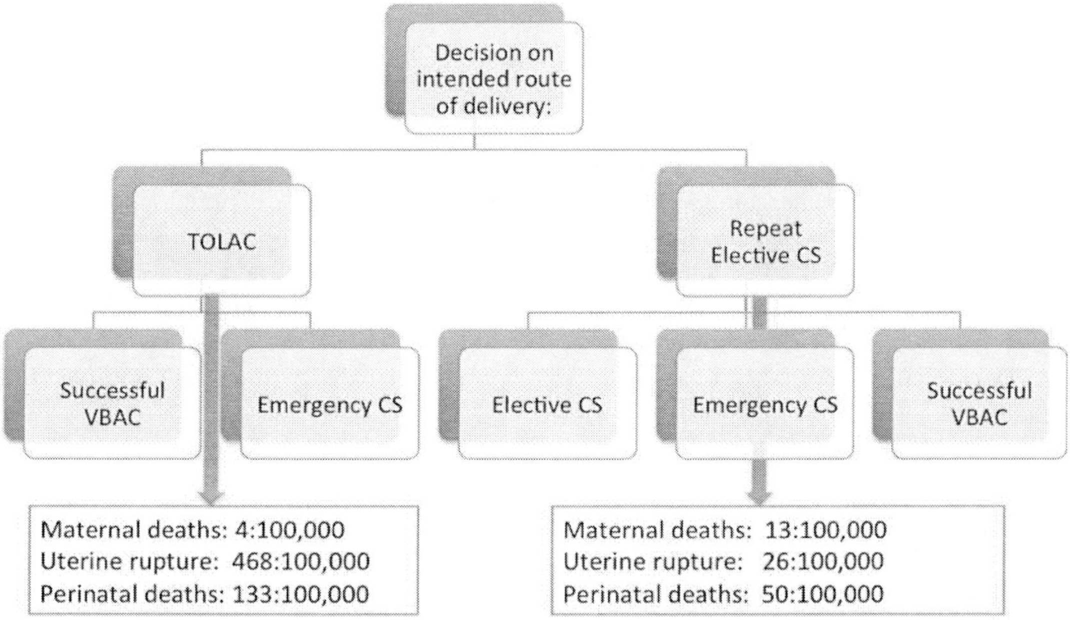

Figure. Decision on delivery route - associated maternal mortality, perinatal mortality and uterine rupture rates.

Trial of Labor after a Cesarean – Risks

For a woman who had a previous cesarean delivery there are three main possible outcomes (see figure): a successful TOLAC resulting in a vaginal birth, an unsuccessful TOLAC resulting in a repeat cesarean delivery, or an elective repeat cesarean delivery (ERCD).

Neither ERCD nor TOLAC are without maternal or neonatal risk. TOLAC resulting in a successful VBAC carries the lowest morbidity. On the other hand, the highest risks for maternal and neonatal morbidity are associated with an unsuccessful TOLAC resulting in an emergency cesarean delivery. [20]

Maternal Death

Maternal mortality rose in the U.S. from 7-9 per 100,000 in the 80s and 90s to 12 -15 per 100,000 since 2003 despite improvement in medical care. [36-38] Understanding whether choices patients and providers make about route of delivery contribute to maternal mortality is, thus, critically important. Advanced maternal age, co-morbidities, a dramatic increase in maternal obesity, and an increase in multiple gestations necessitating operative deliveries are all contributors to the increase in maternal mortality in recent years. In addition, there is the alarming concern of an increased incidence of placenta accreta associated with multiple uterine scars, emergency cesarean hysterectomy, blood transfusion, and maternal mortality due to obstetrical hemorrhage. The strength of evidence regarding the rate of mortality for women with a prior cesarean delivery is high with good consistency and precision. In general, maternal mortality is a rare outcome with an overall rate of 10.1 per 100,000 (0.01%) for all women with a prior cesarean section.

However, the risk of maternal mortality is significantly increased with elective repeat cesarean section (ERCD). For TOLAC the risk of maternal mortality is 3.8 per 100,000 while the risk for women undergoing ERCD is 13.4 per 100,000 – almost 4 fold. While rare for both TOLAC and ERCD, this difference translates to roughly 9 less deaths per 100,000 women attempting TOLAC. Maternal mortality is significantly lower among studies of term populations compared with studies of any gestational age (1.9 per 100,000 for TOLAC and 9.6 per 100,000 for ERCD, both at term).

Thus, maternal mortality is not a risk of TOLAC compared with ERCD but, rather, a benefit.

Uterine Rupture

Catastrophic uterine rupture is the most dreaded complication for women attempting VBAC. Uterine rupture is the complete separation of the uterine wall, through its entire thickness, including the serosa. This potentially life-threatening complication (for both mother and fetus) has been directly attributed to VBAC.

It is important to distinguish uterine rupture from uterine scar dehiscence. Dehiscence most often represents an occult scar separation with intact uterine serosa and thus does not risk for fetal or maternal sequelae. In contrast, uterine rupture carries potential consequences leading to severe fetal and maternal compromise.

The overall risk for uterine rupture is 0.3% for all women with a previous cesarean delivery attempting either VBAC or ERCD. [30,31,33] The reported maternal death rate is 1 per 500 ruptures. [39] The risk of perinatal death in the event of uterine rupture ranges from 0 to 20 percent [30] and the risk of hysterectomy due to uterine rupture ranges from 14 to 33 percent of rupture cases. Naturally, this association with perinatal and maternal morbidity and mortality raises substantial concerns among patients, clinicians, and policymakers. Estimating the risk of uterine rupture for women with a prior cesarean has been challenging because studies often mix true anatomic ruptures with asymptomatic dehiscences. As well, rates are reported on actual rather than intended route of delivery. The combined risk of uterine rupture for women undergoing a TOLAC is 0.47 percent (95 percent CI: 0.28 to 0.77 percent) compared to 0.026 percent (95% CI 0.009-0.082) for women undergoing an ERCD. [30] Thus, women undergoing a TOLAC have a significantly higher risk of uterine rupture with a relative risk of 20.74 (95% CI 9.77 - 44.02) compared to ERCD. Spong et al reported a risk for uterine rupture among women attempting TOLAC that is double that reported by other well designed studies (0.7% versus 0.03-0.4%). [20,40-42]

A review of 10 observational studies providing the best evidence on the rate of symptomatic rupture in women undergoing TOLAC revealed rates ranging from 0/1000 to 7.8/1000. [43] The Maternal Fetal Medicine Units Network Study, in 2004 by Landon et al mentioned earlier, reported a 0.7% incidence with 124 symptomatic ruptures occurring in 18,000 women undergoing TOLAC. [31] Though the studies are limited in number, there does not appear to be a reduction in the occurrence of uterine rupture in recent years. Because uterine rupture is one of the most significant complications of TOLAC, identifying the subgroup of women at increased risk of uterine rupture is of paramount importance (Table 1).

Table 1. Factors associated with uterine rupture in women attempting TOLAC

Factor	*Uterine rupture probability*
Ante-partum	
Term gestation	Increased
Advanced maternal age	Increased
Previous high risk uterine scar (T, classical, low vertical)	Increased
>1 previous cesarean delivery	Increased
Previous preterm cesarean delivery	Increased
Short inter-delivery interval (<18-24 months)	Increased
Previous single layer uterine closure	Increased
Previous vaginal delivery	Decreased
Lower uterine segment thickness >3.5mm	Decreased
Intra-partum	
Low bishop score on admission	Increased
Labor induction with PG	Increased
Use of oxytocin	Increased
Birth weight >4kg	Increased

Both antepartum demographic characteristics and intra-partum factors modify the risk of uterine rupture. However, the ability to reliably predict an individual's risk for uterine rupture remains a challenge. The occurrence of uterine rupture is significantly higher for term patients compared with studies including patients of any gestational age (0.78% versus 0.32%, p=0.033).

Additional risk factors associated with uterine rupture probability are listed in Table 1. Factors related to labor management, including low bishop score on admission, labor induction (with prostaglandins or oxytocin) and the use of oxytocin augmentation, have been shown by some to significantly effect rupture rates. Although multiple factors have been demonstrated to be associated with uterine rupture, such associations even in combination may not allow accurate prediction of this catastrophic outcome. The fact that some risk factors are only weakly associated with uterine rupture further limits development of a risk model.

The most common imaging technique used in an attempt to predict increased risk for uterine rupture is the ultrasound measurement of the lower uterine segment thickness. Various studies used different cutoffs for predicting an increased risk (<2.3mm, <3.5mm). [44-45] Until recently, the 3.5 mm cut-off value for full lower uterine segment thickness was the best validated, with 937 cases analyzed in the literature. This cut-off demonstrated high sensitivity and a strong negative predictive value for uterine scar defect but weak specificity. Bujold et al. suggested that 2.3 mm could be a better cut-off value for the prediction of complete uterine rupture during a trial of vaginal birth. [45]

Perinatal Mortality

Perinatal mortality (including fetal and neonatal death up to 28 days), [46] is an obvious concern when considering the safety of VBAC versus ERCD. Five cohort studies [41,46-49] met the study criteria established in the NIH/AHRQ systematic evidence review. [50] The combined risk of perinatal mortality was significantly higher for the TOLAC group as compared with ERCD with a relative risk of 1.82 (95% CI, 1.24-2.67).

As for *neonatal* mortality (birth up to 28 days of age), the risk is significantly higher for TOLAC compared with ERCD (RR 2.06, 95% CI 1.35-3.1). [50] Importantly, women with high-risk conditions [51] and women with indications for a repeat cesarean delivery appear to have higher rates of neonatal mortality regardless of the actual route of delivery. [41]

Neonatal Morbidity

Evidence has accumulated regarding the timing of ERCD at term and neonatal outcomes. Gestational age at the scheduled ERCD timing has a significant effect on perinatal morbidity. In a retrospective cohort study in 19 academic medical centers involving over 13,000 deliveries, Alan Tita found that over a third (35.8%!) of the ERCDs were performed prior to 39 completed weeks of gestation. This finding was associated with an increase in respiratory and other adverse neonatal outcomes. [52] A study by Wilmink et al included all ERCDs of singleton pregnancies beyond 37 weeks of gestation and concluded that performing an ERCD at less than 39 weeks of gestation jeopardized neonatal outcome and should be avoided whenever possible. [53] In cohort studies evaluating Apgar scores [48,49,54,55] no significant difference in 5-minute Apgar scores was reported between neonates born in TOLAC and ERCD.

Several good-quality cohort studies compared neonatal intensive care unit (NICU) admission rates. [40,48,54-57] Hook and colleagues [54] found significantly more neonates admitted to the NICU if they were born by repeat cesarean following a failed TOLAC compared with those born by VBAC (7% vs 2%, P<.007). Similarly, Kamath and colleagues [56] found that repeat cesarean after failed TOLAC increased the likelihood of NICU admission (OR 2.26; 95% CI: 0.85 to 6.0) but that the greatest likelihood of NICU admission was for term infants who did not experience labor and were born by an ERCD (OR 2.93; 95% CI 1.28-6.72).

The most common adverse respiratory outcome for term infants is transient tachypnea of the newborn (TTN). Results of studies reporting on TTN rates are not consistent. [48,54,55] Hook and colleagues [54] and Richardson and colleagues [48] found greater TTN in the ERCD group, whereas Fisler and colleagues [55] found the opposite. Based on the current body of evidence, it is unclear whether TOLAC is associated with increased or decreased risk of neonatal respiratory morbidity. At present, there are insufficient data comparing risks of respiratory morbidities with TOLAC versus ERCD to be useful when counseling women on mode of delivery.

As mentioned above, one important complication of TOLAC is uterine rupture, which is potentially life threatening for the fetus, and can result in a hypoxic-ischemic injury (HIE). In the landmark paper by Landon and colleagues [31] an increased incidence of uterine rupture during attempted VBAC was demonstrated compared with ERCD (0.7% vs 0%; P<.001) with an associated increase in the incidence of HIE (0.08% vs 0%; P<.001) and odds ratio of 2.90 (95% CI, 1.74 - 4.81). Importantly, adverse perinatal outcomes such as HIE occurred in women without uterine rupture in half of the HIE cases. Others showed similar or borderline results. [48,51] The effects of VBAC versus ERCD on later neurodevelopmental outcomes are unknown.

One of the common indications for admission to the NICU is a concern for neonatal sepsis. Prolonged rupture of membranes and intra-amniotic infection are likely greater in TOLAC versus ERCD. The only study to measure “proven sepsis” (confirmed by a positive blood culture) found no statistically significant differences between VBAC neonates (3 neonates [2%]) and those born by cesarean delivery after failed TOLAC (1 neonate [0.3%]). [58]

In summary, peri/neonatal mortality, while rare, is twice as common in women attempting TOLAC compared to ERCD. Reports on neonatal morbidity rates are conflicting and less conclusive. ERCD performed prior to 39 completed weeks of gestation is undoubtedly associated with increased neonatal morbidity and must be justifiable.

Trial of Labor after a Cesarean – Benefits

The benefits of successful TOLAC are a result of avoidance of the risks associated with a repeat cesarean delivery. A successful TOLAC results in: lower maternal morbidity and mortality, fewer postpartum maternal complications, shortened hospital stay and quicker return to routine activities, as compared with a repeat cesarean delivery.

Importantly, the morbidity associated with multiple repeated cesarean deliveries is avoided. With an increase in cesarean delivery rates, maternal morbidity and mortality has risen. Recent studies have documented an increased incidence of placenta previa and accreta with repeated uterine scaring. Women with two prior cesarean deliveries have a 2% incidence of placenta previa; nearly half of which are associated with placenta accreta. [59] Serious maternal morbidity is increasing progressively with increasing numbers of cesarean deliveries. Women, and physicians, should understand that 9% of women undergoing multiple cesarean deliveries may suffer from major complications and 1% will require hysterectomy, most commonly as a result of abnormal placentation. [60]

Flood et al performed a retrospective cohort study to identify trends in peripartum hysterectomy. [61] The authors found that the percentage of peripartum hysterectomy (in a setting of a previous cesarean delivery) increased significantly and that placenta accreta as an indication of peripartum hysterectomy increased significantly as well (from 5.4% to 46.5%). [61] Thus, avoidance of all the above-mentioned maternal morbidity associated with multiple repeat cesarean deliveries is a major benefit of TOLAC.

On the other hand, the benefits of ERCD are mainly avoidance of the risks associated with *failed* TOLAC. Another benefit of ERCD is scheduling convenience. A patient's desire to schedule the date of delivery to accommodate herself, her partner, and family members is compelling. From the physician perspective, the ability to schedule an ERCD in a suitable timing, without the inconvenience of having to remain in the hospital for countless hours conducting a TOLAC, is a clear benefit.

Patient Counseling

The woman with a history of cesarean delivery who presents for care is common in clinical practice. The counseling physician must remember that a successful VBAC carries the least morbidity for the woman, and that appropriate patient selection for TOLAC is of paramount importance.

Patient counseling is individualized in its nature. Discussion should be focused on individual characteristics that affect the chances of success, and of complications associated with each selected delivery route (see Figure). The patient can then choose her intended route of delivery based on data that is most personally relevant. There are two main options:

1) Trial of labor (TOLAC) – with an overall success rate of approximately 75%. [30] The success rate depends on individual factors, which are detailed ahead.
2) Elective repeat cesarean section (ERCD) – which includes both scheduled and planned cesarean.

The woman's decision is influenced by a variety of factors, some non-medical. The healthcare provider's recommendations have a major influence on the decision, and this fact should be well acknowledged by the counseling physician. [30,33] If possible, the preliminary discussion with the patient should take place as early as possible in the pregnancy course and even pre-conceptionally (Table 2). This is possible as many of the factors that are related to VBAC success rate and uterine rupture probability are known early in pregnancy. [62-64] An early preliminary discussion with the patient allows her more time to consider the options.

Table 2. Topics for discussion during patient counseling

Topic	Comments
Previous cesarean delivery complete medical circumstances	Such as: indication for cesarean, surgical technique, inter-pregnancy interval, etc.
TOLAC success rates	Overall 75% Discuss individual factors - see Table 3
Uterine rupture probability	Overall risk (all women with a previous uterine scar) - 0.3% TOLAC – 0.47% ERCD – 0.026% See Table 1
Maternal mortality	Overall risk (all women with a prior cesarean scar) 10.1 per 100,000 TOLAC - 3.8 per 100,000 ERCD - 13.4 per 100,000
Maternal morbidity	Significantly increased in multiple repeat cesareans Significantly increased in failed TOLAC
Perinatal mortality	Increased in TOLAC with RR ~ 2 TOLAC – 0.13% ERCD – 0.05%
Neonatal morbidity	Conflicting results ERCD prior to 39w increases morbidity
Scheduling convenience	With ERCD
Reproductive plans	Including intended family size
Available facility for delivery	Immediate availability of necessary staff and equipment for an emergency cesarean

A detailed history, indicating the circumstances surrounding the previous cesarean delivery, is crucial for assessing the patient's risk and the likelihood of TOLAC success. Inquiries regarding fetal status and cervical dilation at the time of the previous cesarean are important as well. Attempts should be made to obtain the patient's medical records and specifically the previous uterine incision type, indication for the cesarean and any intra- or post operative complications.

Risks, benefits and probability of a successful TOLAC should be discussed (Table 2). Intended family size and the risks associated with repeated cesarean deliveries should also be included in the discussion. The facilities available to support women electing TOLAC as their intended delivery site must be considered. TOLAC may be safely undertaken in both university and community hospitals. [32,65-68]

Factors Associated with TOLAC Success Rates

Women should understand the factors that influence the success/failure ratio of trial of labor after a cesarean delivery (Table 3): The highest success rate for women attempting TOLAC is in women who have a history of a prior successful vaginal delivery (either prior to, or following, the cesarean delivery) and who present for TOLAC in active labor. Cervical dilatation in late gestation has been consistently reported to be associated with successful TOLAC. [69-73]Another important predicting factor is the indication for the previous cesarean section. Fetal mal-presentation as the indication is a positive predictive factor for future successful TOLAC. Combining these positively predicting factors results in a success rate higher than 80%. [69-72,74-76]

Table 3. Reported TOLAC success rates with some associated factors

Factor	TOLAC success rate	Reference
Prior vaginal delivery	Yes – 86.6% No – 60.9%	Landon et al [71]
	No previous VBAC - 63.3% One previous VBAC – 87.6% Two previous VBACs – 90.9%	Mercer [114]
Previous multiple cesarean deliveries	Previous one – 83% Previous ≥2 – 75.3%	Miller et al [115]
	Previous one - 75.5% Previous two - 74.6%	Macones et al [116]
	Previous one – 76.5% Previous two - 71.1%	Tahseen and Griffiths [117]
	Previous one – 75.5% Previous 3 or more - 79.8%	Cahill et al [118]
Indication for previous cesarean	Non progressive labor –63.8% Entire cohort – 78.1%	Bhal et al [119]
	Labor dystocia - 33%	Holt and Mueller [120]
	Labor dystocia - 54% Other indications - 67%	Peaceman et al [121]
Inter-pregnancy interval	Less than 19 months - 79% More than 19 months - 85.5%	Huang et al [122]
Maternal weight	More than 300 pounds - 13.3% 200–300 pounds - 57.1% Less than 200 pounds - 81.8%	Carroll et al [123]
	Obese - 54.6% Normal BMI - 70.5% Underweight – 84.7%	Durnwald et al [124]
	BMI≥30 - 68.4% BMI<30 - 79.6%	Landon et al [71]
Maternal age	Over 35 years old - 75%	Srinivas et al [125]
Maternal Ethnicity	Caucasian - 79.3% African American - 70.0%	Hollard et al [126]
Fetal birth weight	3.8% decreased success rate for each 100 g increase in birth weight	Peaceman et al [121]

Factors that reduce the likelihood of successful TOLAC include: no previous vaginal delivery, suspected fetal macrosomia, post-term pregnancy and an indication for the previous cesarean being non progressive labor or non reassuring fetal HR monitoring - reducing the TOLAC success rate to 50% or less. [30,71] Labor induction also reduces the likelihood of success. The reported chance of achieving a successful vaginal birth for women with a previous uterine scar following labor induction ranges from 51% to 80%. [77-81] Demographic factors, which negatively influence the success rate, include increasing maternal age (>35 y), lower education, single marital status, and African American ethnicity. [30,71] An inter-pregnancy interval shorter than 6 months is a risk factor for uterine rupture during TOLAC and other maternal morbidity. [82]

Algorithms exist that incorporate these factors and provide individual risk assessments with varying prediction successes. [63,75,83-85] The goal of these algorithms is to identify the patients most likely to deliver vaginally and decrease the chances for failed TOLAC and its associated morbidity. The report by Guise and colleagues [30] outlines a detailed description and evaluation of screening tools and other predictors of VBAC and uterine rupture for women contemplating VBAC. These investigators conclude that VBAC predicting models which include intra-partum factors provide reasonable ability to identify women who have a better chance of a successful VBAC, but none have discriminating ability to consistently identify women who are at risk for cesarean births. [30] One decision model favored a trial of labor if the VBAC success rate was predicted at 50% or more. [85] Table 3 lists some of the reported TOLAC success rates, in association with different factors.

Patient Selection

It is critical for practitioners to realize that for women with a history of a prior low transverse cesarean, the mode of delivery associated with the least maternal morbidity and mortality is successful TOLAC. Therefore, identifying appropriate candidates, namely women likely to experience success in undergoing TOLAC, is most important and clinical judgment remains crucial in identifying those candidates. Some women are inappropriate candidates for TOLAC since the risks of TOLAC clearly outweigh the benefits: [86]

1) Lack of an appropriate facility staffed and equipped for a trial of labor after a cesarean.
2) Standard obstetrical indications for a cesarean section (such as placenta previa) are present.
3) Previous uterine rupture - Case series report a risk of recurrent uterine rupture of 6% for scars that are confined to the lower uterine segment. Repeat rupture rates may be as high as 32% for those that extend to the fundus. [87-88]
4) Women with a high-risk uterine scar – including a classical, T or J previous uterine incision. For women with incisions that extend into the contractile portion of the uterus, the risk of uterine rupture may be as high as 4% - 9%. [89] As well, women who have had various uterine surgeries (such as myomectomy) with extension of the incision into the myometrium are considered to have a high-risk uterine scar.

In contrast, the following high-risk characteristics do not categorically exclude patients from considering TOLAC. Data on the risk of uterine rupture is limited and individualized risk assessment is important and challenging:

Post-term pregnancy, unknown uterine scar, prior low vertical incision, suspected macrosomia, multi-fetal pregnancy, and multiple prior cesarean sections. In contrast to the previous ACOG recommendations, prior cesarean deliveries without a prior vaginal birth are no longer a contraindication for TOLAC. While not contraindicated for a TOLAC, breech presentation and an estimated fetal weight of greater than 5000 g are two examples in which a repeat cesarean delivery may reduce patient morbidity. [90]

Counseling is a dynamic process. Other circumstances and data may arise during the pregnancy course that may change the risks or benefits of TOLAC and the chances for a successful TOLAC (e.g., suspected macrosomia, need for labor induction). These should be addressed. This is especially important for women who are at higher risk for uterine rupture and TOLAC failure. Following counseling, the ultimate decision to undergo TOLAC or an ERCD should be made by the patient together with her health care provider. In all patients, documentation of counseling and the management plan should be included in the medical record.

LABOR AND DELIVERY CONSIDERATIONS

Once labor has begun, continuous electronic fetal monitoring is recommended. [86] More invasive monitoring devices, such as intrauterine pressure catheters or fetal scalp electrodes, were not shown to improve perinatal outcome or increase the prediction of uterine rupture. [91-92]

Signs and symptoms of uterine rupture should be monitored and looked for at all times. The most common sign is non-reassuring fetal heart rate (occurring in up to 70% of rupture cases). [86] Other signs are variable and may include vaginal bleeding, loss of fetal station, new onset of intense uterine pain and more. [93-95]

Induction and Augmentation of Labor

Previous cesarean section is not a contra-indication for labor induction or augmentation. Nevertheless, induction of labor raises the risk of uterine rupture and lowers TOLAC success rate. [21,31,32,80,96-97] With oxytocin, there is a dose response effect: increasing risk of uterine rupture occurs with higher maximum doses of oxytocin. Because studies have not identified a clear threshold for rupture, an upper limit for oxytocin dosing with TOLAC has not been established. Studies of the effects of prostaglandins, grouped together as a class of agents, on uterine rupture in women with a prior cesarean delivery have demonstrated inconsistent results. [21,31-32] However, when compared with women with a uterine scar who enter labor spontaneously, prostaglandin labor induction is associated with an increased risk of rupture. [21,31,98] Evidence from small studies show that the use of prostaglandin E1 in women with a previous cesarean delivery is associated with an increased risk of uterine rupture. [99-102] Thus, prostaglandin E1 should not be used for cervical ripening or labor induction in these patients or in patients who have undergone other major uterine surgery. [99-102] The risk with prostaglandin E2 is less established and definite recommendations are hard to make. One large study found an increased risk of uterine rupture only when oxytocin was used after cervical ripening with prostaglandins. [32] Therefore, selecting women most likely to have successful VBAC while avoiding sequential use of prostaglandins and oxytocin appears to carry the lowest risks of uterine rupture. [86]

The use of oxytocin to augment labor has been repeatedly associated with a reduction in the chance of a woman achieving vaginal birth. [31,73,103-105] It has also been studied, with conflicting results, as to an increased risk for uterine rupture. [31-32,97,106-107] Oxytocin augmentation is reported to increase the risk of uterine rupture by a factor of 2.5 by some investigators, [31,103] increasing to 12.7-fold by others. [108] However, this finding is not uniform, with Rageth and colleagues [104] failing to identify an association between augmentation of labor and risk of uterine rupture. The varying outcomes of available studies, and small absolute magnitude of the risk reported in those studies, support the recommendation that oxytocin augmentation may be used in patients undergoing TOLAC. [86]

There is lack of compelling data regarding mechanical cervical ripening and increased risks. In three reports of trans-cervical placement of Foley catheter for labor induction, two reported no increase in uterine rupture risk [96,109] while the third showed a significant increase. [110] Therefore, mechanical interventions may be an option for TOLAC candidates with an unfavorable cervix. [86]

Analgesia

Adequate pain relief during labor and delivery may encourage more women to choose TOLAC. [11,111] Epidural analgesia does not reduce the likelihood of a successful TOLAC [11,71,112] and does not mask signs of uterine rupture. [95,113]

Delivery

The actual VBAC delivery is not different than other vaginal deliveries. Routine manual exploration of the uterine cavity following VBAC was not shown to improve outcome and is probably not necessary. [86] However, signs of uterine rupture following the delivery such as post partum hemorrhage and hemodynamic instability should prompt complete evaluation of the genital tract.

Facility

TOLAC should be undertaken in facilities with immediate availability of appropriate personnel and equipment. If such resources are not available, a discussion should be held between the patient and the health care provider explaining the possible implications and potential risks of TOLAC in these circumstances. [86] Referral to an appropriate facility is, unfortunately, not always an option.

Conclusion

Millions of women around the world undergo a cesarean section each year, and this number is likely to increase. The appropriate and safe use of cesarean and vaginal birth after cesarean is not only an individual patient concern but also a public health policy concern as well as a financial one. The practice of "once a cesarean, always a cesarean" still resonates despite evidence suggesting otherwise. VBAC is a reasonable and safe choice for the majority of women with a prior cesarean. Vaginal birth after a cesarean section carries the lowest maternal mortality and morbidity rates, compared to the alternatives. Additionally, it is important to consider the morbidity in future pregnancies that would be derived from multiple cesareans, particularly in association with placental abnormalities. If the trial of labor fails, however, maternal morbidity is significantly elevated. Efforts must be directed at identifying optimal candidates for TOLAC. This will serve for both lowering cesarean section rates as well as minimizing maternal morbidity. To reverse the trend of the rising cesarean delivery rate, the primary cesarean delivery rate must also be lowered. For women with a uterine scar, TOLAC should be promoted whenever possible and more so in women who plan future pregnancies.

Acknowledgment

I would like to thank Ms. Ilina Badeva for her help in the preparation of this chapter.

References

[1] Sakala C, CorryM. Evidence-based maternity care: what it is and what it can achieve. New York (NY): The Milbank Memorial Fund; 2008. Available at http://www. milbank.org/ reports/0809 MaternityCare/0809 MaternityCare. html. Accessed March 2009.

[2] Rates of cesarean delivery--United States, 1991. Centers for Disease Control and Prevention (CDC). *MMWR Morb. Mortal. Wkly. Rep.*,, 1993;42:285–9.

[3] Hamilton BE, Martin JA, Ventura SJ. Births: preliminary data for 2007. *Natl. Vital. Stat. Rep.*, 2009;57(12):1–23.

[4] MacDorman M, Declercq E, Menacker F. Recent trends and patterns in cesarean and vaginal birth after cesarean (VBAC) deliveries in the United States. *Clin. Perinatol.*, 2011;38:179-92.

[5] Organization for Economic Cooperation and Development. OECD health data. 2010. Available at: http://www.ecosante.org/index2. php?base5OCDEandlangh5 ENG andlangs5ENGandsessionid. Accessed October 25, 2010.

[6] Clark SL, Hankins GD. Temporal and demographic trends in cerebral palsy-fact and fiction. *Am. J. Obstet. Gynecol.*, 2003;188:628–33.

[7] Lee HC, El-Sayed YY, Gould JB. Population trends in cesarean delivery for breech presentation in the United States, 1997-2003. *Am. J. Obstet. Gynecol.*, 2008;199:59. e1–59.e8.

[8] Goetzinger KR, Macones GA. Operative vaginal delivery: current trends in obstetrics. *Womens Health*, 2008; 4:281–90.

[9] Martin JA, Hamilton BE, Menacker F, Sutton PD, Mathews TJ. Preliminary births for 2004: Infant and maternal health. Health E-stats. Hyattsville, MD: National Center for Health Statistics. Released November 15, 2005.

[10] Agency for Healthcare Research and Quality. Healthcare Cost and Utilization Project (HCUP). http://hcupnet.ahrq.gov/. *Accessed Dec.*, 9, 2009.

[11] Flamm BL, Lim OW, Jones C, et al. Vaginal birth after cesarean section: results of a multicenter study. *Am. J. Obstet. Gynecol.*, 1988;158:1079–84.

[12] Flamm BL, Newman LA, Thomas SJ, et al. Vaginal birth after cesarean delivery: results of a 5-year multicenter collaborative study. *Obstet. Gynecol.*, 1990;76: 750–4.

[13] Cesarean Childbirth. NIH Consensus Statement Online 1980;3:1-30.

[14] College of Obstetricians and Gynecologists. Guidelines for vaginal delivery after previous cesarean birth. Washington, DC: The American College of Obstetricians and Gynecologists; 1988.

[15] Placek PJ, Tafel SM. Vaginal birth after cesarean (VBAC) in the 1980s. *Am. J. Public. Heath.*, 1988;78:512.

[16] Martin, JA, Hamilton, BE, Sutton, PD, et al. Births: Final data for 2004. National Vital Statistic Reports. Vol.55; No.1 National Center for Health Statistics; Hyattsville, MD 2006.

[17] Jones RO, Nagashima AW, Hartnett-Goodman MM, Goodlin RC. Rupture of low transverse cesarean scars during trial of labor. *Obstet. Gynecol.*, 1991; 77:815.

[18] Scott JR. Mandatory trial of labor after cesarean delivery: an alternative viewpoint. *Obstet. Gynecol.*, 1991; 77:811.

[19] Sach BP, Koblin C, Castro MA, et al. The risk of lowering the cesarean-delivery rate. *N. Engl. J. Med.*, 1999; 340:5.

[20] McMahon MJ, Luther ER, Bowes WA, Olshah AF. Comparison of trial labor with an elective second cesarean section. *N. Engl. J. Med.*, 1996; 335:689-95.

[21] Lydon-Rochelle M, Holt VL, Easterling TR, Martin DP. Risk of uterine rupture during labor among women with a prior cesarean delivery. *N. Engl. J. Med.*, 2001; 345:3-8.

[22] American College of Obstetricians and Gynecologists. ACOG practice bulletin No. 2. Vaginal birth after previous cesarean delivery. *Obstet. Gynecol.*, 1998; 92:1–7.

[23] American College of Obstetricians and Gynecologists. ACOG practice bulletin No. 5. Vaginal birth after previous cesarean delivery. *Obstet., Gynecol.*, 1999; 94:1–8.

[24] Greene MF. Vaginal delivery after cesarean section–is the risk acceptable*? N. Engl. J. Med.*, 2001;345:54–5.

[25] Martin JA, Hamilton BE, Sutton PD, Ventura SJ, Menacker F, Munson ML. Births: Final Data for 2006. *Natl. Vital. Stat. Rep.*, 2009; 57:1.

[26] Martin JA, Hamilton BE, Sutton PD, Ventura SJ, Mathews MS, Kirmeyer S, Osterman MJ. Births: final data for 2007. *Natl. Vital. Sta.t Rep.*, 2010; 58:1.

[27] Martin JA, Hamilton BE, Sutton PD, Ventura SJ, Mathews MS, Osterman MJ. Births: final data for 2008. *Natl. Vital. Stat. Rep.*, 2010; 59:1.

[28] American College of Obstetricians and Gynecologist. Overview of the 2009 ACOG Survey on Professional Liability http://acog.org/ departments/professionalLiability/ 2009PLSurveyNational.pd. Accessed October 1,2010.

[29] Clark SL, Belfort MA, Byrum SL, et al. Improved outcomes, fewer cesarean deliveries, and reduced litigation: results of a new paradigm in patient safety. *Am. J. Obstet. Gynecol.*, 2008; 199:105.e1.

[30] Guise JM, Eden K, Emeis C, Denman MA, Marshall N, Fu R, Janik R, Nygren P, Walker M, McDonagh M. Vaginal Birth After Cesarean: New Insights. *Evid. Rep. Technol. Assess.*, (Full Rep) 2010; 191:1-397.

[31] Landon M, Hauth JC, Leveno KJ, et al. Maternal and perinatal outcomes associated with a trial of labor prior cesarean delivery. *N. Eng. J. Med.,* 2004; 351:2581-9.

[32] Macones GA, Peipert J, Nelson DB, Odibo A, Stevens EJ, Stamilio DM, et al. Maternal complications with vaginal birth after cesarean delivery: a multicenter study. *Am. J. Obstet. Gynecol.*, 2005: 193:1656-62.

[33] National Institutes of Health Consensus Development Conference Panel. National Institutes of Health Consensus Development conference statement: vaginal birth after cesarean: new insight March 8-10, 2010. *Obstet. Gynecol.*, 2010; 115:1279.

[34] Resnik R. Can a 29% cesarean delivery rate possibly be justified? *Obstet. Gynecol.*, 2006;107:752–3.

[35] Betran AP, Merialdi M, Lauer JA, et al. Rates of caesarean section: analysis of global, regional and national estimates. *Paediatr. Perinat. Epidemiol.*, 2007;21:98–113.

[36] Hoyert DL, Hoyert DL. Maternal mortality and related concepts. *Vital. Health. Stat.*, 2007:1-13.

[37] Kung HC, Hoyert DL, Xu J, at al. Deaths: final data for 2005. *Natl. Vital. Stat. Rep.*, 2008;56:1-120.

[38] Minino AM, Heron MP, Murphy SL, at al. Deaths: final data for 2004 *Natl. Vital. Stat. Rep.*, 2007;55:1-119.

[39] Wen SW, Huang L, Liston R, et al. Severe maternal morbidity in Canada, 1991-2001. *CMAJ*, 2005;173:759.

[40] Loebel G, Zelop CM, Egan JFX, Wax J. Maternal and neonatal morbidity after elective repeat Cesarean delivery versus a trial of labor after previous Cesarean delivery in a community teaching hospital. *J. Matern. Fetal. Neonatal. Med.*, 2004;15:243-246.

[41] Spong CY, Landon MB, Gilbert S, et al. Risk of uterine rupture and adverse perinatal outcome aterm after cesarean delivery. *Obstet. Gynecol.*, 2007;110:801-807.

[42] Cahill AG, Stamilio DM, Odibo AO, et al. Is vaginal birth after cesarean (VBAC) or elective repeat cesarean safer in women with a prior vaginal delivery*? Am. J. Obstet. Gynecol.*, 2006;195:1143-1147.

[43] Guise JM, McDonagh MS, Osterweil P, et al: Systematic review of the incidence and consequences of uterine rupture in women with previous Cesarean section. *BMJ*, 2004;329:19-25.

[44] Rozenberg P, Goffinet F, Phillipe HJ, Nisand I. Ultrasonographic measurement of lower uterine segment to assess risk of defects of scarred uterus. *Lancet*, 1996; 347:281.

[45] Bujold E, Jastrow N, Simoneau J, Brunet S, Gauthier R.J. Prediction of complete uterine rupture by sonographic evaluation of the lower uterine segment. *Am. J. Obstet. Gynecol.,* 2009;201:320.e1-6.

[46] Sibony O, Alran S, Oury JF. Vaginal birth after cesarean section: X-ray pelvimetry at term is informative. *J. Perinat. Med.*, 2006;34:212–5.

[47] Bujold E, Francoeur D. Neonatal morbidity and decision-delivery interval in patients with uterine rupture. *J. Obstet. Gynaecol. Can.*, 2005;27:671–3.

[48] Richardson BS, Czikk MJ, daSilva O, et al. The impact of labor at term on measures of neonatal outcome. *Am. J. Obstet. Gynecol.*, 2005;192:219–26.

[49] Smith GC, Pell JP, Cameron AD, et al. Risk of perinatal death associated with labor after previous cesarean delivery in uncomplicated term pregnancies. *JAMA*, 2002;287:2684–90.

[50] Guise JM, Denman MA, Emeis C, et al. Vaginal birth after cesarean: new insights on maternal and neonatal outcomes. *Obstet. Gynecol.*, 2010;115:1267–78.

[51] Gregory KD, Korst LM, Fridman M, et al. Vaginal birth after cesarean: clinical risk factors associated with adverse outcome. *Am. J. Obstet. Gynecol.*, 2008;198:452 e1–10.

[52] Tita AT, Landon MB, Spong CY, Lai Y, Leveno KJ, Varner MW, et al. Timing of elective repeat cesarean delivery at tern and neonatal outcomes. *N. Engl. J. Med.*, 2009;360:111–20.

[53] Wilmink FA, Hukkelhoven CW, Lunshof S, Mol BW, van der Post JA, Papatsonis DN. Neonatal outcome following elective cesarean section beyond 37 weeks of gestation: a 7-year retrospective analysis of a national registry. *Am. J. Obstet. Gynecol.*, 2010;202:250.e1– 8.

[54] Hook B, Kiwi R, Amini SB, et al. Neonatal morbidity after elective repeat cesarean section and trial of labor. *Pediatrics*, 1997;100:348–53.

[55] Fisler RE, Cohen A, Ringer SA, et al. Neonatal outcome after trial of labor compared with elective repeat cesarean section. *Birth*, 2003;30:83–8.

[56] Kamath BD, Todd JK, Glazner JE, et al. Neonatal outcomes after elective cesarean delivery. *Obstet. Gynecol.*, 2009;113:1231–8.

[57] Landon MB, Spong CY, Thom E, et al. Risk of uterine rupture with a trial of labor in women with multiple and single prior cesarean delivery. *Obstet. Gynecol*, 2006;108:12–20.

[58] Durnwald C, Mercer B. Vaginal birth after Cesarean delivery: predicting success, risks of failure. *J. Matern. Fetal. Neonatal. Med.*, 2004;15:388–93.

[59] Clark SL, Kooning PP,Phelan JP. Placenta previa/accrete and prior cesarean section. *Obstet. Gynecol.*, 1985;66:88–92.

[60] Nisenblat V, Barak S, Griness OB, Degani S, Ohel G, Gonen R. Maternal complications associated with multiple cesarean deliveries. *Obstet. Gynecol.*, 2006;108:21–6.

[61] Flood KM, Said S, Geary M, Robson M, Fitzpatrick C, Malone FD. Changing trends in peripartum hysterectomy over the last 4 decades. *Am. J. Obstet. Gynecol.*, 2009;200:632.el–6.

[62] Srinivas SK, Stamilio DM, Stevens EJ, Odibo AO,Peipert JF, Macones GA. Predicting failure of a vaginal birth attempt after cesarean delivery. *Obstet. Gynecol.*, 2007;109:800–5.

[63] Grobman WA, Lai Y, Landon MB, Spong CY, Leveno KJ, Rouse DJ, et al. Development of a nomogram for prediction of vaginal birth after cesarean delivery. NICHD Maternal-Fetal Medicine Units Network (MFMU). *Obstet. Gynecol.*, 2007;109:806–12.

[64] Grobman WA, Lai Y, Landon MB, Spong CY, Leveno KJ, Rouse DJ, et al. Prediction of uterine rupture associatedwith attempted vaginal birth after cesarean delivery. National Institute of Child Health and HumanDevelopment Maternal-Fetal Medicine Units Network. Am J *Obstet. Gynecol.*, 2008;199:30.e1–e5.

[65] Gregory KD, Korst LM, Cane P, Platt LD, Kahn K. Vaginal birth after cesarean and uterine rupture rates in California. *Obstet. Gynecol.,* 1999;94:985–9.

[66] Raynor BD. The experience with vaginal birth after cesarean delivery in a small rural community practice. *Am. J. Obstet. Gynecol.*, 1993;168:60–2.

[67] Blanchette H, Blanchette M, McCabe J, Vincent S. Is vaginal birth after cesarean safe? Experience at a community hospital. *Am. J. Obstet. Gynecol.*, 2001;184:147887.

[68] DeFranco EA, Rampersad R, Atkins KL, Odibo AO, Stevens EJ, Peipert JF, et al. Do vaginal birth after cesarean outcomes differ based on hospital setting? *Am. J. Obstet. Gynecol.*, 2007;197:400.e1–e6.

[69] Flamm BL, Geiger AM. Vaginal birth after cesarean delivery: an admissionscoring system. *Obstet. Gynecol.*, 1997;90:907–10.

[70] Gonen R, Tamir A, Degani S, et al. Variables associated with successful vaginal birth after one cesarean section: a proposed vaginal birth after cesarean section score. *Am. J. Perinatol.*, 2004;21:447–53.

[71] Landon MB, Leindecker S, Spong CY, et al. The MFMU Cesarean Registry: factors affecting the success of trial of labor after previous cesarean delivery. *Am. J. Obstet. Gynecol.,* 2005;193:1016–23.

[72] Learman LA, Evertson LR, Shiboski S. Predictors of repeat cesarean delivery after trial of labor: do any exist? *J. Am. Coll Surg.*, 1996;182:257–62.

[73] Macones GA, Hausman N, Edelstein R, et al. Predicting outcomes of trials of labor in women attempting vaginal birth after cesarean delivery: a comparison of multivariate methods with neural networks. *Am. J. Obstet. Gynecol.,* 2001;184:409–13.

[74] Gyamfy C, Juhasz G, Gyamfi P, Stone JL. Increased success of trial of labor after previous vaginal birth after cesarean. *Obstet. Gynecol.,* 2004; 104:715.

[75] Weinstain D, Benshushan A, Tanos V, et al. Predictive score for vaginal birth after cesarean section. *Am. J. Obstet. Gynecol.*, 1996; 174:192-8.

[76] Bujold BL, Blackwell SC, Hendler I, et al. Modified Bishop's score and induction of labor in patients with a previous cesarean delivery. *Am. J. Obstet. Gynecol.*, 2004;191:1644.

[77] McNally OM, Turner MJ. Induction of labour after 1 previous Caesarean section. *Aus. NZJ. Obstet. Gynaecol.*, 1999;39:425–9.

[78] Grinstead J, Grobman WA. Induction of labor after one prior cesarean: predictors of vaginal delivery. *Obstet. Gynecol.*, 2004;103:534–8.

[79] Delaney T, Young DC. Spontaneous versus induced labor after a previous cesarean delivery. Obstet Gynecol. 2003;102:39–44.

[80] Grobman WA, Gilbert S, Landon MB, et al. Outcomes of induction of labor after one prior cesarean. *Obstet. Gynecol.*, 2007;109:262–9.

[81] Zelop CM, Shipp TD, Cohen A, et al. Trial of labor after 40 weeks' gestation in women with prior cesarean. *Obstet. Gynecol.,* 2001;97:391–3.

[82] Stamilio DM, DeFranco E, Pare E, et al. Short inter pregnancy interval: risk of uterine rupture and complications of vaginal birth after cesarean delivery. *Obstet. Gynecol.*, 2007;110:1075.

[83] Jakobi P, Weissman A, Peretz BA, et al. Evaluation of prognostic factors for vaginal delivery after cesarean section. *J. Reprod. Med.*, 1993;38:729–33.

[84] Pickhardt MG, Martin JN Jr, Meydrech EF, et al. Vaginal birth after cesarean delivery: are there useful and valid predictors of success or failure? *Am. J. Obstet. Gynecol.*, 1992;166:1811–9.

[85] Mankuta DD, Leshno MM, Menasche MM, et al. Vaginal birth after cesarean section: trial of labor or repeat cesarean section? A decision analysis. *Am. J. Obstet. Gynecol.*, 2003;189:714–9.

[86] American College of Obstetricians and Gynecologists. ACOG Practice Bulletin no.115: Vaginal birth after previous cesarean delivery. *Obstet. Gynecol.*, 2010;116:450.

[87] Ritchie EH. Pregnancy after rupture of the pregnant uterus. A report of 36 pregnancies and a study of cases reported since 1932. J Obstet Gynaecol *Br. Commonw.*, 1971;78:642–8.

[88] Reyes-Ceja L, Cabrera R, Insfran E, et al. Pregnancy following previous uterine rupture. Study of 19 patients. *Obstet. Gynecol.,* 1969;34:387–9.

[89] Scott JR. Avoiding labor problems during vaginal birth after cesarean delivery. *Clin. Obstet. Gynecol.*, 1997;40:533–41.

[90] ACOG Committee on Obstetric Practice. ACOG Committee Opinion No. 340. Mode of term singleton breech delivery. *Obstet. Gynecol.,* 2006;108:235–7.

[91] Devoe LD, Croom CS, Youssef AA, Murray C. The prediction of "controlled" uterine rupture by the use ofintrauterine pressure catheters. *Obstet. Gynecol.*, 1992;80:626–9.

[92] Rodriguez MH, Masaki DI, Phelan JP, Diaz FG. Uterine rupture: are intrauterine pressure catheters useful in the diagnosis? *Am. J. Obstet. Gynecol.*, 1989;161:666-9.

[93] Yap OW, Kim ES, Laros RK Jr. Maternal and neonatal outcomes after uterine rupture in labor. *Am. J. Obstet. Gynecol.*, 2001;184:1576–81.

[94] Leung AS, Farmer RM, Leung EK, Medearis AL, Paul RH. Risk factors associated with uterine rupture during trial of labor after cesarean delivery: a case-control study. *Am. J. Obstet. Gynecol.,* 1993;168:1358–63.

[95] Ridgeway JJ, Weyrich DL, Benedetti TJ. Fetal heart rate changes associated with uterine rupture. *Obstet. Gynecol.*, 2004;103:506–12.

[96] Ravasia DJ, Wood SL, Pollard JK. Uterine rupture during induced trial of labor among women with previous cesarean delivery. *Am. J. Obstet. Gynecol.*, 2000;183:1176–9.

[97] Zelop CM, Shipp TD, Repke JT, Cohen A, Caughey AB, Lieberman E. Uterine rupture during induced or augmented labor in gravid women with one prior cesarean delivery. *Am. J. Obstet. Gynecol.*, 1999;181:882–6.

[98] Smith GC, White IR, Pell JP, et al. Predicting cesarean section and uterine rupture among women attempting vaginal birth after prior cesarean section. *PLoS Med.*, 2005;2(9):e252.

[99] Bennett BB. Uterine rupture during induction of labor at term with intravaginal misoprostol. *Obstet. Gynecol.*, 1997;89:832–3.

[100] Wing DA, Lovett K, Paul RH. Disruption of prior uterine incision following misoprostol for labor induction in women with previous cesarean delivery. *Obstet. Gynecol.,* 1998;91:828–30.

[101] Plaut MM, Schwartz ML, Lubarsky SL. Uterine rupture associated with the use of misoprostol in the gravid patient with a previous cesarean section. *Am. J. Obstet. Gynecol.*, 1999;180:1535–42.

[102] Aslan H, Unlu E, Agar M, Ceylan Y. Uterine rupture associated with misoprostol labor induction in women with previous cesarean delivery. *Eur. J. Obstet. Gynecol. Reprod. Biol.,* 2004;113:45–8.

[103] Eden KB, McDonagh M, Denman MA, et al. New insights on vaginal birth after cesarean: can it be predicted? *Obstet. Gynecol.,* 2010;116:967–81.

[104] Rageth JC, Juzi C, Grossenbacher H. Delivery after previous cesarean: a risk evaluation. Swiss Working Group of Obstetric and Gynecologic Institutions. *Obstet. Gynecol.*, 1999;93:332–7.

[105] Spaans WA, Sluijs MB, van Roosmalen J, et al. Risk factors at caesarean section and failure of subsequent trial of labour. *Eur. J. Obstet. Gynecol. Reprod. Biol.,* 2002;100:163–6.

[106] Horenstein JM, Phelan JP. Previous cesarean section: the risks and benefits of oxytocin usage in a trial of labor. *Am. J. Obstet. Gynecol.,* 1985;151:564–9.

[107] Flamm BL, Goings JR, Fuelberth NJ, Fischermann E, Jones C, Hersh E. Oxytocin during labor after previous cesarean section: results of a multicenter study. *Obstet. Gynecol.*, 1987;70:709–12.

[108] Dekker GA, Chan A, Luke CG, et al. Risk of uterine rupture in Australian women attempting vaginal birth after one prior caesarean section: a retrospective population-based cohort study. *BJOG*. 2010;117:1358–65.

[109] Bujold E, Blackwell SC, Gauthier RJ. Cervical ripening with transcervical foley catheter and the risk of uterine rapture. *Obstet. Gynecol.*, 2004; 103:18.

[110] Hoffman MK, Sciscione A, Srinivasana M, et al. Uterine rupture in patients with a prior cesarean delivery: the impact of cervical ripening. *Am. J. Perinatol.*, 2004;21:217.

[111] Sakala EP, Kaye S, Murray RD, Munson LJ. Epidural analgesia. Effect on the likelihood of a successful trial of labor after cesarean section. *J. Reprod. Med.*, 1990;35:886–90.

[112] Stovall TG, Shaver DC, Solomon SK, Anderson GD. Trial of labor in previous cesarean section patients, excluding classical cesarean sections. *Obstet. Gynecol.*, 1987;70:713–7.

[113] Kieser KE, Baskett TF. A 10-year population-based study of uterine rupture. *Obstet. Gynecol.,* 2002;100:749–53.

[114] Mercer BM, Gilbert S, Landon MB, et al. Labor outcomes with increasing number of prior vaginal births after cesarean delivery. *Obstet. Gynecol.*, 2008;111:285–91.

[115] Miller DA, Diaz FG, Paul RH. Vaginal birth after cesarean: a 10-year experience. *Obstet. Gynecol.*, 1994;84:255–8.

[116] Macones GA, Cahill A, Pare E, et al. Obstetric outcomes in women with two prior cesarean deliveries: is vaginal birth after cesarean delivery a viable option? *Am. J. Obstet. Gynecol.*, 2005;192:1223–9.

[117] Tahseen S, Griffiths M. Vaginal birth after two caesarean sections (VBAC-2)— a systematic review with meta-analysis of success rate and adverse outcomes of VBAC-2 versus VBAC-1 and repeat (third) caesarean sections. *BJOG*, 2010;117:5–19.

[118] Cahill AG, Tuuli M, Odibo AO, et al. Vaginal birth after caesarean for women with three or more prior cesareans: assessing safety and success. *BJOG*, 2010;117:422–7.

[119] Bhal PS, Sharma A, Asaad K. Vaginal delivery after caesarean section: factors influencing success rates. *Aust. NZJ Obstet. Gynaecol.*, 1996;36:497–8.

[120] Holt VL, Mueller BA. Attempt and success rates for vaginal birth after caesarean section in relation to complications of the previous pregnancy. *Paediatr. Perinat. Epidemiol.*, 1997;11:63–72.

[121] Peaceman AM, Gersnoviez R, Landon MB, et al. The MFMU Cesarean Registry: impact of fetal size on trial of labor success for patients with previous cesarean for dystocia. *Am. J. Obstet. Gynecol.*, 2006;195:1127–31.

[122] Huang WH, Nakashima DK, Rumney PJ, et al. Interdelivery interval and the success of vaginal birth after cesarean delivery. *Obstet. Gynecol.*, 2002;99: 41–4.

[123] Carroll CS Sr, Magann EF, Chauhan SP, et al. Vaginal birth after cesarean section versus elective repeat cesarean delivery: weight-based outcomes. *Am. J. Obstet. Gynecol.,* 2003;188:1516–22.

[124] Durnwald CP, Ehrenberg HM, Mercer BM. The impact of maternal obesity and weight gain on vaginal birth after cesarean section success. *Am. J. Obstet. Gynecol.*, 2004;191:954–7.

[125] Srinivas SK, Stamilio DM, Sammel MD, et al. Vaginal birth after caesarean delivery: does maternal age affect safety and success? *Paediatr. Perinat. Epide- moil.* 2007;21:114–20.

[126] Hollard AL, Wing DA, Chung JH, et al. Ethnic disparity in the success of vaginal birth after cesarean delivery. *J. Matern. Fetal. Neonatal. Med.*, 2006;19:483–7.

In: Cesarean Section: Procedures, Complications and Recovery ISBN: 978-1-62081-214-3
Editor: Eyal Sheiner

Chapter XVII

Diabetes Mellitus: Is it an Indication for Cesarean Delivery?

Kinneret Tenenbaum-Gavish and Yariv Yogev*
Helen Schneider Hospital for Women, Rabin Medical Center, Petah Tiqva, and Sackler Faculty of Medicine, Tel Aviv University, Tel Aviv, Israel

Introduction

Cesarean section (CS) is believed to be the oldest obstetrical surgical operation, though, in the past, excessive maternal mortality rate has limited its application. In 1937, cesarean delivery rate in the United States averaged at 3% [1]. However, this is no longer the case. Cesarean section rate in the United States has risen ten-fold to a formidable 30% in 2005 [2] partly due to evolution in anesthesia and supportive care, which was associated with decrease in maternal and neonatal postoperative complications. This increase in CS rate is a world wide trend shared by both developing and developed countries [3]. Improved surgical techniques and use of antibiotic prophylaxis together with regional anesthesia has caused a dramatic decrease in post operative complications. Notwithstanding this improvement it is imperative to bear in mind that cesarean delivery still carries a significantly higher rate of both short and long term complications in comparison to vaginal delivery [4,5]. This rise in cesarean section rate is accompanied by a dramatic change in characteristics of pregnant women population. Pregnant women of the 21st century are older and heavier and more likely to experience concurrent medical conditions such as chronic hypertension and diabetes [2 32,3].

The prevalence of diabetes is increasing, affecting approximately one in 6-10 pregnant women [6]. The prevalence of Type 1 diabetes is increasing in children, and that of Type 2 diabetes is increasing in all age groups, especially in adolescences. Therefore more women of child bearing age are expected to have pregnancy complicated by diabetes.

* Correspondence address: Yariv Yogev, MD, Department of Obstetrics and Gynecology. Helen Schneider Hospital for Women. Rabin Medical Center. Beilinson Campus. Petah Tiqva 49100. Israel. . Tel: +972-3-9377400. Fax: +972-3-9377409. Email: Yarivyogev@hotmail.com.

These parallel epidemics are kin to one another. Their rapid progression worldwide is like the rampage of the mythical twins Phobos and Deimos changing modern obstetrics. It's likely that cesarean section and diabetes have compounding effects on pregnancy outcomes which highlights the need for a comprehensive strategy to improve clinical outcomes in these pregnancies.

The Complexity of Timing of Delivery in Pregnancy Complicated by Diabetes

Judging how long to carry on a pregnancy around term and how to deliver are key decisions in the management of pregnancies complicated by diabetes for both the diabetic women and their health care providers. The decision to deliver a diabetic patient takes into account maternal and fetal risks and benefits and tries to find the exact balance between them. Fetal risk such as potential intrauterine death, shoulder dystocia and the consequences of premature delivery should be balanced against maternal risks from induction of labor- mainly unplanned or emergent cesarean section and its complications. Additionally, labor related complications such as birth-canal trauma should be taken into consideration as well.

There is a general agreement that all women with pre-gestational diabetes should be delivered by 40 weeks of gestation to minimize the risk of stillbirth. As to women with gestational diabetes mellitus (GDM) the ACOG deems that routine delivery before 40 weeks is not supported by evidence but studies suggest that pharmacologically -treated GDM patients may benefit from induction of labor at 38-39 weeks in terms of increased proportion of AGA babies and decrease in shoulder dystocia rates [7]. The issue of setting a time limit for the delivery date of women with diet-treated GDM with good glycemic control is yet to be decided.

The American Agency for Healthcare Research and Quality (AHRQ) report on GDM from 2008 also concluded that there is lack of conclusive evidence to support an unequivocal recommendation for elective labor induction or cesarean delivery in women with gestational diabetes [8].

The American diabetes association (ADA) recommendations state that prolongation of gestation past 38 weeks increase the risk of fetal macrosomia without reducing cesarean rates, so that delivery during the 38th week is recommended unless obstetric considerations dictate otherwise [9]. In this context, it is important to keep in mind that in this specific population there is a higher prevalence of other maternal complications, such as hypertensive disease, that may necessitate planned delivery.

The two primary motives for setting a time limit for delivery in pregnancies complicated by diabetes are concern about fetal demise during the third trimester of pregnancy and shoulder dystocia. Studies on women with type 1 and type 2 diabetes reported a statistically significant increase in the risk for fetal mortality among these women in comparison with non-diabetic controls10,11]. Higher perinatal mortality rates were also reported in women with GDM managed with diet alone [12,13]. Most cases of late-pregnancy fetal demise occurred in large-for-gestational age (LGA) infants and in pregnancies with poor glycemic control [14,15].

Identifying the Fetus at Risk for Shoulder Dystocia

There are several epidemiologic recognized risk factors for shoulder dystocia. These include macrosomia and fetal adiposity, maternal diabetes, maternal obesity, operative vaginal delivery, precipitous delivery and prolonged second stage of labor, previous delivery of a macrosomic infant, previous delivery complicated by shoulder dystocia, post term pregnancy, and advanced maternal age. Although these factors have been suggested in univariant design studies as contributors for the risk of shoulder dystocia, most of them are also associated with fetal macrosomia.

Women with diabetes are at increased risk of fetal macrosomia and shoulder dystocia [16]. The risk for shoulder dystocia is increased six-fold in pregnancies complicated by diabetes compared to general population [17]. Any increase in birth weight above 3750gr in infants of diabetic mothers raises further the risk for shoulder dystocia. Furthermore, perinatal mortality rate, incidence of birth injuries, and incidence of shoulder dystocia are increase in diabetic mothers compared to similar-weight fetuses of non-diabetic pregnancies [18].

Infants to diabetic mothers are also more likely to suffer from brachial plexus injury once shoulder dystocia has occurred compared to infants of non-diabetic mothers [18]. Should we therefore deliver all diabetic pregnancies by cesarean section and thus prevent all cases of shoulder dystocia and brachial plexus injury to infants of diabetic mothers? Although not common, brachial plexus injury after cesarean deliveries has been described, and may account for 1% to 4% of cases [19,20]. There are even descriptions of in-utero brachial plexus injury [20]. It is therefore clear that cesarean section is not an absolute "cure" for obstetric brachial plexus injury. The overall risk of brachial plexus injury for a macrosomic (over 4000gr) infant of a diabetic mother during a vaginal delivery is estimated at 2-5% [18]. Further assessment indicates that 6.7% of brachial plexus injuries cause persistent (rather than transient) neurological damage. Based on those calculations, 13-33 cases of persistent brachial plexus injury are expected if we allow 10,000 vaginal deliveries of macrosomic infants [21]. Among infants with persistent obstetric brachial plexus palsy, 70-75% of those who were treated operatively a few months after delivery regained shoulder and elbow function [22].

Rouse et al [21,23] constructed a decision analysis model to compare labor and delivery management policies in both diabetic and non-diabetic patients. The study compared rates of shoulder dystocia, rates of permanent brachial plexus injury, the number and cost of additional cesarean births, and the potential cost savings for averting permanent brachial plexus injury. Analysis in the diabetic population, applying a macrosomia threshold of 4500gr, concluded that 443 cesarean deliveries and $930,000 are required to prevent one case of permanent brachial plexus injury.

This is not meant to belittle the fact that shoulder dystocia is still one of the most terrifying obstetric emergencies, and that brachial plexus injury may cause severe disability for infants. It is not meant to diminish the related medico-legal issues regarding litigation due to shoulder dystocia, but only to highlight the evidence behind this issue. Furthermore, brachial plexus injury is not the only possible complication of shoulder dystocia. Shoulder dystocia without Erb's palsy remains a serious complication involving bone fractures, asphyxia and even fetal death. Above all it is important to emphasize that intensive treatment of diabetes and good glycemic control reduces the risk of both macrosomia and shoulder dystocia with its related fetal injuries [17,24].

In the desire to avoid this horrifying event we are left with only the crude measure of antenatal detection of the large fetus, who is more likely to suffer a shoulder dystocia and nerve injury. There are several widely accepted methods used to detect large for date fetuses. The American College of Obstetricians and Gynecologists (ACOG) acknowledged either ultrasound measurements or clinical weight estimation preformed by physician or an experienced expecting mother as legitimate methods [25].

The macrosomic offspring of the obese and diabetic women manifests an increased fat mass and not lean body mass. However, most conventional ultrasonographic weight estimation models do not take into account the significance of fetal soft tissue (or adiposity) in the pathophysiology of birth trauma and shoulder dystocia. Some degree of correlation between prenatal ultrasound fetal biometry, such as abdominal circumference (AC), and infant (neonatal) body fat percentage was noted by some investigators [26] but we are still very lacking in our ability to distinguish between constitutionally large fetuses and those who are pathologically or disproportionately grown.

Taking into account the inborn inaccuracy of fetal weight estimation methods- there are some studies that indicate that using ultrasound-derived fetal weight estimates may help make inform decisions regarding timing and route of delivery in diabetic women and those may decrease rates of shoulder dystocia [27]. Langer et al [16] reviewed 75,979 vaginal deliveries from 1970 to 1985 (diabetic and non-diabetic pregnancies) which were subdivided by weight categories at 250 gm intervals. They found that for diabetic patients, using a 4000gr or greater threshold for cesarean delivery would prevent 84% of shoulder dystocia cases. Using a higher threshold of 4500 gm recommended by ACOG [28] will increase the cesarean section rate by 0.14% but will still leave 46% of shoulder dystocia cases unidentified. Applying a 4000gr estimated weight limit for vaginal delivery in diabetic population may resulted in a small but significant increase in the overall cesarean delivery rate among diabetic women [27 27,29] it still prevents the majority of fetuses at greatest risk for shoulder dystocia to avoid the hazards of vaginal delivery.

Labor Management Options for Diabetic Patients

Labor Management options for diabetic patients include expectant management, labor induction, or elective cesarean delivery. The clinician's choice of the preferred route of management and mode of delivery should take into account such factors as estimates of fetal weight, gestational age, and maternal glucose control along with other factor including the presence of a uterine scar, maternal pre-eclampsia etc.

It is not surprising therefore that the CEMACH report from 2005 [66] found that only a minority (18.0%) of women with diabetes went into spontaneous labor compared with 69% of general population and that pregnant women with pre-gestational diabetes were twice as likely to be induced (38.9% compared with 21% in the general maternity population) [30]. The CEMACH also reported that spontaneous vaginal delivery accounted for a mere 24% of deliveries in women with diabetes compared with 67% in the general maternity population. The cesarean section rate in the diabetic population was 3 times that of the general population. Furthermore, induction of labor for women with diabetes is more likely to result in emergency caesarean section (43.0%, compared with 19% for mothers in general) although the risk of cesarean section for non-progressive labor was comparable to that of general obstetric population [66].

The key question is essentially this: when is the risk of severe maternal morbidity from cesarean section outweighed by the risk of intrauterine fetal demise or severe fetal birth trauma such as shoulder dystocia and brachial plexus injury? Lucky enough both major maternal complications from cesarean delivery and severe fetal birth-related trauma are catastrophic events which are rare occasions in usual obstetric practice.

Specific Complication Related to Cesarean Section in the Diabetic (and Most Often Obese) Patient

As a general assumption, it is factual that cesarean delivery results in a 2-7 fold increased risk of maternal mortality than vaginal delivery [31,32]. However, in most reports, all cesarean deliveries were compared to all vaginal deliveries regardless of circumstance of delivery. It is only logical to assume that pre-labor cesarean section complication rates are not comparable with those of intrapartum cesarean deliveries, although few clinical trials have addressed this issue specifically. Furthermore, women suffering from complications such as severe hypertensive disease, disruption of placentation (placental abruption or previa) or life-threatening infections are often delivered by cesarean section which makes it more difficult to distinguish between complications related to cesarean delivery per se and those resulting from circumstances leading to it.

In contras, cesarean delivery for suspected macrosomia is more likely to occur under more ideal pre-labor and controlled conditions. What are the potential complications that clinicians and expectant mothers should take into account when considering an elective CS? Review of the available literature indicates that the most prevalent post operative complications after CS are: post partum endometritis, surgical wound infection (with its related complications of scar dehiscence) and postpartum anemia. Other complications worth mentioning are post operative thromboembolic complications such as deep vein thrombosis (including pelvic vein thrombosis), endometritis and abdominal wound infection

Gregory et al [33] reviewed the state of Washington's birth event records database for 1990. The researchers used CDC codes in birth certificates to estimate the general population risks of maternal and infant complications with the birth of macrosomic (at least 4000 gr) infants. They found that the overall complication rate for women who had cesarean section without labor were low (less than 3%). The women who delivered a macrosomic infant by pre-labor CS had a threefold greater risk of postpartum infection, an 11-fold greater risk of wound complications, but an 80% lower risk of postpartum hemorrhage than women experiencing a vaginal delivery of a macrosomic infant. Lydon-Rochelle and colleagues [34] reviewed 256,795 singleton deliveries of primiparous women with no chronic medical conditions in a retrospective cohort study of data from the Washington State Birth Events Record Database. They used maternal postpartum re-hospitalization as a measure of maternal complication rate. They found that women who had cesarean delivery were more likely to be re-hospitalized with uterine infection compared to women who had spontaneous vaginal delivery, (RR=2.0; 95% CI, 1.7-2.4) and more likely to have thromboembolic conditions (RR=2.5; 95% CI, 1.5-3.5). They also reported an increased risk of re-hospitalization for other indications in the CS group.

However, these studies do not sufficiently address the issue of cesarean section complications in the diabetic population. Chaim et al. [35] conducted a cross-sectional study of the outcome of 75,947 term and preterm singleton deliveries; vaginally and by cesarean section from 1989-1997. In that study the rate of post partum endometritis (PPE) after cesarean section was found to be 15 times higher than that after vaginal delivery (2.6% vs. 0.17%). Gestational diabetes mellitus did not increase the risk of PPE in that study's population. The researchers also reported a rate of wound infection after cesarean section of 3.97% (318/7,995). Women who suffered from post-operative wound infection were more likely to have suffered from GDM (rather than pre GDM).

Women with diabetes and obese pregnant women appear to have increased morbidity and mortality associated with caesarean delivery and from anesthesia-related complications in particular those of general anesthesia for caesarean delivery [2020]. Leth et al [36] addressed this issue in a prospective cohort study that reviewed 2,492 women who delivered by cesarean section (CS). They reported an 18.4% post-cesarean infection rate within 30 days of delivery. Among diabetic women, obesity increased the risk of post-cesarean infections more than twofold; the adjusted ORs were 2.06 (95%CI: 1.13-3.75) for infections. Schneid-Kofman and colleagues [37] reported that combined obesity and diabetes (gestational and pregestational) increased the risk for wound infection 9.3-fold (95% CI, 4.5-19.2; P < .001). Obesity is also a risk factor for anesthesia related maternal mortality. Obese patients present the anesthesiologist with a significant technical difficulty in administering epidural analgesia on the one hand and an exceedingly high risk for difficult or failed intubation on the other [38,39]. Post operative morbidity is further increased in the obese patient by prolonged operating time, increased blood loss and a higher risk of thromboembolic events [40].

The conclusion drawn from these reports is that post cesarean section complication in the diabetic and obese population are not negligible or trifle even in the setting of pre-labor cesarean delivery. Health care providers should also take into account the consequences of repeated cesarean deliveries. Previous cesarean deliveries increase maternal risks for serious adverse events in subsequent pregnancies which are not liable to happen to women without uterine scar such as placenta previa, placenta accreta, postpartum hysterectomy, and uterine rupture. These disastrous events may also have a deleterious effect on fetuses and neonates of subsequent pregnancies with profound neonatal depression or death whether or not a trial of labor is attempted.

CONCLUSION

The main principal in modern obstetrics is the achievement of a high-quality pregnancy outcome for both mother and child. With this standard in mind it is important to consider the welfare of both and to find the proper balance between them when considering the appropriate timing and mode of delivery for pregnancies complicated by diabetes. There is no single route of delivery that is appropriate for all pregnancies complicated by diabetes but rather a personalized strategy tailored to suit each pregnant patient's need according to glycemic control, obstetric history and fetal assessment. Patients and clinicians should use all available data regarding the risk and benefits that each delivery strategy carries in order help individualize treatment.

REFERENCES

[1] Duncan CJ, Doyle JB. Cesarean section: a ten-year study of 703 cases at the Boston City Hospital. *N. Engl. J. Med.*, 1937; 216:1-5.

[2] Hamilton BE, Martin JA, Ventura SJ. Births: preliminary data for 2005. Health e-stats. Hyattsville, MD: National Center for Health Statistics, November 21, 2006. (Accessed February 8, 2007, at http://www.cdc.gov/nchs/products/pubs/pubd/hestats/prelimbirths05/prelimbirths05.htm.)

[3] Jeffrey L. Ecker, M.D., and Fredric D. Frigoletto, Jr., M.D. Cesarean Delivery and the Risk–Benefit Calculus. *N. Engl. J. Med.,* 2007;356;9.

[4] Cunningham F, Leveno KJ, Bloom SL. Cesarean delivery and peripartum hysterectomy. In: Cunningham F, Leveno K, Bloom N, Hauth J, Gilstrap L, Wenstrom K, editors. Williams's obstetrics, 22nd edition, New York: McGraw-Hill, 2005; pp 587-606.

[5] Burrows LJ, Meyn LA, Weber AM. Maternal morbidity associated with vaginal versus cesarean delivery. *Obstet. Gynecol.*, 2004; 103:907-912.

[6] Confidential Enquiry into Maternal and Child Health: Pregnancy in Women with Type 1 and Type 2 Diabetes in 2002–03, England, Wales and Northern Ireland.London: CEMACH; 2005.

[7] ACOG Practice Bulletin. Clinical management guidelines for obstetrician-gynecologists. Number 30, September 2001 (replaces Technical Bulletin Number 200, December 1994). Gestational diabetes. *Obstet. Gynecol.*, 2001; 98(3):525-38.

[8] Nicholson WK, Wilson LM, Witkop CT, Baptiste-Roberts K, Bennett WL, Bolen S, Barone BB, Golden SH, Gary TL, Neale DM, Bass EB. Therapeutic Management, Delivery, and Postpartum Risk Assessment and Screening in Gestational Diabetes. Evidence Report/Technology Assessment No. 162 (Prepared by the Johns Hopkins University Evidence-based Practice Center under Contract No. 290-02-0018.) AHRQ Publication No. 08-E004. Rockville, MD: Agency for Healthcare Research and Quality. March 2008.

[9] Gestational diabetes mellitus. Diabetes Care January 2004 vol. 27 no. suppl 1 s88-s90.

[10] Casson IF, Clarke CA, Howard CV, McKendrick O, Pennycook S, Pharoah PO, Platt MJ, Stanisstreet M, van Velszen D, Walkinshaw S. Outcomes of pregnancy in insulin dependent diabetic women: results of a five year population cohort study. *BMJ.* 1997 2;315(7103):275-8.

[11] Cundy T, Gamble G, Townend K, Henley PG, MacPherson P, Roberts AB. Perinatal mortality in Type 2 diabetes mellitus. *Diabet Med.*, 2000; 17(1):33-9.

[12] Schmidt MI, Duncan BB, Reichelt AJ, Branchtein L, Matos MC, Costa e Forti A, Spichler ER, Pousada JM, Teixeira MM, Yamashita T; Brazilian Gestational Diabetes Study Group. Gestational diabetes mellitus diagnosed with a 2-h 75-g oral glucose tolerance test and adverse pregnancy outcomes. *Diabetes Care*, 2001;24(7):1151-5.

[13] Pettitt DJ, Knowler WC, Baird HR, Bennett PH. Gestational diabetes: infant and maternal complications of pregnancy in relation to third-trimester glucose tolerance in the Pima Indians. *Diabetes Care*, 1980;3(3):458-64.

[14] Langer O, Conway DL. Level of glycemia and perinatal outcome in pregestational diabetes. *J. Matern. Fetal. Med.*, 2000;9(1):35-41

[15] Langer O, Yogev Y, Most O, Xenakis EM. Gestational diabetes: the consequences of not treating. *Am. J. Obstet. Gynecol.*, 2005; 192(4):989-97.

[16] Langer O, Berkus MD, Huff RW, Samueloff A. Shoulder dystocia: should the fetus weighing greater than or equal to 4000 grams be delivered by cesarean section? *Am. J. Obstet. Gynecol.*, 1991; 165(4 Pt 1):831-7.

[17] Langer O, Rodriguez DA, Xenakis EM, McFarland MB, Berkus MD, Arrendondo F. Intensified versus conventional management of gestational diabetes. *Am. J. Obstet. Gynecol.*, 1994;170(4):1036-46; discussion 1046-7.

[18] Conway D, Obstetric Management in Gestational Diabetes Care, 30, *Supll*,(2) 2007:10.2337-s212.

[19] Bar J, Dvir A, Hod M, Orvieto R, Merlob P, Neri A. Brachial plexus injury and obstetrical risk factors. *Int. J. Gynaecol. Obstet.,* 2001 Apr;73(1):21-5.

[20] Doumouchtsis SK, Arulkumaran S. Are all brachial plexus injuries caused by shoulder dystocia? *Obstet. Gynecol. Surv.,* 2009; 64(9):615-23.

[21] Rouse DJ, Owen J: Prophylactic cesarean delivery for fetal macrosomia diagnosed by means of ultrasonography: a Faustian bargain? *Am. J. Obstet. Gynecol.*, 1999 181:332–338.

[22] Dumont CE, Forin V, Asfazadourian H, Romana C. Function of the upper limb after surgery for obstetric brachial plexus palsy. *J. Bone Joint. Surg. Br.*, 2001;83(6):894-900.

[23] Rouse DJ, Owen J, Goldenberg RL, Cliver SP. The effectiveness and costs of elective cesarean delivery for fetal macrosomia diagnosed by ultrasound. *JAMA*, 1996 13;276(18):1480-6.

[24] Crowther CA, Hiller JE, Moss JR, McPhee AJ, Jeffries WS, Robinson JS; Australian Carbohydrate Intolerance Study in Pregnant Women (ACHOIS) Trial Group. Effect of treatment of gestational diabetes mellitus on pregnancy outcomes. *N. Engl. J. Med.,* 2005 16;352(24):2477-86.

[25] American College of Obstetricians and Gynecologists (ACOG). Fetal macrosomia. Washington, DC; 2000. ACOG practice bulletin; no. 22.

[26] Moyer-Mileur LJ, Slater H, Thomson JA, Mihalopoulos N, Byrne J, Varner MW. Newborn adiposity measured by plethysmography is not predicted by late gestation two-dimensional ultrasound measures of fetal growth. *J. Nutr.*, 2009;139(9):1772-8. E.

[27] Conway DL, Langer O: Elective delivery of infants with macrosomia in diabetic women: reduced shoulder dystocia versus increased cesarean deliveries. *Am. J. Obstet. Gynecol.*, 1998, 178:922–925.

[28] ACOG Practice Bulletin: Clinical management guidelines for obstetrician gynecologists: *shoulder dystocia*. 2002; 40(100):1045-9.

[29] Yogev Y, Ben-Haroush A, Chen R, Glickman H, Kaplan B, Hod M. Active induction management of labor for diabetic pregnancies at term; mode of delivery and fetal outcome--a single center experience. *Eur. J. Obstet. Gynecol. Reprod. Biol.*, 2004 15;114(2):166-70.

[30] Department of Health. NHS Maternity Statistics, England 2002–03. Statistical Bulletin 2004/10.

[31] Miller JM Jr: Maternal and neonatal morbidity and mortality in cesarean section. *Obstet. Gynecol. Clin. North. Am.*,1988, 15: 629–638.

[32] American College of Obstetricians and Gynecologists Task Force on Cesarean Delivery T Rates: Evaluation of cesarean delivery, Washington, DC, American College Obstetricians and Gynecologists, 2000.

[33] Gregory KD, Henry OA, Ramicone E, Chan LS, Platt LD. Maternal and infant complications in high and normal weight infants by method of delivery. *Obstet. Gynecol.*, 1998;92(4 Pt 1):507-13.

[34] Lydon-Rochelle M, Holt VL, Martin DP, Easterling TR. Association between method of delivery and maternal rehospitalization. *JAMA*. 2000 10;283(18):2411-6.

[35] Chaim W, Bashiri A, Bar-David J, Shoham-Vardi I, Mazor M. Prevalence and clinical significance of postpartum endometritis and wound infection. *Infect. Dis. Obstet. Gynecol.*, 2000;8(2):77-82.

[36] Leth RA, Uldbjerg N, Nørgaard M, Møller JK, Thomsen RW. Obesity, diabetes, and the risk of infections diagnosed in hospital and post-discharge infections after cesarean section: a prospective cohort study. *Acta. Obstet. Gynecol. Scand.*, 2011; 90(5):501-9.

[37] Schneid-Kofman N, Sheiner E, Levy A, Holcberg G. Risk factors for wound infection following cesarean deliveries; *Int. J. Gynaecol. Obstet.,* 2005;90(1):10-5.

[38] Saravanakumar K, Rao SG, Cooper GM. Obesity and obstetric anaesthesia. *Anaesthesia*, 2006;61(1):36-48

[39] Galtier F, Raingeard I, Renard E, Boulot P, Bringer J. Optimizing the outcome of pregnancy in obese women: from pregestational to long-term management. *Diabetes Metab.*, 2008;34(1):19-25.

[40] Hall LF, Neubert AG. Obesity and pregnancy; *Obstet. Gynecol. Surv.*, 2005;60(4):253-60.

In: Cesarean Section: Procedures, Complications and Recovery ISBN: 978-1-62081-214-3
Editor: Eyal Sheiner

Chapter XVIII

Cesarean Section and HIV Transmission

David Kulak and Anatte Karmon*
Albert Einstein College of Medicine
Department of Obstetrics, Gynecology and Women's Health, Bronx, NY, US

Introduction

There are currently 33.3 million people worldwide with HIV or AIDS, of which 15.8 million are women and 2.5 million are children [1].

Maternal to child transmission (MTCT) is the most common source for pediatric infection with more than 2000 children infected through this method on a daily basis, totaling nearly 750,000 a year [2]. Thus, preventing it is of vital importance to curb the spread of HIV.

Without medical intervention, the MTCT rate is between 15-25 percent; including breastfeeding this rate is as high as 40 percent [3].

Treatment for HIV Reduces Transmission

In 1994, the landmark protocol 076 trial showed that zidovudine treatment given prior to and during labor to HIV seropositive mothers and for 6 months to their newborn infants decreased the MTCT rate dramatically from 25 percent to nearly 8 percent [4].Still, studies were done to find mechanisms to further lower the rate of transmission. Observational studies found that the risk of transmission was directly related to viral load[5] and time in labor or time with ruptured membranes [6,7]. Interestingly, studies also found that the risk of transmission in twin pregnancies was significantly higher for twin A than for twin B [8,9]. In a study by Duliege et al. [9] HIV transmission occurred with 35% of vaginally delivered firstborn twins and 15% of vaginally delivered second born twins, with an adjusted odds ratio of 2.8 for HIV infection of A versus B twins (95% confidence interval 1.6 - 5.0). These observations led many to believe that labor, ruptured membranes, and passage through the vaginal canal were

* Corresponding author: Anatte Karmon, MD, Albert Einstein College of Medicine, Department of Obstetrics, Gynecology and Women's Health, 1300 Morris Park Avenue, Bronx, NY 10461, Email: anatte@gmail.com.

risk factors for MTCT via placental microtransfusion [10,11], rising vaginal infections and infected vaginal secretions [12,13] respectively. Thus it was postulated that MTCT would be lower if cesarean delivery was performed as compared to vaginal delivery; however, numerous observational studies compared vaginal and cesarean deliveries and found no significant difference in the rates of MTCT [6,14,15].

HIV Transmission: Is Cesarean Section the Preferred Mode of Delivery?

In 1999, a study from 6 European countries randomized patients to elective cesarean delivery (ECD), meaning before the onset of labor or rupture of membranes, or to normal labor management. This study enrolled 436 women and had final infection status on 370 infants; patients were randomized to ECD before labor thus avoiding the potential transmission modes of placental microtransfusions and rising infections. The study showed an 80 percent reduction in MTCT with elective cesarean delivery (odds ratio 0.3; 95percent CI 0.1-0.8) [16]. It also demonstrated that non-elective cesarean deliveries (i.e. those performed after the onset of labor or subsequent to rupture of membranes) had a non-significant improvement of MTCT from the vaginal delivery rate of 10.2 percent to 8.8 percent (odds ratio 1.0; 95 percent CI, 0.3-3.7).

That same year a meta-analysis of individual-patient data from 15 prospective cohort studies totaling 8533 mother-child pairs from North America and Europe showed a 50 percent reduction in MTCT if ECD was performed. The study was unique compared to the European study in that it controlled for zidovudine use and also demonstrated that there was no decrease in MTCT in vaginal deliveries with rupture of membranes just before delivery. Because of the large number of patients in the study, there was enough power to show with statistical significance that when antiretroviral therapy during prenatal, intrapartum and neonatal periods was used in conjunction with elective cesarean delivery the MTCT rate decreased by 87 percent to a transmission rate of 2 percent (adjusted odds ratio 0.13; 95 percent confidence interval 0.09 to 0.19). The study also showed that in the absence of antiretroviral therapy, elective cesarean delivery decreases the rate of transmission to 10.4 percent [17].

A limitation of these two major studies is that they did not segregate or control for HIV maternal serum viral load. HIV viral load is known to be directly correlated to the transmissibility of the disease [18]. Subsequent studies defined the HIV-1 viral load at which the transmission rate is unaffected by mode of delivery. Two large studies were then published that compared specific viral loads with transmission rate. The first study (480 women) compared maternal plasma levels of CD4+ lymphocyte counts, HIV-1 p24 antibody levels and, total HIV-1 RNA level (viral load). Through multivariate analysis it was found that only HIV-1 RNA levels were correlated to MTCT, and that there was no transmission if the HIV-1 RNA levels were undetectable at the time of delivery; the cutoff for detectability at that time was 500 copies per milliliter [19]. Another study by Garcia et al [5] measured maternal plasma HIV-1 RNA levels at the time of delivery and rate of transmission.

The study showed that below 1000 copies per milliliter, there was no vertical transmission even with vaginal deliveries. The authors further analyzed these results and showed that the MTCT is 16.6 percent among women with 1000 to 10,000 copies per milliliter (32 of 193), 21.3 percent among women with 10,001 to 50,000 copies per milliliter (39 of 183), 30.9 percent among women with 50,001 to 100,000 copies per milliliter (17 of 54), and 40.6 percent among women with more than 100,000 copies per milliliter (26 of 64, P<0.001). Interestingly, they also showed that among women with more than 100,000 copies per milliliter who did not receive AZT prophylaxis the MTCT rate was 63.3 percent [5].

Consensus Guidelines

Based on the combination of the above findings, ACOG [20] and the US preventive task force [21] issued guidelines in 2000 with new recommendations for the management of HIV positive patients in labor. The committee opinion had five major points:

All HIV positive women should be counseled on the role of AZT therapy in pregnancy, and offered this therapy.

Women with viral loads greater than 1000 copies per milliliter should be counseled on the benefits of elective (scheduled) cesarean delivery to reduce the MTCT rate.

Delivery should occur after 38 weeks of gestation in order to avoid spontaneous labor or rupture of membranes. Although it is before 39 weeks, an amniocentesis for assessment of fetal lung maturity should be avoided in all HIV positive patients.

Zidovudine infusion should begin three hours preoperatively to ensure adequate serum level at the time of delivery. Highly active antiretroviral therapy should be continued during this period.

To decrease risk of infection in these patients with baseline impaired immunity, prophylactic antibiotics should be given (although subsequent practice guidelines state that all patients should receive prophylactic antibiotics at the time of cesarean delivery).

Since 1999 and the publishing of the two foundational studies on ECD, the cesarean section rate among HIV positive women has risen at a higher rate than that of the general population. In the US, the rate of cesarean delivery rose from 22 to 33 percent in that time period, however the rate among HIV seropositive patients rose from 33 percent to 40 percent [22] and the total cesarean delivery rate including non-elective cases was as high as 50 percent; similar trends were found in Europe [23]. In Sweden, the total cesarean delivery rate (elective and non elective) for HIV-infected women increased from 8 percent in 1985-1993 to 44 percent in 1994-1998, and to 80 percent in 1999-2003 [24].

Consequences of Cesarean Delivery

With the increasing rate of cesarean delivery came increased morbidity. Multiple studies have shown that women infected with HIV undergoing cesarean delivery are at higher risk for minor postoperative complications. The risk is between 2.5-4 times more likely to occur when compared with similar HIV seronegative patients [25-27]. The most common complication was post-operative fever, but also included endometritis, wound infection, and post-operative anemia. However, there is no statistically significant difference in rates of major complications between the two groups (9.3% vs 3.4%; odds ratio 2.84; 95% confidence interval 0.65-14.06) [28]. These risks are highest when cesarean deliveries are performed in non-elective settings [29]. RNA viral load level greater than 1000 confers increased risk of maternal morbidity [30]. There is no evidence of increased fetal risk from cesarean deliveries in HIV seropositive mothers compared to HIV negative mothers, however the risk of fetal laceration in an HIV positive mother does raise the risk of transmission [31].

Elective cesarean delivery increases the risk of fetal respiratory distress; however there is no additional increase in the rate of this morbidity among HIV positive patients [32,33]. Although the gestational age of the fetus is inversely correlated with the risk of respiratory distress, this risk must be balanced with the increasing risk of labor or rupture of membranes with increasing gestational age. Additionally, it is more difficult to establish fetal lung maturity in HIV positive patients as amniocentesis is avoided in this population secondary to the theoretical risk of MTCT. Although the maternal risks of any form of cesarean delivery and implications for future pregnancies are manifold these risks are magnified greatly in the developing world and resource limited locations, and thus for both fetal and maternal reasons ECD in HIV positive women is often not the recommended mode of delivery in these locations [34].

Unanswered Questions

Even with the guidelines set by multiple organizations and the extensive literature available there are still unanswered questions and clinical "gray areas" where optimal mode of delivery is still uncertain. For patients with preterm premature rupture of membranes before 34 weeks of gestation, guidelines recommend delaying delivery until 34 weeks of gestation; in the HIV infected population this recommendation must be weighed against the increasing risk of MTCT in the setting of vaginal delivery after prolonged rupture of membranes. There is no strong evidence that weighs the respective risks [35]. For patients that present immediately after rupture of membranes there is no definitive evidence or guidelines as to optimal mode of delivery and transmission rates; this is critical as there is strong evidence to show that both in HIV positive and negative patients the maternal and fetal risks are highest in non-elective cesarean delivery. Although currently elective cesarean delivery is recommended for patients with a viral load of 1000 or greater, there is new evidence to say that ECD decreases MTCT for patients with a viral load of less then one thousand [36]. Finally, there are no clear data showing MTCT rates in patients diagnosed with HIV at the time of delivery when there is no available viral load, although many clinicians would offer or recommend cesarean delivery to their patients in such a situation [37].

References

[1] A.M. Duliege, C.I. Amos, S. Felton, R.J. Biggar and J.J. Goedert, Birth order, delivery route, and concordance in the transmission of human immunodeficiency virus type 1 from mothers to twins: International Registry of HIV-Exposed Twins. *J. Pediatr.*, 126 (1995), pp. 625–632.

[2] Aagaard-Tillery KM, Lin MG, Lupo V, Buchbinder A, Ramsey PS. Preterm premature rupture of membranes in human immunodeficiency virus-infected women: a novel case series. *Infect. Dis. Obstet. Gynecol.*, 2006;2006:53234.

[3] American College of Obstetricians and Gynecologists, Scheduled cesarean delivery and the prevention of vertical transmission of HIV infection: ACOG committee opinion no.: 234 (replaces no.: 219). *Int. J. Gynaecol. Obstet.*, 73 (2001), pp. 279–281.

[4] Bjorklund K, Mutyaba T, Nabunya E, et al. Incidence of postcesarean infections in relation to HIV status in a setting with limited resources. *Acta. Obstet. Gynecol. Scand.*, 2005;84(10):967–71.

[5] C. Hutto, W.P. Parks and S.H. Lai, et al. A hospital-based prospective study of perinatal infection with human immunodeficiency virus type 1. *J. Pediatr.*, 118 (1991), pp. 347–353.

[6] Centers for Disease Control and Prevention, US Public Health Service Task Force recommendations for use of antiretroviral drugs in pregnant HIV-1-infected women for maternal health and interventions to reduce perinatal HIV-1 transmission in the United States. *MMWR Recomm. Rep.*, 51 (2002), pp. 1–38.

[7] Centers for Disease Control and Prevention. Enhanced perinatal surveillanceparticipating areas in thc United States and dependent areas, 2000–2003. HIV/AIDS Surveillance Supplement Report, 2008. Available at: http://www.cdc.gov/hiv/topics/surveillance_HIVAIDS_SSR_Vol13_No4.pdf.

[8] Clemetson DB, Moss GB, Willerford DM, et al. Detection of HIV DNA in cervical and vaginal secretions: prevalence and correlates among women in Nairobi, Kenya. *JAMA*, 269:2860-4, 1993.

[9] Connor EM, Sperling RS, Gelber R, et al. Reduction of maternal-infant transmission of human immunodeficiency virus type 1 with zidovudine treatment: Pediatric AIDS Clinical Trials Group Protocol 076 Study Group. *N. Engl. J. Med.*, 331:1173-80, 1994.

[10] E.J. Rodriguez, C. Spann, D. Jamieson and M. Lindsay, Postoperative morbidity associated with cesarean delivery among human immunodeficiency virus-seropositive women. *Am. J. Obstet. Gynecol,*, 184 (2001), pp. 1108–1111.

[11] European Mode of Delivery Collaboration, Elective caesarean-section versus vaginal delivery in prevention of vertical HIV-1 transmission: a randomized clinical trial. *Lancet*, 353 (1999), pp. 1035–1039.

[12] Garcia PM, Kalish LA, Pitt J, Minkoff H, Quinn T, Burchett SK, et al. Maternal levels of plasma human immunodeficiency virus type 1 RNA and the risk of perinatal transmission. Women and Infants Transmission Study Group. *N. Engl. J. Med.*, 1999;341:394-402.

[13] International Perinatal HIV Group, Duration of ruptured membranes and vertical transmission of HIV-1: a meta-analysis from 15 prospective cohort studies. *AIDS*, 15 (2001), pp. 357–368.

[14] International Perinatal HIV Group, The mode of delivery and the risk of vertical transmission of human immunodeficiency virus type 1: a meta-analysis of 15 prospective cohort studies. *N. Engl. J. Med.*, 340 (1999), pp. 977–987.

[15] J.J. Goedert, A.M. Duliege, C.I. Amos, S. Felton and R.J. Biggar, High risk of HIV-1 infection for first-born twins: the International Registry of HIV-exposed Twins. *Lancet*, 338 (1991), pp. 1471–1475.

[16] Jamieson DJ, Read JS, Kourtis AP, et al. Cesarean delivery for HIV-infected women: recommendations and controversies. *Am. J. Obstet. Gynecol.*, 2007;197 (Suppl 3):S96–100.
[17] K.L. Dominguez, M.L. Lindegren and P.J. D'Almada, et al. Increasing trend of cesarean deliveries in HIV-infected women in the United States from 1994 to 2000. *J. Acquir. Immune. Defic. Syndr.,* 33 (2003), pp. 232–238.
[18] Kalish LA, Pitt J, Lew J, et al. Defining the time of fetal or perinatal acquisition of human immunodeficiency virus type 1 infection on the basis of age at first positive culture. Women and Infants Transmission Study (WITS). *J. Infect. Dis.*, 1997;175(3): 712–5.
[19] Kaneda T, Shiraki K, Hirano K, et al. Detection of maternofetal transfusion by placental alkaline phosphatase levels. *J. Pediatr.*, 1997;130(5):730–5.
[20] Kreitchmann R, Cohen R, Pinto J, et al. Mode of delivery and neonatal respiratory morbidity among HIV-exposed infants from Latin America and the Caribbean: the NISDI perinatal study [abstract 929]. 17th Conference on Retroviruses and Opportunistic Infections. Infant Outcome after Prenatal ART Exposure. San Francisco (CA), February 16–19, 2010.
[21] L. Naver, S. Lindgren and E. Belfrage, et al. Children born to HIV-1-infected women in Sweden in 1982-2003: trends in epidemiology and vertical transmission. *J. Acquir. Immune. Defic. Syndr.,* 42 (2006), pp. 484–489.
[22] Landesman SH, Kalish LA, Burns DN, et al. Obstetrical factors and the transmission of human immunodeficiency virus type 1 from mother to child. *N. Engl. J. Med.*, 334:1617-23, 1996.
[23] Livingston E, Huo Y, Patel K, et al. Mode of delivery and infant respiratory morbidity among infants born to HIV-1-infected women. *Obstet. Gynecol.*, 2010; 116(2 Pt 1):335–43.
[24] Marcollet A, Goffinet F, Firtion G, Pannier E, Le Bret T, Brival ML, Mandelbrot L. Differences in postpartum morbidity in women who are infected with the human immunodeficiency virus after elective cesarean delivery, emergency cesarean delivery, or vaginal delivery.*Am. J. Obstet. Gynecol.,* 2002 Apr;186(4):784-9.
[25] Mayaux M-J, Dussaix E, Isopet J, et al. Maternal virus load during pregnancy and mother-to-child transmission of human immunodeficiency virus type 1: the French Perinatal Cohort studies. *J. Infect. Dis.*, 1997;175:172-5.
[26] Moczygemba CK, Paramsothy P, Meikle S, et al. Route of delivery and neonatal birth trauma. *Am. J. Obstet. Gynecol.*, 2010;202(4):361–6.
[27] Mofenson L. Epidemiology and determinants of vertical HIV transmission. *Semin. Pediatr. Infect. Dis.,* 1994;5:252-265.
[28] Mofenson LM, Lambert JS, Stiehm ER, Bethel J, Meyer WA 3rd, Whitehouse J, et al. Risk factors for perinatal transmission of human immunodeficiency virus type 1 in women treated with zidovudine. Pediatric AIDS Clinical Trials Group Study 185 Team. *N. Engl. J. Med.,* 1999;341:385-393.
[29] Newell ML. Current issues in the prevention of mother-to-child transmission of HIV-1infection. Trans R *Soc. Trop. Med. Hyg.*, 2006;100:1–5.
[30] O. Coll, S. Fiore and M. Floridia, et al. Pregnancy and HIV infection: a European consensus on management. AIDS, 16 suppl (2002), pp. S1–S18.

[31] Panel on treatment of HIV-infected pregnant women and prevention of perinatal transmission. Recommendations for use of antiretroviral drugs in pregnant HIV-1-infected women for maternal health and interventions to reduce perinatal HIV.

[32] R.J. Simonds, R. Steketee and S. Nesheim, et al. Impact of zidovudine use on risk and risk factors for perinatal transmission of HIV: perinatal AIDS Collaborative Transmission studies. *AIDS*, 12 (1998), pp. 301–308.

[33] T.A. Grubert, D. Reindell, R. Kastner, R. Lutz-Friedrich, B.H. Belohradsky and O. Dathe, Complications after caesarean section in HIV-1-infected women not taking antiretroviral treatment. *Lancet*, 354 (1999), pp. 1612–1613.

[34] transmission in the United States. May 29, 2010. p. 1–117 NIH. Available at: http://aidsinfo.nih.gov/ContentFiles/PerinatalGL.pdf.

[35] Tuomola RE, O'Driscoll PT, Bremer JW and the Women and Infants Transmission Study. Cell-associated genital tract virus and vertical transmission of human immunodeficiency virus type 1 in antiretroviral-experienced women. *J. Infect. Dis.*, 187:375-84, 2003.

[36] UNAIDS (2010) 'Unite for universal access: Overview brochure on 2011 High Level Meeting on AIDS'.

[37] V. Maiques-Montesinos, J. Cervera-Sanchez, J. Bellver-Pradas, A. bad-Carrascosa and V. Serra-Serra, Post-cesarean section morbidity in HIV-positive women. *Acta. Obstet. Gynecol. Scand.,* 78 (1999), pp. 789–792.

[38] Warszawski J, Tubiana R, Le Chenadec J, et al. Mother-to-child HIV transmission despite antiretroviral therapy in the ANRS French Perinatal Cohort. *AIDS*, 2008;22:289–99.

In: Cesarean Section: Procedures, Complications and Recovery ISBN: 978-1-62081-214-3
Editor: Eyal Sheiner

Chapter XIX

CAN WE PREVENT ADHESIONS DURING CESAREAN DELIVERY?

***Charles R. S. Baker*[1] *and Ying Cheong*[2]**
[1]Specialty Trainee in Obstetrics and Gynecology, Salisbury District Hospital, Salisbury, Wiltshire, UK
[2]Senior Lecturer and Hon Consultant in Obstetrics and Gynecology, Academic Unit of Human Development and Health, Faculty of Medicine University of Southampton, UK
Clinical Director, Complete Fertility Centre, Southampton, Level F, Princess Anne Hospital, Coxford Road, Southampton, UK

INTRODUCTION

Peritoneal adhesions are a predictable side-effect of cesarean section (CS) and other abdominal and pelvic surgery. Though most are asymptomatic, adhesions are implicated in a spectrum of disease including chronic pelvic pain, infertility, bowel obstruction and a higher risk of organ injury at repeat cesarean or other abdomino-pelvic operation.

This chapter focuses on the pathogenesis of adhesions; the size of the problem and on strategies that might be employed to reduce the burden of morbidity caused by adhesions due to one of the most commonly performed surgical procedures in the world – cesarean section.

CAUSES AND PATHOGENESIS

Causes

Although peritoneal adhesions are most often caused by previous surgery [1], they can also be caused by other non-surgical insults to the peritoneal surfaces including endometriosis, pelvic inflammatory disease, peritonitis and radiotherapy. Other rarer causes of adhesions are foreign bodies which may include perforated intra-uterine contraceptive devices, surgical suture material or exposed mesh used in urogynecological or colorectal 'pexy' procedures (sacrocolpopexy, rectopexy etc).

The peritoneum is a serous membrane lining the abdominal cavity. It is a single cell layer thick, and the mesothelial cells that constitute the peritoneum sit on a basement membrane supported by loose connective tissue relatively sparsely supplied with blood and lymphatics. Peritoneum is particularly susceptible to trauma, with only very loose intercellular connections, but has the remarkable property of being able to regenerate by mesothelial cell migration and differentiation directly from the basement membrane rather than having to heal from the edges in like other epithelial surfaces. Because of this, and the fact that it is only one cell layer thick, denuded and injured surfaces are able to reperitonealise in less than seven days.

Pathogenesis

Adhesions are defined as abnormal fibrous connections between two anatomically different surfaces. The development of adhesions occurs as part of a disordered healing process when trauma or other injurious agent disrupts the mesothelial continuity, and the basement membrane is allowed contact with abdominal organs [2]. These injuries cause an outpouring of fibrin-rich exudate from the injured site depositing fibrinogen onto the peritoneal surfaces. The coagulation cascade turns this fibrinogen into a fibrin matrix that acts as a structure into which immune cells and fibroblasts can invade. Here they act to clear pathogens and lay down scar tissue to heal the damaged structure. Regulation of this deposition of fibrin is performed by plasminogen, cleaved to plasmin by tissue plasminogen activator (tPA). This system of fibrinolysis acts to clear fibrin once it has performed its function, and in turn is regulated by plasminogen activator inhibitor (PAI). When fibrin deposition outweighs fibrinolysis, neovascularisation and organisation into permanent adhesions occurs.

The classical concept of adhesion formation [3] implies that the main reason for this imbalance and subsequent persistence of fibrin leading to adhesions is suppression of fibrinolysis in injured tissues. It is known, for example that tissue ischemia in peritoneum – an inevitable consequence of surgical trauma – causes fibroblasts to down-regulate expression of tPA thus promoting persistence of fibrin matrix [4]. Though there is no doubt that fibrinolysis is suppressed by inflammatory and traumatic insults in the peritoneum, it has been widely shown that this is not always the case, and fibrinolysis is, in fact up-regulated in some circumstances postoperatively [5], especially in the presence of infection and inflammation, yet these patients still develop adhesions.

Therefore formation of adhesions is not as simple as the 'classical concept' originally implied. It has also been suggested that hypoxia is the primary cause of adhesions by the above mechanism, though this assertion ignores the potential for non-ischemic, infected or endometriotic peritoneum to cause adhesions without any direct trauma, or causes of hypoxia at all.

Rather, the enzymes responsible for regulating the formation and removal of fibrin are up- and down-regulated by a multitude of factors. Though hypoxia and inflammation [2] seem to be potent in adhesiogenesis, the presence of infection, blood cells, and the extent and anatomical location of peritoneal trauma as well as other factors (Table 1) are clearly also responsible.

Table 1. Identify some presurgical, intraoperative and post surgical factors that might influence adhesion formation/reformation [2]

Pre-surgical	Intra-operative	Postsurgical
Age Sex Genetic factors Body mass index Medication Infection Smoking Diabetes Stress Phase of menstrual cycle/Pregnancy Oral contraceptives Alcohol intake History of cardiovascular disease Hypercholesterolemia Benign versus malignant disease Exercise	Anesthetics of other medication Type and duration of surgery Laparoscopy versus laparotomy Extent of peritoneal damage Blood loss Antibiotics Use of irrigation Infection Time of surgery (diurnal variation in fibrinolytic activity) Blood transfusion	Antibiotics Medication Infection Individual fibrinolytic response to trauma

It is a complex interplay between these factors that will lead to fibrin clearance and restoration of anatomy, or fibrin persistence and the development of adhesions. These discoveries have led to attempts to reduce the incidence of adhesions by altering these factors with pharmacological and surgical treatments (see below).

While cesarean-related adhesions are clearly a significant problem, adhesion formation is not seen as significant after cesarean section when compared with gynaecological laparotomy [6]. This is unexpected given that in pregnancy a woman's propensity to clot is significantly enhanced, and it is logical to expect that this might push the balance of fibrin deposition and fibrinolysis towards increased fibrin matrix deposition and adhesion formation. Indeed the levels of the fibrin precursor fibrinogen, as well as some clotting factors are increased during pregnancy, while levels of activity of the anticoagulant protein S are decreased [7].

Some of this counter-intuitive effect might be explained by anatomical considerations; it is not usual to handle the bowel at CS (as it is prevented from entering the operative field by the gravid uterus) while it routinely needs to be 'packed away' into the upper abdomen during a gynecological procedure. In addition the posterior structures often involved in adhesion-related disease (ovaries, Fallopian tubes, pouch of Douglas and rectum) are not encountered during a routine cesarean procedure, whereas these structures bear the bulk of benign gynecological pathology. Another theory that has some experimental evidence [8] to support it is that spillage of amniotic fluid (which is rich in factors that augment fibrinolysis) into the abdominal cavity can assist in the clearance of fibrin.

This disparity in the risk of adhesions between CS and gynecological laparotomy has not been adequately explained and might be the subject of further research in the future that might increase our knowledge of, and ability to combat adhesions at cesarean delivery and in gynecology in the future.

The Burden of Disease from Cesarean-related Adhesions

Asymptomatic Adhesions

It follows that short- and long-term morbidity associated with cesarean delivery will increase in proportion with the ever-rising proportion of deliveries conducted abdominally. Estimates of the incidence of adhesions related to CS are variable, and only a small proportion of these patients will require medical consultation or treatment.

The risk of developing significant adhesions at first CS is quoted as high as 70% [9] but it is clear that though many of these patients will have a more complex subsequent CS, most will never develop symptoms from their adhesions.

A large Swedish study [10] looking for diagnoses of adhesions outside of the context of pregnancy showed that the number of women of all ages with a diagnosis of adhesions was 3.1 per thousand in those women that had previous CS, compared with 1.5 per thousand in women with vaginal deliveries alone. The same study found a similar association between cesarean delivery and subsequent bowel obstruction, with 2.2 cases per thousand women that had previous cesarean affected by bowel obstruction compared with 1.2 per thousand in those with vaginal delivery alone. These figures are perhaps a better estimate of the burden of disease caused by cesarean-related adhesions than an "overall adhesion rate", but as this study looked specifically at hospital codes in relation to adhesions, this is likely to be an underestimation of the whole problem when one takes into account consultations carried out in primary care, symptoms left undiagnosed or misdiagnosed, and unreported symptoms.

Increase in Operative Morbidity with Repeat Cesarean Section

It is clear that the number and density of adhesions increases with increasing number of repeat cesarean deliveries [11,12]. Along with this increase in adhesion rate and severity, there is an incremental increase in rate of operative morbidity with increasing number of procedures. The risks of inadvertent cystotomy, enterotomy and ureteric injury, placenta accreta, postoperative paralytic ileus, intensive care admission, blood transfusion of more than 4 units, hysterectomy, and operative time due to distortion of the anatomy by these adhesions are all increased with increasing number of abdominal deliveries [13]. There are other potential adverse intraoperative events that may be caused by adhesions. There is evidence [14,15] that time to delivery of the baby at repeat cesarean can be increased through time taken to dissect through dense abdominal adhesions in order to access the lower uterine segment. This is a potential cause of morbidity and mortality to the fetus when time-sensitive emergency cesarean is performed.

Tubal Infertility and Adhesions

Adhesions causing tubal disease are the leading cause of secondary infertility, accounting for approximately 18% of all infertility cases [16]. Many of these adhesions will be a result of pelvic inflammatory disease, gynecological surgery and endometriosis. It is not clear if previous cesarean delivery is an independent risk factor for adhesion-related infertility. It has been shown that fertility rates are reduced after CS, with women taking on average 6 months longer to conceive after cesarean delivery, a 50% increase in women taking longer than a year to conceive after cesarean [17] and a 9% decrease in any subsequent pregnancy compared to vaginal delivery [18. It is difficult to ascribe this effect to adhesions entirely, as there will be an effect from endometritis, intrauterine adhesions, scarring of the myometrium and confounding factors such as traumatic delivery leading to cesarean that prevents further attempts at conception. In fact there is some evidence that tubal disease is not increased after CS. Some more persuasive evidence for cesarean related tubal disease is that the risk of ectopic pregnancy appears to be slightly increased after cesarean delivery' [18,20] indicating scarring and distortion of tubal anatomy. Whatever the link between cesarean-related adhesions and infertility, it appears to be small.

Small Bowel Obstruction

Small bowel obstruction is a common cause of surgical admission, and is potentially very serious, with an estimated mortality rate of as high as 15% [21]. Most cases of small bowel obstruction are caused by peritoneal adhesions, and the rate of small bowel obstruction after CS reflects reduced adhesion formation compared with gynecological and bowel surgery, with estimates of incidence from 0.5 per thousand [22] after a single cesarean to 9 per thousand after three cesarean deliveries [10]. Though the absolute numbers of this complication are small, the increasing number of women now having multiple repeat cesarean delivery will surely lead to a significant increase in the number of cases of cesarean related small bowel obstruction on the surgical wards.

Chronic Pain and Adhesions

It is well accepted that intra-abdominal adhesions can cause pain (and that adhesiolysis improves pain) [23], and the rates of chronic pelvic pain are higher in women with previous CS compared to vaginal delivery alone with approximately twice as many women affected. The incidence of chronic pain after cesarean is as high as 18% [24] but it is not clear how many of these women have their symptoms caused by adhesions, and how many others by anterior abdominal wall scarring and involvement of the ilio-inguinal and ilio-hypogastric nerves. As attempts to reduce adhesions at cesarean delivery are attempted (see below) the picture should become clearer.

What Can be Done to Reduce the Risk of Cesarean-Related Adhesions?

The burden of morbidity from cesarean-related adhesions is significant (see above) and likely to become greater as the proportion of abdominal deliveries increases. This is not a linear increase as those with one cesarean are more likely to need a second, third or fourth abdominal delivery. This section focuses on methods that can be employed to reduce the risk of adhesions at cesarean delivery, and thus reduce the physiological and socioeconomic burden of these adhesions.

Peritoneal Closure

The subject of peritoneal closure versus non-closure at cesarean delivery has been one of intense debate and research in recent years. Historically both the visceral peritoneum (uterovesical fold) and the parietal peritoneum were closed after the uterine incision was closed following delivery. This technique [25] was used to restore anatomy, act as a barrier to infection, secure hemostasis from the peritoneal edges and reduce the risk of raw tissue edges adhering to surrounding abdomino-pelvic organs.

This practice has come into question in the last decade, with the widespread adoption of non-closure of both peritoneal layers. The UK Royal College of Obstetrics and Gynecologists and National Institute of Clinical Excellence [26] (NICE) have recommended non-closure of the peritoneum. The stated reason for this change in well-established practice is that there is a reduction in short-term morbidity with non-closure of the peritoneum [27]. Research shows that there is a reduction in operating time, as well as reduced analgesic requirements and a reduction in febrile morbidity when the peritoneum is left open [28-31].(table 2).

This evidence seems to suggest that the effects on short-term morbidity are predominantly caused by closure of the parietal peritoneum, as there seems to be no difference between closure of the visceral peritoneum (uterovesical fold) only and non-closure of both layers.

Table 2. Short-term advantages of non-closure of the peritoneum at cesarean delivery [31, 32]

Effect of non-closure of peritoneum	Size of effect
Reduced operation time	6-7 minutes
Reduced analgesic requirements	20%-60%
Reduced early postoperative fever	27%-38%
Reduced hospital Stay	0.4 days

This evidence is compelling, and as stated above has led to widespread adoption of non-closure of both layers of peritoneum by the majority of practitioners, with two-thirds of obstetricians in the UK now routinely leaving both layers of peritoneum open [26]. This evidence does not take into account long-term morbidity – in fact only one of the studies included in the above meta-analysis attempted to demonstrate long-term effect [32], and though it failed to demonstrate any differences between the two groups in terms of urinary symptoms, adhesions, pain and fertility, it was underpowered for this purpose especially when one considers the small numbers of patients likely to be affected as alluded to above. More recently, increasing evidence is emerging that there is a significant increase in the numbers of patients developing adhesions after having a CS with the peritoneum left open [33]. In fact the evidence suggests that not only are the number of adhesions increased by leaving the peritoneum open, but the increase in the number of adhesions is greatest for the denser adhesions [34], with a four-fold rise in the number of grade III (dense and vascular) adhesions with non-closure of both layers of peritoneum compared with closure of both layers.

There is further evidence that the number of adhesion-related complications is increasing in line with the widespread adoption of non-closure. There has been a rise in the number of adhesion-related episodes of small bowel obstruction in women that had previous CS that has occurred in parallel with the change in practice to non-closure of the peritoneum [10].

Surgical Anti-Adhesive Barriers

A more recent development in attempts to reduce adhesions is the trial of barrier substances, which prevent adhesions by preventing injured surfaces coming into contact with each other. These products are in widespread use in general surgery and gynecology [36,35], and the evidence base for their use is increasing.

Evidence for the use of barrier substances, however is limited at CS. Two recent trials [37,38] of sodium hyaluronate and carboxymethylcellulose film (the most-studied of the commercially-available barrier substances) have demonstrated reductions in the numbers of adhesions at second cesarean when women were given a barrier substance at first cesarean compared with controls. The first trial showed that 74% (n=112) of women had no adhesions at second cesarean in the treatment group compared with 22% in the control group (p=0.011), and the second showed a reduction in the incidence of adhesions from 48% to 7% (n=52, p=0.001) with the use of the same barrier. In both studies, the time from incision to delivery was measured at second cesarean and was significantly reduced when barrier had been used in the first procedure. These results are very persuasive, and by themselves might indicate that there is a clear advantage to be had. However, when one considers that only two in a thousand of these adhesions are likely to require hospital treatment, and each barrier application costs approximately £100 for each patient, the argument for use of this treatment becomes less clear. Recent cost analysis [39] has suggested that these products would only be cost-effective if the rate of small bowel-related bowel obstruction was as high as 2.4% - many times higher than the actual rate. This analysis contradicts cost analysis for these barrier substances in gynecology [40], where the incidence of adhesions-related morbidity is higher.

Other barrier substances are available, but the only other barrier with evidence for reducing adhesions at cesarean section is oxidised-regenerated cellulose [41]. Although this study showed a reduction in the number of adhesions similar to the sodium hyaluronate and carboxymethylcellulose studies above, this preparation has the disadvantage that there is evidence that it becomes ineffective in the presence of blood, and in this situation may even be adhesiogenic [42]. In view of the likelihood of significant blood loss at cesarean delivery, this makes carboxymethylcellulose a suboptimal candidate for an anti-adhesive at cesarean.

Expanded polytetrafluorethylene membrane has been trialled directly against oxidised-regenerated cellulose in gynecology with superior results for the former [43], but since this product is non-absorbable and needs to be sutured in place, it is unlikely to have a place in CS because of the high risk that repeat CS might become necessary.

Other Anti-Adhesion Agents and the Future

To date no other anti-adhesion agents have an evidence-base in adhesion reduction at CS. There is an increasing body of evidence in animal models and pilot studies for many other topical and non-barrier anti-adhesives [44]. Evidence is emerging that statins (HMG CoA-reductase inhibitors) – usually used for primary and secondary prevention of cardiovascular disease – are effective at preventing adhesions. Oral and intraperitoneal atovastatin and oral fluvastatin [45] have both been shown to reduce the incidence of adhesions in animal models. In fact, intraperitoneal atorvastatin has been shown to be equally as effective as sodium hyaluronate and carboxymethylcellulose film in a rat model [46] and a study of patients with a diagnosis of small bowel obstruction demonstrated that patients on statins required less operative intervention [47]compared with patients not taking a statin. These drugs seem to act by upregulating expression of tPA[48] which is responsible for 95% of the conversion of plasminogen to plasmin, therefore increasing fibrinolytic activity, while leaving levels of PAI (which reduces fibrinolytic activity) unchanged. Reassuringly, there seems to be no reduction in the strength of a surgical repair with this increase in fibrinolytic activity, with the 'burst pressure' of intestinal anastomosis unaffected [48] in a group of rats who had a reduction in adhesion formation due to statins compared to rats with no statin treatment.

Another, perhaps more intriguing discovery is that medical honey seems to have potent anti-adhesive properties. It has been shown in rat models to be equally as effective as hyaluronate and carboxymethylcellulose film at reducing adhesions in rats when used at laparotomy [49], and has actually been shown to be superior to another commercially available barrier anti-adhesive [50]. Honey does not work only as a simple barrier as it seems effective at reducing adhesions when taken orally [51] but clearly research will need to be confirmed by human trials.

NSAIDs, steroids, linezolid, collagen and gonadotrophin-releasing hormone agonists have all been tested with some effect, and this is sure to be an area of intensive research over the next years given the enormous cost-savings that any of these treatments would have over the barrier substances mentioned earlier.

However, none of the current methods of adhesion prevention/reduction can replace good surgical technique; meticulous haemostasis, gentle tissue handling, adequate irrigation to prevent tissue desiccation and careful use of energy sources during surgery.

Conclusion

This evidence should prompt practitioners to review their practice with regards to cesarean techniques. Severity of adhesions and the morbidity of repeated cesarean delivery increase with increasing number of abdominal deliveries. Therefore careful consideration needs to be given to non-closure of the peritoneum taking into account; the initial findings on entering the abdomen, parity, age, likelihood of further conception and co-morbidities. These factors need to be weighed up against the short-term advantages of non-closure of the peritoneum. The woman certainly needs to be informed of the risks of adhesions when giving consent for a cesarean, and it is important to highlight these risks when discussing the advantages and disadvantages of vaginal birth after cesarean (VBAC) versus elective repeat CS, again in light of increased morbidity with higher order cesarean deliveries. In this age patients are becoming more informed (and sometimes ill-informed) regarding medical practice. A short web search by the authors has demonstrated dozens of patient's internet forums discussing cesarean technique and complications, so one should not assume that patients do not have an opinion. It may be necessary in some cases to ask the patient pre-operatively about her views on this issue.

Whilst investment in anti-adhesion products may not be repaid in the short term, no studies have taken into account the cost of long term morbidities including increasing medico-legal costs.

Until we have an anti-adhesion method which is highly effective, clinically trialled and easily affordable, our recommendation with regard to the reduction of adhesions during CS is a practical one; treatment to patients should be individualised, and aspects of care with regards to adhesion formation/reformation carefully discussed pre-operatively. Most importantly, surgeons should be mindful of the adhesiogenic potential of their surgery and the long-term implications of adhesions. Where possible, the use a suitable available anti-adhesion agent may be of benefit.

REFERENCES

[1] Studer P, Mennicke M, Inderbitzin D. Adhesions and abdominal pain Ther Umsch. 2011 Aug;68(8):468-72.

[2] Hellebrekers BW, Kooistra T. Pathogenesis of postoperative adhesion formation. *Br. J. Surg.*, 2011 Nov;98(11):1503-16.

[3] Bakkum EA, Emeis JJ, Dalmeijer RA, van Blitterswijk CA, Trimbos JB, Trimbos-Kemper TC. Long-term analysis of peritoneal plasminogen activator activity and adhesion formation after surgical trauma in the rat model. *Fertil. Steril.*, 1996 Dec;66(6):1018-22.

[4] Saed GM, Diamond MP. Modulation of the expression of tissue plasminogen activator and its inhibitor by hypoxia in human peritoneal and adhesion fibroblasts. *Fertil. Steril.*, 2003;79(1):164-168.

[5] Hellebrekers BW, Trimbos-Kemper TC, Boesten L, Jansen FW, Kolkman W, Trimbos JB, Press RR, van Poelgeest MI, Emeis SJ, Kooistra T. Preoperative predictors of postsurgical adhesion formation and the Prevention of Adhesions with Plasminogen Activator (PAPA-study): results of a clinical pilot study. *Fertil. Steril.*, 2009 Apr;91(4):1204-14.

[6] Awonuga AO, Fletcher NM, Saed GM, Diamond MP. Postoperative Adhesion Development Following Cesarean and Open Intra-Abdominal Gynecological Operation: A Review. *Reprod. Sci.*, 2011 Jul 20.

[7] Szecsi PB, Jørgensen M, Klajnbard A, Andersen MR, Colov NP, Stender S. Haemostatic reference intervals in pregnancy. *Thromb. Haemost.*, 2010 Apr;103(4):718-27.
[8] Pschera H, Kjaeldgaard A, Larsson B. Fibrinolytic activity in amniotic fluid during late pregnancy. *Acta. Obstet. Gynecol. Scand.*, 1986;65:417–20.
[9] Hamel KJ. Incidence of adhesions at repeat cesarean delivery. *Am. J. Obstet. Gynecol.*, 2007 May;196(5):e31-2.
[10] Andolf E, Thorsell M, and Källén K. Cesarean delivery and risk for postoperative adhesions and intestinal obstruction: a nested case-control study of the Swedish Medical Birth Registry. *Am. J. Obstet. Gynecol.*, 2010;203:406.e1-6.
[11] Makoha FW, Felimban HM, Fathuddien MA, et al: Multiple Cesarean section morbidity. *Int. J. Gynecol. Obstet.*, 87:227-232, 2004)(Nisenblat V, Barak S, Barnett Griness O, et al: Maternal complications associated with multiple Cesarean deliveries. *Obstet. Gynecol.*, 108:21-26, 2006.
[12] Tulandi T, Agdi M, Zarei A, Miner L, Sikirica V. Adhesion development and morbidity after repeat cesarean delivery. *Am. J. Obstet. Gynecol.*, 2009 Jul;201(1):56.e1-6.
[13] Silver RM, Landon MB, Rouse DJ, Leveno KJ, Spong CY, Thom EA, Moawad AH, Caritis SN, Harper M, Wapner RJ, Sorokin Y, Miodovnik M, Carpenter M, Peaceman AM, O'Sullivan MJ, Sibai B, Langer O, Thorp JM, Ramin SM, Mercer BM; National Institute of Child Health and Human Development Maternal-Fetal Medicine Units Network. Maternal morbidity associated with multiple repeat cesarean deliveries. *Obstet. Gynecol.*, 2006 Jun;107(6):1226-32.
[14] Greenberg MB, Daniels K, Blumenfeld YJ, Caughey AB, Lyell DJ. Do adhesions at repeat cesarean delay delivery of the newborn? *Am. J. Obstet. Gynecol.*, 2011 Jun 29.
[15] Morales KJ, Gordon MC, Bates GW Jr. Am J Obstet Gynecol. *Postcesarean delivery adhesions associated with delayed delivery of infant*, 2007 May;196(5):461.e1-6.
[16] Farhi J, Ben-Haroush A. Distribution of causes of infertility in patients attending primary fertility clinics in Israel. *Isr. Med. Assoc. J.*, 2011 Jan;13(1):51-4.
[17] Murphy DJ, Stirrat GM, Heron J, et al: The relationship between Cesarean section and subfertility in a population based sample of 14,541 pregnancies. *Hum. Reprod.*, 17:1914-1917, 2002.
[18] Mollison J, Porter M, Campbell D, et al: Primary mode of delivery and subsequent pregnancy. *Br. J. Obstet. Gynaecol.*, 112:1061-1065, 2005.
[19] Saraswat L, Porter M, Bhattacharya S, Bhattacharya S. Caesarean section and tubal infertility: is there an association? *Reprod. Biomed. Online*, 2008 Aug;17(2):259-64.
[20] Hemminki E: Impact of Caesarian section on future pregnancy—A review of cohort studies. *Paediatr. Perinat. Epidemiol.*, 1996;10:366-379.
[21] O'Connor DB, Winter DC. The role of laparoscopy in the management of acute small-bowel obstruction: a review of over 2,000 cases. *Surg. Endosc.*, 2011 Sep 5 [Epub ahead of print].
[22] Al-Took S, Platt R, Tulandi T. Adhesion-related small-bowel obstruction after gynecologic operations. *Am. J. Obstet. Gynecol.*, 1999;180(2 Pt 1):313-5.
[23] McClain GD, Redan JA, McCarus SD, Caceres A, Kim J. JSLS. Diagnostic laparoscopy and adhesiolysis: does it help with complex abdominal and pelvic pain syndrome (CAPPS) in general surgery? 2011 Jan-Mar;15(1):1-5.

[24] Kainu JP, Sarvela J, Tiippana E, Halmesmäki E, Korttila KT. Int J Obstet Anesth. Persistent pain after caesarean section and vaginal birth: a cohort study. 2010 Jan;19(1):4-9.
[25] Duffy DM, diZerega GS. Is peritoneal closure necessary? *Obstet. Gynecol. Suv.*, 1994;49:817–22.
[26] National Institute for Health and Clinical Excellence (2004). Caesarean section. CG13. London: National Institute for Health and Clinical Excellence.
[27] Fatušić Z, Hudić I, Sinanović O, Kapidžić M, Hotić N, Musić A. Short-term postnatal quality of life in women with previous Misgav Ladach caesarean section compared to Pfannenstiel-Dorffler caesarean section method. *J. Matern. Fetal. Neonatal. Med.,* 2011 Sep;24(9):1138-42.
[28] Bamigboye AA, Hofmeyr GJ. Non-closure of peritoneal surfaces at caesarean section – a systemic review. *S. Afr. Med. J.,* 2005 Feb;95(2):123-6.
[29] Atabekoğlu CS, Türkçüoğlu I, Duru B, Sönmezer M, Süer G, Uysalel A, Koç A, Söylemez F. Closure vs. non-closure of peritoneum at caesarean section: evaluation of pain. *J. Obstet. Gynaecol.,* 2011 May;31(4):307-10.
[30] van Bogaert LJ, Misra A. Peritoneal closure or non-closure at caesarean section. *J. Obstet. Gynaecol.,* 2009 Apr;29(3):217-9.
[31] Malek-Mellouli M, Ibrahima S, Ben Amara F, Néji K, Bouchneck M, Youssef A, Nasr M, Zouari B, Reziga H. J Gynecol Obstet Biol Reprod (Paris). Towards a simplification of caesarean section technique: *Non-closure of peritoneum*? 2011 Oct;40(6):541-8.
[32] Roset E, Boulvain M, Irion O.Eur J Obstet Gynecol Reprod Biol. Nonclosure of the peritoneum during caesarean section: long-term follow-up of a randomised controlled trial. 2003 May 1;108(1):40-4.
[33] Cheong YC, Premkumar G, Metwally M, Peacock JL, Li TC. To close or not to close? A systematic review and a meta-analysis of peritoneal non-closure and adhesion formation after caesarean section. *Eur. J. Obstet. Gynecol. Reprod. Biol.*, 2009 Nov;147(1):3-8.
[34] Shi Z, Ma L, Yang Y, Wang H, Schreiber A, Li X, Tai S, Zhao X, Teng J, Zhang L, Lu W, An Y, Alla N, Cui T. Adhesion formation after previous caesarean section—a meta-analysis and systematic review. *BJOG.* 2011;118:410–422.
[35] Ahmad G, Duffy JM, Farquhar C, Vail A, Vandekerckhove P, Watson A, Wiseman D. Barrier agents for adhesion prevention after gynaecological surgery. *Cochrane Database Syst Rev.,* 2008 Apr 16;(2):CD000475.
[36] Robertson D, Lefebvre G, Leyland N, Wolfman W, Allaire C, Awadalla A, Best C, Contestabile E, Dunn S, Heywood M, Leroux N, Potestio F, Rittenberg D, Senikas V, Soucy R, Singh S; Society of Obstetricians and Gynaecologists of Canada. Adhesion prevention in gynaecological surgery. *J. Obstet. Gynaecol. Can.,*2010 Jun;32(6):598-608.
[37] Chapa HO, Venegas G, Vanduyne CP, Antonetti AG, Sandate JP, Silver L. Peritoneal adhesion prevention at cesarean section: an analysis of the effectiveness of an absorbable adhesion barrier. *J. Reprod. Med.,* 2011 Mar-Apr;56(3-4):103-9.
[38] Fushiki H, Ikoma T, Kobayashi H, Yoshimoto H. Efficacy of Seprafilm as an adhesion prevention barrier in cesarean sections. *Obstet. Gynecol. Treatment.,* 2005;91:557-561.
[39] Albright CM, Rouse DJ. Adhesion barriers at cesarean delivery: advertising compared with the evidence. *Obstet. Gynecol.*, 2011 Jul;118(1):157-60.

[40] Cheong Y, Sadek K, Watson A, Metwally M, Li TC.Adhesion reduction agents in gynaecological procedures: can NHS afford it? An economic cost efficiency analysis. *J. Obstet. Gynaecol.*, 2011 Oct;31(7):631-5.

[41] Kim TH, Kim JS, Lee HH, Nam KH, Lee JJ. Prevention of vesicouterine adhesions after cesarean with Interceed [abstract]. *Korean. Soc. Fetal. Med.*, 2006;2:194.

[42] González-Quintero VH, Cruz-Pachano FE. Preventing adhesions in obstetric and gynecologic surgical procedures. *Rev. Obstet. Gynecol.*, 2009 Winter;2(1):38-45.

[43] Haney AF, Hesla J, Hurst BS, Kettel LM, Murphy AA, Rock JA, Rowe G, Schlaff WD. Expanded polytetrafluoroethylene (Gore-Tex Surgical Membrane) is superior to oxidized regenerated cellulose (Interceed TC7+) in preventing adhesions. *Fertil. Steril.*, 1995 May;63(5):1021-6.

[44] Imai A, Suzuki N. Topical non-barrier agents for postoperative adhesion prevention in animal models. *Eur. J. Obstet. Gynecol. Reprod. Biol.*,. 2010 Apr;149(2):131-5.

[45] Hoşcan Y, Karabulut Z, Hoşcan MB, Arikan S, Oğüş E, Müderrisoğlu H. Oral fluvastatin reduces the severity of peritoneal adhesions in rats. *Acta. Chir. Belg.*, 2010 Jan-Feb;110(1):66-70.

[46] Lalountas MA, Ballas KD, Skouras C, Asteriou C, Kontoulis T, Pissas D, Triantafyllou A, Sakantamis AK. Preventing intraperitoneal adhesions with atorvastatin and sodium hyaluronate/ carboxy methylcellulose: a comparative study in rats. *Am. J. Surg.*, 2010 Jul;200(1):118-23.

[47] Srinivasa S, Kahokehr AA, Sammour T, Yu TC, Abbas SM, Hill AG. Use of statins in adhesive small bowel obstruction. *J. Surg. Res.,* 2010 Jul;162(1):17-21.

[48] Aarons CB, Cohen PA, Gower A, Reed KL, Leeman SE, Stucchi AF, Becker JM. Statins (HMG-CoA reductase inhibitors) decrease postoperative adhesions by increasing peritoneal fibrinolytic activity. *Ann. Surg.*, 2007 Feb;245(2):176-84.

[49] Emre A, Akin M, Isikgonul I, Yuksel O, Anadol AZ, Cifter C. Comparison of intraperitoneal honey and sodium hyaluronate-carboxymethylcellulose (Seprafilm) for the prevention of postoperative intra-abdominal adhesions. *Clinics* (Sao Paulo). 2009;64(4):363-8.

[50] Saber A. Effect of honey versus intergel in intraperitoneal adhesion prevention and colonic anastomotic healing: a randomized controlled study in rats. *Int. J. Surg.*, 2010;8(2):121-7.

[51] Celeplı S, Kismet K, Kaptanoğlu B, Erel S, Ozer S, Celeplı P, Kaygusuz G, Devrım E, Gencay O, Sorkun K, Durak I, Akkuş MA. The effect of oral honey and pollen on postoperative intraabdominal adhesions. *Turk. J. Gastroenterol.*, 2011 Feb;22(1):65-72.

In: Cesarean Section: Procedures, Complications and Recovery ISBN: 978-1-62081-214-3
Editor: Eyal Sheiner

Chapter XX

Ethics of Maternal-Choice Cesarean Delivery

***Frank A. Chervenak*[1,*] *and Laurence B. McCullough*[2]**

[1]Department of Obstetrics and Gynecology, Weill Medical College of Cornell University, New York, US

[2]Center for Medical Ethics and Health Policy, Baylor College of Medicine, Houston, Texas, US

Introduction

Maternal-choice cesarean delivery has become controversial throughout the world. In the United States, for example, the American College of Obstetrics and Gynecologists (ACOG) stated in a committee opinion in 2003 that while, the right of patients to refuse unwanted surgery is well known, less clear is the right of patients to have a surgical procedure when scientific evidence supporting it is incomplete, of poor quality, or totally lacking. [1] The committee concluded that the evidence to support the benefit of elective cesarean is still incomplete and that there is not yet extensive morbidity and mortality data to compare elective cesarean delivery with planned vaginal delivery. In addition, the United States National Institutes of Health (NIH) convened a 2006 conference regarding this issue that concluded that there is insufficient evidence to evaluate fully the benefits and risks of primary elective cesarean delivery as compared to vaginal delivery, and that more research is needed. [2] The NIH conference concluded: "The magnitude of cesarean delivery on maternal request is difficult to quantify. There is insufficient evidence to evaluate fully the benefits and risks of cesarean delivery on maternal request compared with planned vaginal delivery. Any decision to perform a cesarean delivery on maternal request should be carefully individualized and consistent with ethical principles." [2]

As is clear from this statement, ethics is an essential component of maternal-choice cesarean delivery. [3] The purposes of this chapter is to provide ethical justified, practical

* Correspondence: Frank A. Chervenak, M.D. Weill Cornell Medical Center, 525 East 68th Street - J130, New York, N.Y. 10065, Telephone: (212) 746-3045, FAX: (212) 746-8727, Email: fac2001@med.cornell.edu.

guidance for obstetricians in response the maternal-choice cesarean delivery controversy based on ethical principles. We provide define medical ethics and key ethical principles and then show how these ethical principles should guide the clinical judgment and decision making of obstetricians.

MEDICAL ETHICS AND ETHICAL PRINCIPLES

Medical Ethics

Ethics is the disciplined study of morality. Medical ethics is the disciplined study of morality in medicine and concerns the obligations of physicians and health care organizations to patients as well as the obligations of patients. [4,5] It is important not to confuse medical ethics with the many sources of morality in a pluralistic society. These include, but are not limited to, law, our political heritage as a free people, the world's religions (most of which now exist in our country), ethnic and cultural traditions, families, the traditions and practices of medicine (including medical education and training), and personal experience. Medical ethics since the eighteenth century European and American Enlightenments has been secular. [6] It makes no reference to God or revealed tradition, but to what rational discourse requires and produces. At the same time, secular medical ethics is not intrinsically hostile to religious beliefs. Therefore, ethical principles and virtues should be understood to apply to all physicians, regardless of their personal religious and spiritual beliefs. [4]

The traditions and practices of medicine constitute an obvious source of morality for physicians. They provide an important reference point for medical ethics because they are based on the obligation to protect and promote the health-related interests of the patient. This obligation tells physicians what morality in medicine ought to be, but in very general, abstract terms. Providing a more concrete, clinically applicable account of that obligation is the central task of medical ethics, using ethical principles. [4]

The Principle of Beneficence

The principle of beneficence in its general meaning and application requires one to act in a way that is expected reliably to produce the greater balance of benefits over harms in the lives of others. [4,5] To put this principle into clinical practice requires a reliable account of the benefits and harms relevant to the care of the patient, and of how those goods and harms should be reasonably balanced against each other when not all of them can be achieved in a particular clinical situation, such as a request for an elective cesarean delivery. In medicine, the principle of beneficence requires the physician to act in a way that is reliably expected to produce the greater balance of clinical benefits over harms for the patient. [4]

Beneficence-based clinical judgment has an ancient pedigree, with its first expression found in the Hippocratic Oath and accompanying texts. [7] It makes an important claim: to interpret reliably the health related interests of the patient from medicine's perspective. This perspective is provided by accumulated scientific research, clinical experience, and reasoned responses to uncertainty. As rigorously evidence-based, beneficence-based judgment is thus not the function of the individual clinical perspective of any particular physician and therefore should not be based merely on the clinical impression or intuition of an individual physician. On the basis of this rigorous clinical perspective, focused on the best available evidence, beneficence-based clinical judgment identifies the benefits that can be achieved for the patient in clinical practice based on the competencies of medicine. The benefits that medicine is competent to seek for patients are the prevention and management of disease, injury, handicap, and unnecessary pain and suffering, and the prevention of premature or unnecessary death. Pain and suffering become unnecessary when they do not result in achieving the other goods of medical care, e.g., allowing a woman to labor without effective analgesia. [4]

Nonmaleficence means that the physician should prevent causing harm and is best understood as expressing the limits of beneficence. This is also known as *"Primum non nocere"* or "first do no harm." This commonly invoked dogma is really a Latinized misinterpretation of the Hippocratic texts, which emphasized beneficence while avoiding harm when approaching the limits of medicine. [4,5] Nonmaleficence should be incorporated into beneficence-based clinical judgment: when the physician approaches the limits of beneficence-based clinical judgment, i.e., when the evidence for expected benefit diminishes and the risks of clinical harm increase, then the physician should proceed with great caution. The physician should be especially concerned to prevent serious, far-reaching, and irreversible clinical harm to the patient. It is important to note that there is an inherent risk of paternalism in beneficence-based clinical judgment. By this we mean that beneficence-based clinical judgment, if it is mistakenly considered to be the sole source of moral responsibility and therefore moral authority in medical care, invites the unwary physician to conclude that beneficence-based judgments can be imposed on the patient in violation of her autonomy. Paternalism is a dehumanizing response to the patient and, therefore, should be avoided in the practice of obstetrics and gynecology.

In clinical practice the preventive ethics response to this inherent paternalism is for the physician to explain the diagnostic, therapeutic, and prognostic reasoning that leads to his or her clinical judgment about what is in the interest of the patient so that the patient can assess that judgment for herself. This general rule can be put into clinical practice in the following way: The physician should disclose and explain to the patient the major factors of this reasoning process, including matters of uncertainty. The physician should then explain how and why other clinicians might reasonably differ from his or her clinical judgment. The physician should then present a well-reasoned response to this critique. The outcome of this process is that beneficence-based clinical judgments take on a rigor that they sometimes lack, and the process of their formulation includes explaining them to the patient. It should be apparent that beneficence-based clinical judgment will frequently result in the identification of a continuum of clinical strategies that protect and promote the patient's health-related interests. Awareness of this feature of beneficence-based clinical judgment provides an important preventive ethics antidote to paternalism by increasing the likelihood that one or more of these medically reasonable, evidence-based alternatives will be acceptable to the patient.

The Principle of Respect for Autonomy

In contrast to the principle of beneficence, there has been increasing emphasis in the literature of medical ethics on the principle of respect for autonomy. [4,5] This principle requires one always to acknowledge and carry out the value-based preferences of the adult, competent patient, unless there is compelling ethical justification for not doing so, e.g., prescribing antibiotics for viral respiratory infections. The female or pregnant patient increasingly brings to her medical care her own perspective on what is in her interest. The principle of respect for autonomy translates this fact into autonomy-based clinical judgment. Because each patient's perspective on her interests is a function of her values and beliefs, it is impossible to specify the benefits and harms of autonomy-based clinical judgment in advance. Indeed, it would be inappropriate for the physician to do so, because the definition of her benefits and harms and their balancing are the prerogative of the patient. Not surprisingly, autonomy-based clinical judgment is strongly antipaternalistic in nature. [4,5]

To understand the moral demands of this principle in clinical practice, we need an operationalized concept of autonomy to make it relevant to clinical practice. To do this, we identify three sequential autonomy-based behaviors on the part of the patient: 1) absorbing and retaining information about her condition and alternative diagnostic and therapeutic responses to it; 2) understanding that information (i.e., evaluating and rank-ordering those responses and appreciating that she could experience the risks of treatment; and 3) expressing a value-based preference. The physician has a role to play in each of these. They are, respectively, 1) to recognize the capacity of each patient to deal with medical information (and not to underestimate that capacity), provide information (i.e., disclose and explain all medically reasonable alternatives, i.e., supported in beneficence-based clinical judgment), and recognize the validity of the values and beliefs of the patient; 2) not to interfere with but, when necessary, to assist the patient in her evaluation and ranking of diagnostic and therapeutic alternatives for managing her condition; and 3) to elicit and implement the patient's value-based preference. [4]

The Principle of Justice

The ethical principle of justice requires both a fair process of allocating benefits and burdens and a fair outcome of this process. [5] Thus, the benefits and burdens must be distributed fairly. The concept of justice is a population-based ethical principle that obligates the physician not to exploit a population of patients by making recommendations that would benefit only a few patients but at the expense of the majority of patients who bear the burden without experiencing the benefit being sought.

Ethically Guided Clinical Judgment and Decision Making about Maternal-choice Cesarean Delivery

Beneficence-Based Considerations

Cesarean delivery has become safer over time with the advancement in surgical techniques, anesthetic options, antimicrobial availability and blood banking techniques. There are several potential maternal and fetal benefits of undergoing elective cesarean delivery versus planned vaginal delivery. Comprehensive beneficence-based clinical judgment requires that the potential benefits of elective cesarean delivery be balanced against the benefits of planned vaginal delivery and the risks of elective cesarean delivery.

Currently, beneficence-based clinical judgment still favors vaginal delivery, a view shared by most obstetricians. [8] Hence, counseling should be directive, as opposed to non-directive counseling, clearly recommending vaginal delivery where appropriate. [9]

Autonomy-Based Considerations

The ethical principle of respect for autonomy remains the rationale for promotion of elective cesarean delivery. While respect for autonomy surely is a core ethical obligation, it does not create an absolute obligation, i.e., an obligation that admits of no exceptions. Therefore, autonomy-based obligations must be balanced against beneficence-based obligations to the pregnant woman and fetus. A physician should not conclude that every request for an elective cesarean delivery should be implemented routinely. The act of routinely acceding to a patient's demands in the hopes of avoiding unnecessary paternalism is unwarranted as it fails to distinguish between negative and positive rights. Rights are claims that the patient makes to be treated in a certain way. Negative rights involve claims for noninterference and affect the individual patient. Positive rights involve claims to achieve a goal that requires the resources of others. Thus, while respecting negative rights has few limits as it does not require the resources of others, positive rights may involve sacrifice of others and must have limits.

Respect for autonomy is implemented by adherence to the informed consent process, as described above. The obstetrician is expected to exercise professional, beneficence-based clinical judgment when making clinical recommendations and present the medically reasonable alternatives as well as the alternative of nonintervention. The patient can then exercise her rights to accept or refuse intervention. The right for autonomy does not warrant routine offering of elective cesarean delivery, because doing so is not supported in beneficence-based clinical judgment.

Justice-Based Considerations

Regarding elective cesarean delivery, the principle of justice should be considered when evaluating the number of cesarean deliveries that would have to be done to prevent any of the potential morbid events associated with vaginal delivery. For example, one study showed that

539 elective cesarean deliveries would be required to prevent just one single case of anal incontinence. [10] Such a large number-needed-to-treat subjects women to an invasive procedure for the benefit of a tiny number, which is exploitative and prohibited by justice.

Beneficence, Autonomy, and Justice Considered Together

Considering beneficence-based, justice-based and autonomy-based appeals together, there is no ethical obligation to offer non-indicated cesarean delivery in an appropriate informed consent process. The impact of proffering elective cesarean delivery to all patients, as well as the individual and public health consequences of rising rates of elective cesarean delivery may be substantial. Physicians must rigorously adhere to the requirements of professional integrity, to prevent potential bias from influencing the physician's discussion with the patient introduced by economic gain or other forms of self-interest.

As stated earlier, it is important not to misinterpret the ethical principle of respect for patient autonomy. The physician's medical expertise and authority should not be marshaled to convince a patient to choose cesarean delivery. Respect for patients' autonomy should not be used as an excuse to persuade more women to undergo cesarean delivery for reasons such as the physician's convenience or desire to reduce professional liability. When patients request elective cesarean delivery, obstetricians—in their capacity as patients' advocates—must guide patients through the labyrinth of medical information toward a decision that respects the patient's autonomy under the constraint of the physician's obligation to optimize maternal-fetal health.

Responding to Requests for Cesarean Delivery

Although the risk-benefit paradigm for cesarean delivery has evolved, vaginal delivery as a rule is still considered the safest mode of delivery as the short- and long-term safety issues of elective cesarean delivery need further study. However, physicians do need to respond to requests for counseling regarding elective cesarean delivery. In fact, current evidence supports a physician's decision to accede to a patient's request for such a delivery but only after a thorough informed consent process and vigorous attempts to persuade her to accept vaginal delivery. [11,12]

When counseling the patient, adopting a strategy of shared decision-making will help to prevent unjustifiable paternalism. A particular plan of action should not be mandated unless it can be justified by its benefits or even potential benefits on the basis of the best available evidence. Obstetricians must engage in conversation with the patient, in order not to neglect an important implication of patient autonomy: when there is real uncertainty about clinical benefits and risks of reasonable alternatives, competent adult patients should be given the opportunity to make their own decisions about how to manage such uncertainty.

In cases with the highest levels of evidence, such as placenta previa or even breech presentation, cesarean delivery can be recommended with confidence. However, when levels of uncertainty are high, as in using mid-forceps or allowing a prolonged second stage of labor, the pregnant woman's autonomy should be given prominence in the decision-making process. The physician is obligated to take the time to provide her with information and advice, elicit her values, explore her concerns and emotional and social needs and work with her to make a thoughtful decision.

While the physician is obligated to offer this guidance and outline available clinically reasonable choices, the decision should ultimately come from the patient who will live with the consequences of her choice. And, if the patient persists in her request for elective cesarean delivery after this counseling, it meets the test of being well supported in autonomy-based clinical judgment. However, spontaneous and uninformed requests do not meet this ethical standard.

Physicians are not obligated to perform elective cesarean deliveries if they morally disagree. In this case, the physician should arrange for a second-opinion or arrange for the woman's care to be transferred to a physician willing to respect her request.

CONCLUSION

Maternal-choice cesarean delivery is an ethically controversial topic in obstetrics. This controversy has renewed interest in the right of pregnant women to choose the mode of delivery regardless of an accepted medical indication. Respect for autonomy is a core ethical obligation of the physician, but it is not an absolute obligation.

It must be balanced against beneficence-based obligations to the pregnant woman and fetal patient. Obstetricians should adhere to the professional responsibility model of obstetric ethics. [13] Autonomy-based, beneficence-based, and justice-based considerations do not support routinely recommending or offering elective cesarean delivery.

The challenge for the medical profession is to study and define groups of women at high risk who may benefit from planned cesarean delivery. Once identified, such women can then be offered elective cesarean delivery consistent with beneficence-based clinical judgment about what is medically reasonable.

Simplistic, "all-or-none" thinking on the part of obstetrician is clinically and ethically not justified, and a more nuanced approach is more appropriate for managing patients with regard to elective cesarean delivery.[12] In addition, the role of patient-choice cesarean delivery during the intrapartum period needs further exploration as well. We have previously shown that 1 in 8 intrapartum cesarean deliveries at our institution had an element of patient or physician choice. [12] While there is ethical justification in rare cases for a physician to accede to a thoroughly informed patient's request for such a delivery, it does not follow that physicians should routinely offer elective cesarean delivery to all patients.

REFERENCES

[1] NIOH State-of-the Science Conference Statement on Cesarean Delivery on Maternal Request. *NIH Consens State Sci. Statements*. 2006 Mar 27-29;23(1):1-29.

[2] American College of Obstetrics and Gynecology. ACOG Committee Opinion. Surgery and patient choice: the ethics of decision making. *Obstet. Gynecol.*, 2003;102:1101-6.

[3] Beauchamp TL, Childress JF. Principles of Biomedical Ethics, 6th ed. New York: Oxford University Press, 2009.

[4] Chervenak FA, McCullough LB. An ethically justified algorithm for offering, recommending, and performing cesarean delivery and its application in managed care practice. *Obstet. Gynecol.*, 1996; 87: 302–305.

[5] Culligan PJ, Myers JA, Goldberg RP, Blackwell L, Gohmann SF, Abell TD. Elective cesarean section to prevent anal incontinence and brachial plexus injuries associated with macrosomia-a decision analysis. *Int. Urogynecol. J. Pelvic. Floor Dysfunct.*, 2005;16:19-28.

[6] Hippocrates. Oath of Hippocrates. In: Temkin O, Temkin CL, eds. Ancient Medicine: Selected Papers of Ludwig Edelstein. Baltimore, MD: Johns Hopkins University Press; 1976: 6.

[7] Kalish RB, McCullough LB, Chervenak FA. Decision-making about caesarean delivery. *Lancet*, 2006;367:883-45.

[8] Kalish RB, McCullough LB, Gupta M, Thaler HT, Chervenak FA. Intrapartum elective cesarean delivery: a previously unrecognized clinical entity. *Obstet. Gynecol.*, 2004;103:1137-41.

[9] McCullough LB, Chervenak FA. Ethics in Obstetrics and Gynecology. New York: Oxford University Press, 1994.

[10] McCullough LB. The discourses of practitioners in eighteenth-century Britain. In Baker RB, McCullough LB, eds. The Cambridge World History of Medical Ethics. Cambridge: Cambridge University Press, 2009: 403-413.

[11] Minkoff H, Chervenak FA. Elective primary cesarean delivery. *N. Engl. J. Med.*, 2003; 348: 946-950.

[12] Minkoff H. Powederly KR, Chervenak FA, McCullough LB. Ethical dimensions of elective primary cesarean delivery. *Obstet. Gynecol.*, 2004; 103: 387-392.

[13] Chervenak FA, McCullough LB. The professional responsibility model of obstetric ethics: avoiding the perils of clashing rights. *Am. J. Obstet. Gynecol.* 2011; 205: 315.e1-5.

INDEX

F

N

Q

R

T